NEUROSCIENCES RESEARCH PROGRAM BULLETIN

Volume Fourteen

NEUROSCIENCES RESEARCH PROGRAM BULLETIN

Volume Fourteen

Work Session Reports by
Frederic G. Worden, Barton Childs, Steven Matthysse, and Elliot S. Gershon
William E. Bunney, Jr., and Dennis L. Murphy
Barry H. Smith and Georg W. Kreutzberg
Fred Plum, Albert Gjedde, and Fred E. Samson

The MIT Press
Cambridge, Massachusetts, and London, England

ACKNOWLEDGMENTS OF SPONSORSHIP AND SUPPORT

The Neurosciences Research Program, a research center of the Massachusetts Institute of Technology, is an interdisciplinary, interuniversity organization with the primary goal of facilitating the investigation of how the nervous system mediates behavior including the mental processes of man. To this end, the NRP, as one of its activities, conducts scientific meetings to explore crucial problems in the neurosciences and publishes reports of these Work Sessions in the *Neurosciences Research Program Bulletin.* NRP is supported in part through Massachusetts Institute of Technology by National Institute of Mental Health Grant No. MH23132, National Institute of Neurological and Communicative Disorders and Stroke Contract No. NO1-NS-6-2343, National Science Foundation, The Grant Foundation, Max-Planck-Gesellschaft, Surdna Foundation, and through the Neurosciences Research Foundation, by The Arthur Vining Davis Foundations, The Rogosin Foundation, The Alfred P. Sloan Foundation, van Ameringen Foundation, Inc., and Vollmer Foundation, Inc. At the time of the Work Sessions published herein the NRP was also supported in part by the following organizations: National Aeronautics and Space Administration and U.S. Office of Naval Research.

CONTENTS

PARTICIPANTS IN REPORTED WORK SESSIONS

Albuquerque, Edson X.
Arnason, Barry

Benfari, Robert C.
Bisby, Mark A.
Black, Ira B.
Bloom, Floyd E.
Blout, Elkan R.
Bodmer, Walter F.
Bunney, William E., Jr.

Cavalli-Sforza, L. Luka
Childs, Barton
Clausen, John A.
Collins, Robert C.
Costa, Jonathan L.

Diamond, Jack
Dilger, William C.
Duffy, Thomas E.

Edds, Mac V., Jr.
Edwards, John H.
Eigen, Manfred
Eisenman, George
Essen-Möller, Erik
Evarts, Edward V.

Gershon, Elliot S.
Gjedde, Albert
Gottesman, Irving I.
Grafstein, Bernice
Graybiel, Ann M.
Greene, Lloyd A.
Gruenberg, Ernest M.
Guth, Lloyd

Herrup, Karl
Hille, Bertil
Hirano, Asao
Hubel, David H.

Karnovsky, Manfred L.
Kauer, John S.
Kety, Seymour S.
Kreutzberg, Georg W.
Kringlen, Einar

La Du, Bert N.
Landmesser, Lynn T.
LaVail, Jennifer
Leaf, Alexander
Lehn, Jean-Marie
Leighton, Alexander H.
Lentz, Thomas L.
Livingston, Robert B.
Lynch, Gary

Mandell, Arnold J.
Matthysse, Steven
Mosher, Loren R.
Moskowitz, Michael A.
Mountcastle, Vernon B.
Murphy, Dennis L.
Murphy, Jane M.

Nauta, Walle J.H.

Onsager, Lars

Patterson, Paul
Ploog, Detlev

Plum, Fred
Polletti, Charles E.

Quarton, Gardner C.

Raisman, Geoffrey
Reivich, Martin
Rosenthal, David
Ross, Virginia
Rudolph, Stephen A.

Sakalosky, George
Samson, Fred E.
Schmitt, Francis O.
Schou, Mogens
Schubert, Peter
Schulsinger, Fini
Sharp, Frank R.
Shepherd, Gordon M.
Singer, Irwin
Smith, Barry H.
Sokoloff, Louis
Strömgren, Eric
Suelter, C.H.

Thoenen, Hans

Wender, Paul H.
Wiesel, Torsten
Williams, R.J.P.
Winkler, Ruthild
Winokur, George
Wolff, Jan
Worden, Frederic G.
Wurtman, Richard J.
Wyatt, Richard J.

FRONTIERS OF PSYCHIATRIC GENETICS

Based on an NRP Work Session
held December 1-3, 1974, and updated by participants

by

Frederic G. Worden
Neurosciences Research Program
Boston, Massachusetts

Barton Childs
The Johns Hopkins Hospital
Baltimore, Maryland

Steven Matthysse
Massachusetts General Hospital
Boston, Massachusetts

Elliot S. Gershon
National Institute of Mental Health
Bethesda, Maryland

Joyce Taylor
NRP Writer-Editor

CONTENTS

PARTICIPANTS

Robert C. Benfari
Department of Behavioral Sciences
Harvard School of Public Health
667 Huntington Avenue
Boston, Massachusetts 02115

Walter F. Bodmer
Department of Biochemistry
Genetics Laboratory
University of Oxford
South Parks Road
Oxford OX1 3QU, England

William E. Bunney, Jr.
Adult Psychiatry Branch, IRP
National Institute of Mental Health
Building 10, Room 3N-212
9000 Rockville Pike
Bethesda, Maryland 20014

L. Luka Cavalli-Sforza
Department of Genetics
Stanford University School
    of Medicine
Stanford, California 94305

Barton Childs
Department of Pediatrics
The Johns Hopkins Hospital
Baltimore, Maryland 21205

John A. Clausen
Institute of Human Development
University of California, Berkeley
Edward Chace Tolman Hall
Berkeley, California 94720

William C. Dilger
Lidell Laboratory
Cornell University
Ithaca, New York 14850

Mac V. Edds, Jr.*
Neurosciences Research Program
165 Allandale Street
Jamaica Plain, Massachusetts 02130

John H. Edwards
The Infant Development Unit
Queen Elizabeth Medical Centre
Central Birmingham Health District
Edgbaston Birmingham B15 2TG,
England

Erik Essen-Möller
Alsbäck 453 00
Lysekil, Sweden

Elliot S. Gershon
National Institute of Mental Health
Building 10, Room 3N-218
9000 Rockville Pike
Bethesda, Maryland 20014

Irving I. Gottesman
Department of Psychology
University of Minnesota
Elliott Hall
Minneapolis, Minnesota 55455

Ernest M. Gruenberg
Department of Mental Hygiene
The Johns Hopkins University
615 North Wolfe Street
Baltimore, Maryland 21205

Seymour S. Kety
Psychiatric Research Laboratory
Massachusetts Genera Hospital
Boston, Massachusetts 02114

*Dr. Edds died November 29, 1975.

Einar Kringlen
Psykiatrisk Institutt
Universitetet I Oslo
Vinderen, Olso 3, Norway

Bert N. La Du
Department of Pharmacology
University of Michigan
Ann Arbor, Michigan 48104

Alexander H. Leighton
Department of Behavioral Sciences
Harvard School of Public Health
677 Huntington Avenue
Boston, Massachusetts 02115

Steven Matthysse
Psychiatric Research Laboratory
Massachusetts General Hospital
Boston, Massachusetts 01224

Loren R. Mosher
Center for Studies of Schizophrenia
National Institute of Mental Health
5600 Fishers Lane
Rockville, Maryland 20852

Jane M. Murphy
Department of Behavioral Sciences
Harvard School of Public Health
677 Huntington Avenue
Boston, Massachusetts 02115

Detlev Ploog
Max-Planck-Institut für Psychiatrie
Klinisches Institut
Kraepelinstrasse 10
8 Munich 40, West Germany

David Rosenthal
Laboratory of Psychology and
    Psychopharmacology, IRP
National Institute of Mental Health
Bethesda, Maryland 20014

Fred E. Samson
Ralph L. Smith Mental Retardation
    Research Center
University of Kansas Medical Center
Kansas City, Kansas 66103

Francis O. Schmitt
Neurosciences Research Program
165 Allandale Street
Jamaica Plain, Massachusetts 02130

Fini Schulsinger
Psykiatrisk Afdeling
Kommunehospitalet, Psykologisk Institut
1399 København K, Denmark

Eric Strömgren
Psychiatric Hospital
Univerisity of Aarhus
DK-8240 Risskov, Denmark

Paul H. Wender
Department of Psychiatry
The University of Utah
    Medical Center
50 North Medical Drive
Salt Lake City, Utah 84132

George Winokur
Department of Psychiatry
University of Iowa
500 Newton Road
Iowa City, Iowa 52243

Frederic G. Worden
Neurosciences Research Program
165 Allandale Street
Jamaica Plain, Massachusetts 02130

Richard J. Wyatt
National Institute of Mental Health
Building 10, Room 4N206
Bethesda, Maryland 20014

Note: NRP Work Session reports are reviewed and revised by participants prior to publication.

FOREWORD

This report grew out of a Work Session that was held December 1-3, 1974, to evaluate current research in psychiatric genetics and to explore ways in which new methods from other areas of genetic and behavioral research might be applied to psychiatric problems. Leading contributors to research on genetic factors in psychiatric disorders participated in a multidisciplinary discussion with scientists from related disciplines including general, population, and medical genetics, biology, biochemistry, pharmacology, animal behavior, anthropology, sociology, psychology, and psychiatry.

The proceedings of the Work Session have been substantially reorganized with regard to both sequence and emphasis in order to achieve the most effective and succinct treatment of important issues and opportunities in research on psychiatric genetics. The purpose here is not to give a chronological account of the proceedings of the Work Session; rather it is an attempt to synthesize the scientific issues and topics that were discussed. Attribution to participants has been kept to a minimum in the text to promote a smooth flow of thought; however, the names of the leading participants in the discussion are listed at the beginning of each section.

I. INTRODUCTION

Psychiatric genetics is a part of medical genetics, but it has been shaped by phenomenological characteristics peculiar to mental, or psychiatric, illness as well as by conceptual problems about the fundamental nature of mental illness. For example, much of this report concerns studies of the two major psychiatric illnesses, schizophrenic and manic-depressive psychoses, because these two illnesses have been more amenable to genetic research than the broad range of nonpsychotic disorders such as psychoneuroses, character disorders, and other impairments of personality function that are less dramatically disruptive of the adaptive resources of the patient. It is difficult to defend the argument that psychotic patients are not "ill" and do not fit into the traditional medical model of illness (which includes heart disease, cancer, and cirrhosis of the liver) because the disruption of mental processes (e.g., hallucinations and delusions in schizophrenia) and of affective experience (manic excitement and depression) is so grossly crippling of physiological, behavioral, and social adaptation. In contrast, the nonpsychotic disorders range all the way from borderline psychosis to syndromes that are difficult to differentiate from the "normal" range of problems in living. For these, a question arises as to whether the traditional medical-biological view of illness is as appropriate as alternative views, such as that they are disorders of learning stemming from faulty training or faulty habit patterns. Whatever such ideas may mean, there is in them a less compelling implication of disordered biological substrates. A simplistic analogy is the differentiation between a violin sonata that sounds bad because of defects in the violin and one that sounds bad because the violinist plays it poorly. For psychotic illnesses, impairments in the biological substrates (the violin) are increasingly evident, whereas for many of the nonpsychotic disorders, it is still plausible to hold that the main problem is not in the biological apparatus but rather in the acquired and habitual way the individual adapts to normal problems in living. Thus, a person, heavily overindulged in childhood ("spoiled"), and who suffers mainly from unrealistic expectations of the adult world, seems to be a less promising subject for research on genetic factors in psychiatric disorders than the patient with major psychotic symptoms.

Implications of Mental Illness for Neuroscience

A preliminary note on schizophrenia and manic-depressive illness may be useful in providing some perspective on the implications of these disorders for the neuroscientist.

It is a useful oversimplification to categorize schizophrenia as primarily a disorder of thought processes and manic-depressive illness as primarily a disorder of emotional processes manifested by abnormal mood. The organization of thought processes and the regulation of affective tone are both high-level aspects of human brain function. In this context, "high-level" refers not merely to the hierarchical level of organization of neurophysiological processes in the brain, but also to high-level experiential factors that shape brain processes, including interpersonal, social, and cultural influences. It follows that a scientific understanding of these disorders would require a model of brain function explicating the specificity and the interaction of genetic and environmental factors and their influence on the maturation of the brain and the human personality. Because both disorders involve substantial disturbances of subjective experience, investigation of the neural mechanisms producing these disorders bears, at least indirectly, on the question of how the brain mediates conscious experience including perception, discrimination, attention, emotion, learning, and memory. Symptoms such as hallucinations and delusions may reflect pathological brain processes that are more accessible to research than those brain processes mediating normal higher mental processes. At least it is clear from the history of medical science that study of pathological phenomena often illuminates the understanding of normal functions.

By the term "schizophrenia," Eugen Bleuler intended to signify a splitting between thought and emotional processes suggested by the observation that the emotional reaction of schizophrenics is often incongruous with their thought processes and with external circumstances. Obviously, schizophrenia is not only a disorder of thought but also of emotional processes. Similarly, in manic-depressive illness, both thought and mood are distorted. During depression, for example, thought processes may become self-critical to a degree that involves a break with generally accepted judgments about reality. The patient may think he is the greatest sinner in history and that certain of his actions are the most heinous examples of moral turpitude. Conversely, during manic excitement, thought processes may be grandiose and elated, the

patient speaking expansively about his outstanding charms, his un-
equalled virtues, and his unlimited powers.

Bleuler differentiated between primary symptoms that are
fundamental to schizophrenia and secondary symptoms, such as
delusions and hallucinations, that develop as a consequence of the
primary ones. Bleuler's primary symptoms, the four "A's," are autism
(a withdrawal from external to internal reality), ambivalence (simultaneously held contradictory affects or attitudes), affective disorder
(flattening of affective tone and incongruity between affective quality
and content of intellectual processes), and finally, a disorder of the
associative process that lends a bizarre quality to schizophrenic
thinking. Thought becomes illogical, disorganized, and often incompre-
hensible.

Discussing his concept of the associative process, Bleuler wrote:

> The direction of our associations is determined not by
> any single force but by an almost infinite number of influences.
> In the thought processes of schizophrenia, however, all the
> associative threads indicated [above], whether singly or in
> haphazard groupings, may remain totally ineffective. [Bleuler,
> 1911, p. 17]

An example of disordered associative processes taken from
Bleuler may convey the nature of the cognitive disturbance better than
descriptive phrases. (In this excerpt, Bleuler used an asterisk "*" to
mark sudden leaps in thought, some of which Bleuler explained by
environmental influences and the distractibility of the patient.)

> One must have arisen sufficiently early and then there is
> usually the necessary "appetite" present. *"L'appétit vient en
> mangeant,"* says the Frenchman. * With time and years the
> individual becomes so lazy in public life that he is not even
> capable of writing any more. On such a sheet of paper, one can
> squeeze many letters if one is careful not to transgress by one
> "square shoe." * In such fine weather one should be able to take
> a walk in the woods. Naturally, not alone, but with a girl. * At
> the end of a year one always renders the annual accounting. *
> The sun is now in the sky yet it is not yet 10 o'clock. In
> Burgholzli, too? I don't know since I have no watch with me as I
> used to have! *Après le manger, On va p. . . . !* There are also
> plenty of entertainments for people who do not and never did
> belong to this hospital. In Switzerland it is not permitted to do
> mischief with human flesh!! * *Le foin,* hay, *L'herbe* grass,

mordre-bite, etc. etc. etc. and so on! R. K. In any event, much
"merchandise" comes to Burgholzli from Zurich. Otherwise we
would not have to stay in "bed" until it may please this or that
person to "tell" who is to blame that one is no longer permitted
to go about freely. O . . . * 1000 hundredweights. * Appendage
to acorns!!! [Bleuler, 1911, p. 20]

The central role of attentional disorders in schizophrenia was
first emphasized by Kraepelin in 1919, building on the first scientific
studies of attention in the laboratories of Wundt, Lange, and Külpe:

> The patients digress, do not stick to the point, let their thoughts
> wander without voluntary control in the most varied directions.
> On the other hand the attention is often rigidly fixed for a long
> time . . . . Further it happens that they deliberately turn away
> their attention from those things to which it is desired to attract
> it . . . . But in the end there is occasionally noticed a kind of
> irresistible attraction of the attention to casual external impres-
> sions. [Quoted in Chapman and Chapman, 1974, pp. 8-9]

Dysfunction of attentional control is of special interest to the
neuroscientist because this process may be more amenable to neurophysiological and neurochemical analysis than some of the ideational
and interpersonal aspects of psychosis. Pharmacological and lesion
experiments on attention are too numerous to review here, but it may
be useful to mention recent work by Mountcastle suggesting that the
study of attention at a single neuronal level is possible. He observed
neurons in monkey parietal cortex that are activated "before and
during those movements aimed at objects previously identified as
desirable," and others that "increase their discharge rates abruptly
when the animal fixates with his eyes objects of interest in his
immediate surround" (Mountcastle, 1975, 1976).

II. CONTEMPORARY MEDICAL GENETICS

Medical Genetics: B. Childs

Genetics is the study of the hereditary components of variation; medical genetics consists of the discovery and uses of genetic knowledge for the advancement of conventional medical missions. The latter are: (1) diagnosis, which is most helpful when based on an understanding of cause; (2) management, including both specific treatment and supportive care; and (3) prevention. Genetic knowledge can best serve the latter, and it is likely that within a decade or so medical genetics will be more concerned with prevention than with either diagnosis or management.

The Genetic Method

The genetic method involves, first, the assignment of the origin of a phenotype to a specific representative of the genetic material, or allele, that occupies a specific locus in a defined chromosome. This is an analysis of the genetic composition of an individual. A second aim of the genetic method consists of an analysis of the distribution of genes in populations, the study of the factors that account for such distributions, and the frequencies in which the genes are found. This is an analysis of the genetic composition of populations. The genetic method also uses such other disciplines as biochemistry and physiology in characterizing the actions of genes and in describing genetic control over metabolic pathways.

Pedigree Genetics

In accomplishing the first aim of the genetic method, we are, of course, unable to use the breeding test in human beings and so must make inferences based on our knowledge and understanding of gene action. For example, the existence of a protein defines at least one locus even in the absence of variants, and our knowledge of mutation, and its constancy and randomness, suggests that genetic variation exists in all systems where proteins are involved. Second, discovery of a protein variant, whether by electrophoresis or other technique, suggests the segregation of an allele even without family study. Although a family study would be preferable, success so far in finding a genetic basis for protein variance suggests that the probability is high that most of the variants will eventually be shown to be hereditary. If the variant is associated with clinical expression, a relationship of some kind is established even though it may be impossible to describe in detail. At the least, the presence of the variant may be used for diagnostic purposes, and at best, it may point to the cause of the clinical expression. Third, a biochemical difference not subject to day-to-day variation may be suspected of being inherited even in the absence of affected relatives. Tolerance tests of parents, for example, have often shown such differences to be the recessive expression of genes in heterozygotes; such a biochemical characterization may lead to identification of the protein involved. Fourth, when the biochemical variation is rare, the discovery that the parents of the individual are genetically related (for example, first cousins) is additional evidence for heritability of the character. Fifth, evidence for the inheritance of a character is given by an examination of the distribution of affected persons in families—that is, by pedigree inspection—and various modes of inheritance are suggested depending on whether or not the parents of affected children are themselves affected or whether both parents are able equally to transmit the character. When large numbers of families are studied, segregation analysis can be carried out to calculate the agreement or disagreement with various Mendelian hypotheses.

The use of these ideas and analytical methods has resulted in the rapid identification of a large number of inborn errors, protein variants, malformations, and other human characteristics that can be assigned to a specific locus. The virtues of such discoveries lie in the elucidation both of normal human differences and of disease. In the latter, the discovery of cause has often led to effective treatment.

Genetic Heterogeneity. If treatment is to be directed to specific cause, it is necessary to establish the degree to which all examples of a particular phenotype are ascribable to the same cause. There are two kinds of genetic heterogeneity. One accounts for the variations of severity, age of onset, frequency of exacerbations, and so on, by the segregation in populations of different mutants (alleles) for the same locus; whereas in the second type of heterogeneity, similar phenotypes are seen to be due to mutants at different loci that accomplish the same ends by diverse biochemical means. The general method to detect heterogeneity is to compare phenotypes within and between families on the assumption that all members of the same family possess the same gene. The detection of particular alleles in families may be important for prognosis because they may determine whether the disease is mild, moderate, or severe; the detection of genes at separate loci causing single phenotypes has particular implications for treatment because the biochemical mechanisms must differ according to the locus of the gene.

Linkage. The ultimate aim of genetic analysis in individuals and families is the assignment of a phenotype to a specific locus in a definite chromosome. This can now be done in some instances due to the rapidly increasing number of genetic markers and to progress in the assignment of specific genes to numbered chromosomes owing to improvements in chromosome definition and somatic cell hybridization techniques. In the future, there may be diagnostic value in linkage because a gene without manifestation may be detected by the constancy of its association or dissociation with other, detectable genes in families, which also provides useful prognostic or counseling information. In addition, linkage may also be used as evidence favoring the inheritance of a character and may be a way to cut through the fog of environmental factors, which introduce so much variability.

Multifactorial Disorders. There are many common diseases that are sometimes aggregated in families, but not in distributions that suggest origin in genes at a single locus. Examples are malformations, diabetes mellitus, gout, emphysema, chronic bronchitis, as well as schizophrenia and affective psychosis. These disorders may be treated as unitary phenotypes, and empirical risks can be calculated for counseling purposes. Diseases of this type are called multifactorial; that is, they involve both genes and special experiences. They may also be multigenic; that is, they may involve an unspecified number of genes at unspecified loci. The probability of multigenic origin of a character can be treated mathematically, but the usefulness of such information in the accomplishment of medical missions is small. It is perhaps more rewarding to assume that the phenotype is heterogeneous in origin, being sometimes caused by the effects of single mutants operating in specific environments and, in other cases, the combined effects of genes at more than one locus.

One example of such a phenotype is the hemolysis and anemia that are produced by twenty or thirty frequently used drugs and chemicals in persons whose erythrocytes are deficient in glucose 6-phosphate dehydrogenase (Beutler, 1972). The genetic origin of the hemolytic anemia is seldom evident because there may be only one person in a family who has had a hemolytic episode. Another example is given by the association between deficiency of α_1-antitrypsin and emphysema (Talamo, 1975). Persons homozygous for the Z allele of this multiallelic system of mutants may have a rapidly developing emphysema beginning in young adult life; other homozygotes develop cirrhosis of the liver as infants. Because the Z allele has a frequency in the general population of 2% or 3%, these disorders, although not common, are not rare. Of perhaps more interest is the possibility that persons who are heterozygous for the Z allele and who smoke may be especially prone to develop emphysema. A further example is the observation of Kellermann and his co-workers (1973b) that persons homozygous for a gene contributing to an easily inducible form of the enzyme aryl hydrocarbon hydroxylase develop bronchogenic carcinoma if they are heavy smokers. In all of these instances, the gene is distributed in families in a Mendelian way; but because special experiences, such as the ingestion of drugs or smoking, are required to produce the disease, the character does not segregate even though there may be familial aggregations of cases.

A more complex condition is seen in premature myocardial infarctions—that is, heart attacks that develop in individuals before ages 55 to 60. Such persons are more likely than others to come from families in which other members have also experienced myocardial infarctions, but the distribution is certainly not Mendelian (Goldstein and Brown, 1975). Students of this disease speak of several risk factors, each of which appears to play a part in predisposing persons to myocardial infarction. The risk factors most commonly mentioned are hyperlipidemia, hypertension, diabetes, obesity, and smoking. Heredity is also said to be a risk factor, but it seems probable that the genetic element is acting through the hereditary components of the other risk factors. For example, it has been demonstrated recently that, although most hyperlipidemia is dietary in origin, some is the result of possession of mutants at single loci (Goldstein and Brown, 1975); that is, to be heterozygous or homozygous for these mutants at single loci strongly predisposes an individual to early myocardial infarction. If, in addition, such genetic hyperlipidemia is accompanied by hypertension, heavy smoking, and obesity, the probability that such a person will have a heart attack is proportionately increased.

There is some evidence that hypertension is familial and that there is strong genetic control over blood pressure (Murphy, 1973);

diabetes is also a genetic disorder, although the precise numbers and qualities of the genes involved are not clear. Obesity is surely the result of caloric intake exceeding use, although there are constitutional differences in the way in which this balance is managed. Nothing is known of any genetic differences in responses of the vascular system to smoking tobacco, but it seems entirely reasonable to suppose that they exist. Thus, it is apparent that, if one would understand the genetic contribution to premature myocardial infarction, it is necessary to study the genetics of the risk factors and to look, in the first instance, for single gene influences. The medical mission here is to prevent the arteriosclerosis that predisposes to coronary occlusion. And to do that the genetic properties of the individual that predispose him to that disorder should be discovered and nullified by appropriate dietary or other changes in living conditions. The virtue of such knowledge is not only that it may prevent this distressing disease in susceptible persons, but it may also allow nonsusceptible individuals to indulge in habits whose pleasures are attested to by the numbers of people who indulge in them. The genetic contribution to heart attacks will differ in different families so that each man's coronary occlusion may have slightly different genetic causes. Thus, it is not coronary occlusion that is inherited, but only one or a number of genes whose actions fail to support homeostasis in the face of special experiences. There should be some lessons here for the detailed analysis of genetic contributions to psychiatric disease.

Population Genetics

The second genetic method of importance to medicine consists of the analysis of the distributions and frequencies of genes in populations. The laws governing the distributions of genes in populations are simply extensions of Mendel's laws of segregation and independent assortment, but the outcomes in terms of the frequencies of the genes depend upon the contribution of such genes to differential fertility as well as random factors. The probability of the concatenation of specific alleles in single individuals, on the other hand, depends upon whether or not mating is random and upon the frequency with which the specific genes exist in the population. The applications of such knowledge in medicine are limited, at present, to genetic counseling and the various forms of genetic screening. The genetic aspect of such counseling consists of providing persons with the medical properties of the diseases in which they are interested, the probabilities that their relatives may have the disease, their own reproductive outcomes, and the risk in mating with other individuals in the population who have similar genotypes. Screening involves the discovery in the population of persons with incipient or overt disease whose adverse effects can be averted or corrected and finding persons who have particular genes who might like to know about them when making reproductive decisions. Such a decision may be to avoid having children altogether, or, as it is now possible to make a prenatal diagnosis of a number of disorders providing the genotypes of the parents are known, the parents may choose to terminate the pregnancy when a fetus is found to be affected. Such a measure means that all children in that family will be spared that particular disease. It is probable that, in the future, genetic knowledge will be more widely used in screening than in diagnosis and treatment, since prevention is regarded by everyone as more desirable than intervention after the onset of disease.

Cytogenetics

Advances in cytogenetics of interest may be briefly summarized. First, although abnormalities of chromosomes produce a good deal of disease, much of it is lethal, causing abortions and stillbirths. Second, postzygotic aberrations, of which mongolism is an example, are not, strictly speaking, inherited; however, prezygotic abnormalities are distributed in families according to Mendel's laws. Third, the pathogenesis of the diseases caused by chromosome abnormalities is very poorly understood; it is not known why additions or deletions of chromosomal material cause malformation or death. Perhaps more will be known when very large numbers of gene loci are known to belong to specific chromosomes and the effects of having abnormal numbers of particular genes can be studied.

Sex chromosome disorders, on the other hand, are the most frequent and may have some relevance to psychiatric variation. In general, the human organism appears to tolerate extra X chromosomes better than extra autosomes, perhaps because all but one X is inactivated. Again, the pathogenesis of the disorders is not known, nor do we know how many of the possessors of these supernumerary chromosomes are, in fact, abnormal. In general, the more supernumerary X's an individual has, the lower will be the IQ, and although other behavioral effects of these chromosome abnormalities may well have been exaggerated, it is possible that some possessors of extra X's and Y's will be shown, at the least, to have learning disabilities (Polani, 1969).

Is Schizophrenia "Inherited"?

It has been said that schizophrenia may not be inherited at all, but that it is a learned behavior like being a Republican or a Democrat. A geneticist might counter this idea with an analogy. It is now generally agreed by psycholinguists that there is a universal grammar that is subject to the constraints of the central nervous system; the brain makes use of sounds abstracted from the environment to formulate a language, but always according to the same rules. Thus, the substrate of language is not learned but is inherited. What is learned is the particular sounds and words that are arranged into Chinese or German or English; what is inherited is how the language is learned and how much. Perhaps the capacity to become schizophrenic is inherited, but the details of the phenotype are the result of the affected person's special experiences.

For research seeking to clarify the nature of the genetic factor in schizophrenia, it is important to make a clear distinction between the concept of a monogenic disorder and that of a multigenic effect. Schizophrenia has been said by some to be the result of genes at a single locus with incomplete penetrance and by others to be a multigenic effect. In both instances, it is acknowledged that the phenotype is produced only when the genes are acting in a context favorable for its appearance. Mathematical tests of these hypotheses have been carried out; however, because no one knows anything about the putative genes, it has been impossible to decide between the monogenic and multigenic hypotheses. In addition, the possibility of genetic heterogeneity has been raised; that is, some cases may be monogenic, others multigenic.

Perhaps because of the difficulties in defining schizophrenia and in measuring its various attributes, it has not been possible to approach the important genetic question of which loci are involved and what the alleles occupying those loci might be doing. If one knew that, it might be seen that there is little difference between the multigenic and monogenic viewpoints. Multigenic systems are made up of two or more loci, each with its own constellation of alleles, perhaps a few of them common, but most of them rare. A single phenotype may be the outcome of one or of several genetic defects in a metabolic pathway. The affected person may be homozygous for mutants of large effect at one locus or heterozygous for mutants of lesser effects at several loci. Other combinations are possible depending upon the qualities of the mutants themselves, their zygosity, and the number of loci involved; and in the final analysis, which of these possibilities is actually encountered will depend upon the frequencies of each of the mutants.

Although the phenotypes are similar, segregation would appear only in those in which the effects of the genes at one locus overrode those at others. The affected individual might be homozygous for mutants of moderate effect at one locus and heterozygous for mutants at others. In this case, the phenotype might be described as monogenic, while the genes occupying the other loci would be called modifiers. Segregation of the phenotype might be irregular because of the segregation of the modifiers, and if so, penetrance might be invoked.

To characterize a phenotype as multigenic is to define it as being influenced by genes at more than one locus and to admit ignorance of which ones they are. To characterize a phenotype as monogenic means that one has some chance of discovering the biochemical action of the gene and, therefore, of nullifying its bad effects. The discovery of the loci involved in the genetic contribution to common multifactorial diseases is not hopeless. The genes contributing to common diseases must be, by definition, common alleles. Mathematical treatment cannot help in making decisions about which loci and which alleles are important in schizophrenia. For this we must look for (1) better definition of the specific characteristics of schizophrenia, which, in turn, might lead to the discovery of segregating characters that may be given biochemical characterization and (2) biochemical markers representing the effects of polymorphic genes in appropriate metabolic pathways that might then be correlated with cognitive or other characteristics of the disease.

Critical Issues in Psychiatric Genetics:
F.G. Worden and S.S. Kety

Many questions and issues in psychiatric genetics are common to any branch of genetic research, but some problems are especially prominent in psychiatric genetics and constitute special, if not unique, difficulties for it. Some of these issues will be listed here, with a brief preliminary discussion that may be useful for the reader who is unfamiliar with the topic.

The Phenomenological Basis of Psychiatric Diagnosis

One serious problem for psychiatric genetics is the question of how to group patients and their nonpatient relatives into meaningful categories of mental status. Both schizophrenic and manic-depressive psychoses are diagnosed on the basis of observations of phenomenological manifestations rather than of etiological mechanisms. On the basis of behavioral observations, including verbal reports, a cluster of signs and symptoms is identified that corresponds with the criteria for a particular psychiatric syndrome. Much of the disturbance in psychiatric illness involves abnormalities of the subjective life, and these are not directly observable, taking forms such as delusional thinking, hallucinations, distorted self-images, and pathological affective responses—depression, elation, or an inadequate, flat emotional response to life circumstances. Inferences about such experiences are based upon behavioral observation. It follows that simulation of psychopathology is not easy to discriminate from real psychopathology. A person who claims falsely to be hearing voices and who acts as if in response to the messages allegedly conveyed by these voices is difficult to differentiate from a person who is having genuine hallucinatory experiences.

Criteria for psychiatric diagnosis vary from psychiatrist to psychiatrist and from country to country. Criteria for the diagnosis of schizophrenia may be very strict, as is common in European countries, or very broad, as is common in the United States. (For details about the nature of criteria used in clinical psychiatric diagnosis, see Meehl, 1972.) It is important to note that the diagnostic difficulty is not only in the accuracy with which a given cluster of manifestations can be described and recognized, but also in differences of opinion as to whether a given syndrome should be labeled schizophrenia or manic-depressive psychosis. Schizophrenia is diagnosed more frequently in the United States than in Britain, whereas the reverse is true for manic-depressive psychosis. Collaborative studies between British and American psychiatrists have established that this is largely a difference in labeling, rather than a difference in the description of the manifestations or in the prevalence of the two psychoses.

Another bias in psychiatric genetics is that the chance of being discovered by psychiatrists depends not just on the severity of illness but also on the tolerance of the society; in urban cultures, psychiatric illness is detected much more frequently than in rural cultures because psychiatric illness and rural life are more amenable. In studies where interviews of a whole population are carried out, more instances of schizophrenia are found than had previously been seen by a psychiatrist. This is especially true of the less severe forms of illness. If a significant proportion of schizophrenia is not ascertained, this provides a selective bias favoring the finding of a familial tendency because families with two or more schizophrenics have a greater likelihood of being discovered than those with a solitary incidence.

The Problem of Heterogeneity

Although interrater reliability for global diagnostic categories is fairly high in trained psychiatric researchers, it is also well known that within a given category of patients phenotypic homogeneity of the disease is limited largely to those symptoms and signs making up the diagnostic syndrome, whereas in other respects, the patients may demonstrate a great diversity of personality and physiological functioning not relevant for the diagnostic label. The more thoroughly persons within a diagnostic category are investigated, the more impressive these differences are seen to be, reflecting a shift of the observer's attention from psychopathological manifestations to other aspects of the person who has the psychopathology. These differences presumably reflect genotypic and environmental variables that could be important for the etiological understanding of an individual patient. It is, of course, equally true for all diseases that great personality heterogeneity exists within a population of patients with a given disease, but the importance of this personality variable for treatment and prognosis may vary from trivial (e.g., infectious diseases responsive to antibiotics) to substantial (e.g., hypertension, duodenal ulcer, asthma) to critical, in a condition like schizophrenia where personality functions are the main domain of the pathological symptoms. In other words the description of the pathological signs and symptoms does not tell what kind of person has the syndrome. One patient may have considerable unimpaired personality functions, including a drive to get well and to seek help and the capacity for interpersonal relationships that may be quite successful in areas not distorted by delusional, hallucinatory, or other psychotic trends. Another patient, with similar pathological symptoms and signs, may be so complacently passive and accepting of his condition that the schizophrenia appears more like a way of life than an illness. Indeed, the history of such a patient may reveal such a lack of success in coping with life at every developmental stage that "way of life" is not necessarily an inappropriate term. That is, to "cure" such a patient means not to restore a former state of health but rather to initiate a state that has not previously existed.

In other words, psychiatric diagnoses are weak in descriptive value of the normal capacities that are still operative in persons manifesting psychopathology. Patients with similar psychiatric symptoms may differ enormously in the degree to which normal personality functions are spared or impaired, and consequently prognosis will be more accurate if these remaining personal adaptive capacities are evaluated along with the quality and intensity of psychopathology per se. For example, does a paranoid delusional system preempt most of the patient's waking energies, or does it exist in an "encapsulated" form that interferes little with social adaptation and subjective function?

Differences in the quality and strength of unaffected adaptive capacities may have important implications for underlying genetic and environmental factors, yet the psychiatric label tells almost nothing about this variable, either in the cross-sectional view of the patient at a given time or in the longitudinal view of the course of the patient's illness, both of which focus largely on presence or absence of psychopathology.

A further complication is that a reliable cluster of psychopathological symptoms does not necessarily mean that there is an underlying homogeneous etiology; the reliable association of fever, headache, and vomiting does not define a group of patients having a single underlying etiological mechanism. Even if that combination were shown to have a high concordance in monozygotic (MZ) twins or in the biological relatives of adoptees who showed the triad, one could still be dealing with a heterogeneous group of illnesses in which genetic factors varied in importance and mode of transmission.

The Nature-Nurture Issue

A developmental perspective is necessary for understanding the interaction of genetic and environmental factors. Genetic expression can occur only as an intrinsic interaction with environmental factors that are diverse, complex, and, to varying degrees, difficult to differentiate from genetic factors. For example, when a virus particle from the environment enters a cell and joins the genetic material of that cell, it can be seen that a bit of environment has become a bit of genetic material. It is a tenable hypothesis that organelles such as mitochondria became part of the intracellular apparatus by invading the cell as alien organisms at some point in evolutionary development.

In the ovum and sperm, genetic material interacts with its cytoplasmic environment that, in turn, interacts with its tissue, organ, and organismic environment. During embryogenesis, environmental influences range from cytoplasmic and cell population factors to intrauterine variables such as the structure of the placenta, the position and number of embryos, and the character of the maternal blood supply. Perinatal factors include complications of birth and immediate postnatal life, which lead into the developmental interaction between the genetic endowment and the physical and sociocultural milieu. These environmental variables include malnutrition, toxins, infections, interpersonal relationships, education, etc.

For schizophrenic and manic-depressive psychoses, the important questions should not try to specify the cause as either genetic or environmental. More relevant to an understanding of cause are such questions as: How much of the variance is attributed to each? To what extent can genetic and environmental factors be isolated and specified in the interaction producing the phenotypic manifestation of the psychiatric disorder? What factors trigger phenotypic manifestations? And conversely, what factors inhibit phenotypic expression? How many chromosome disorders or gene loci are involved, and in what constellation or patterns? Are there critical environmental factors, or are there critical stages of development during which particular environmental factors acquire a special potency?

The Question of Animal Models

Obviously it is not possible to use human subjects in classical genetic research such as breeding experiments. To what extent can animal models of psychiatric illness be useful? Since lithium, an effective treatment for human mania, also blocks amphetamine hyperactivity in animals, what interpretations are justifiable? Do animals have subjective experience that is analogous to such human experience as depression, euphoria, hallucination, delusion, and feelings of depersonalization or derealization? Although answers to these questions are not possible, it is clear that animal studies have been extremely productive in the development and testing of psychopharmacologically active agents.

With regard to animal models of schizophrenia, Matthysse and Haber (1975) have proposed four criteria that animal behavior should satisfy if it is to be a useful model for testing antipsychotic drugs and formulating hypotheses about pathophysiology: (1) The aberrant animal behavior ought to be restored to normal, at least in part, by drugs that are known to be effective in the treatment of schizophrenia. (2) Drugs closely related in chemical structure to the phenothiazines and butyrophenones, but without efficacy in the treatment of psychosis, ought also to be without normalizing effect in the animal model. (3) Tolerance should not develop to the effect of antipsychotic drugs in the animal model, since tolerance does not develop to their antipsychotic action (sedative effects can frequently be ruled out in this way). (4) The normalizing effect should not be blocked by the simultaneous administration of anticholinergic agents, since the latter are frequently used as an adjunct to phenothiazine treatment in order to counteract the parkinsonian side effects of these drugs, without apparently diminishing their antipsychotic activity. As knowledge of animal social behavior, communication, and cognitive processes advances, the usefulness of animal studies may be enhanced. For example, Dilger's report (see below, "Animal Behavior Patterns") on the behavioral genetics of African parrots and Benzer's (1971, 1973) studies of behavioral genetics in the fruit fly represent promising frontiers.

Psychiatric genetics thus differs from animal genetics and medical genetics in having more serious problems with the reliability and validity of psychiatric diagnostic categories, the relationship of these phenomenological syndromes to unknown underlying etiological mechanisms, and the difficulty in analyzing, for given diagnostic categories, the relationships of genotypic and phenotypic heterogeneity to complex environmental factors.

III. PERSPECTIVES IN PSYCHIATRIC GENETICS

Historical Overview: E. Essen-Möller and E. Strömgren

The Early Studies

The first major systematic study of the genetic risk of schizophrenia in relatives of schizophrenics was published by Rüdin (1916b) in Munich. Using statistical methods introduced by Weinberg, Rüdin attempted to apply Mendelian principles to the families of over 700 index cases, many of whom had also been diagnosed by Kraepelin. Many family studies followed in Europe, the largest single contribution being that of Kallmann (1938). Thus, the data base concerning familial factors in the etiology of schizophrenia gradually became established on the basis of an extensive pool of observations.

The findings in families of index cases were compared with the prevalence and incidence of schizophrenia in the general population (e.g., Schulz, 1927; Luxenburger, 1928b; Brugger, 1929; Klemperer, 1933; Sjögren, 1935; Strömgren, 1938; and Fremming, 1951). These early studies in psychiatric genetics, which employed various techniques for avoiding selective biases, may well be considered to have pioneered our present medical epidemiology. The main finding of the family and population studies was that schizophrenia occurs about 10 to 15 times more frequently in siblings and in children of schizophrenics than in the corresponding general population, where its incidence is about 1%. In second-degree relatives, the incidence is about 2% to 3%, and in children of two schizophrenic parents, about 40%.

Monozygotic co-twins of schizophrenic index cases were first systematically investigated by Luxenburger (1928a). The first round of additional samples were studied by Rosanoff and his co-workers (1934), Kallmann (1946, 1950), Essen-Möller (1941), and Slater (1953). Kallmann again contributed the largest sample, which, together with his family study (1938), did much to stimulate genetic interest among American psychiatrists.

If a wide definition of schizophrenia in the co-twins of the index cases was adopted, these twin studies showed about 60% to 70% concordance in monozygotic twins; even higher rates were obtained if the studies were age-corrected. With a stricter diagnosis, the concordance rates came out somewhat lower. Luxenburger (1934) gave 33% concordance for his enlarged and diagnostically revised sample, and

Essen-Möller, in his small sample of seven schizophrenic index cases, found none of the co-twins to be strictly schizophrenic, although five were judged psychotic or borderline with certain symptoms reminiscent of schizophrenia and the remaining two revealed minor character traits thought to be genetically related to schizophrenia. Rosanoff had previously been interested in this clinical variation in degree of concordance in twins, a phenomenon called "schizophrener Kreis" and more recently described as "spectrum disorders," which has long been recognized from the study of ordinary relatives.

The Antigenetic Period

The findings in families and twins were taken to indicate the powerful contribution of genetic factors to the etiology of schizophrenia. However, the experiential and psychodynamic outlook, which expanded particularly after the war, eclipsed or minimized the importance of the genetic view in many quarters (e.g., Jackson, 1960). The increased risk to close relatives was no longer attributed to shared genes but rather to shared environment. The risk was seen in terms of psychological stress exerted by the ill upon the other family members or of communicated morbid behavior and thinking. Reinforcing this neglect of genetic factors, especially in America, was a postwar increase in the influence of the idea, pioneered by Watson and the behaviorist school, that one can shape the individual by shaping his environment during early development. A similar influence came from the psychoanalytic concept that early life experiences shape personality maturation and could have etiological significance for psychiatric illness. A third factor was the misconception that labeling a disorder as genetically determined implied a nihilistic attitude toward therapy.

At the high tide of these antigenetic opinions, a number of papers appeared that seemed to offer strong empirical support for them. Thus, in an interesting series of papers, Rosenthal (see, e.g., 1962b) produced some evidence that the early monozygotic twin concordance rate might have been too high because of the composition of the hospital populations from which the index cases had been taken. Tienari (1963), starting from a twin population rather than from hospitals, found no concordance for schizophrenia among sixteen monozygotic pairs; and Kringlen (1964b) described a sample of eight cases, only two of which were concordant for schizophrenia. A later report by Pollin and his collaborators (1969) gave 14% concordance.

Recent Studies

These striking results incited great interest and stimulated the collection of new, more rigorous samples by Kringlen (1967), Gottesman and Shields (1972), and Fischer (1973). Their concordance rates, 41% to 51% on an average (36% to 61% in the individual samples when calculated uniformly as risk to co-twins of index cases, the higher rates corresponding to wider diagnoses), obviously come closer to the older samples than to the low figures of the intermediate period. As for the latter, they have been partly adjusted by follow-up studies, and certain methodological peculiarities explain at least some of the remaining deviation.

Another response to the antigenetic challenge was the initiation of adoption studies. Here genetic and environmental factors can be more successfully separated than in twin and family studies because the rearing experience is specifically identified with the adoptive parents and is separated from the influence of the biological parents. The first studies of this kind were reported by Heston (1966) and Karlsson (1966). Presently, extensive investigations of adoptees have been and are being conducted by Kety, Rosenthal, Wender, and Schulsinger (see below, "Adoption Studies of Schizophrenia"). The adoption studies have strengthened the argument for the importance of genetic factors in the etiology of schizophrenia. However, because monozygotic twins are far from 100% concordant for schizophrenia (present studies give about 50% concordance), there is no doubt that environmental factors are also powerful. But there is nothing to prove that these factors are psychological in nature; they could also be caused by the intrauterine, dietary, or chemical environment.

Monozygotic twins discordant for schizophrenia would seem an ideal group for studying important environmental factors retrospectively. In fact most twin researchers have attempted to separate out environmental factors on the basis of discordance, but largely without striking results. Special attention was attracted to reports of more perinatal complications and abnormal neurological signs in the ill twin (e.g., Pollin et al., 1966; Mosher et al., 1971b; Mosher, 1972). However, since the risk of falling ill with schizophrenia is about the same for the siblings of discordant twins as it is for those of concordant twins, it would seem that discordant pairs, rather than being examples of sporadic cases, might be instances of low penetrance in the well twin. A complex and continuous interaction between genetic and environmental factors seems to be the most plausible explanation.

Another way of studying such possible interaction is prospective. Here children of schizophrenics (high-risk subjects) are followed in detail during their development in the hope that informative differences in reactivity and environment will emerge between those who eventually become schizophrenic and those who do not (see the discussion by Schulsinger in the section below, "The New Research Strategies—A Critique").

An overrepresentation of single cases in families was observed by Schulz (1934), and certain schizophrenics with a plausible history of eliciting factors, psychological or somatic, were found to show a low risk rate in their families (Schulz, 1932). Slater and his colleagues (1963) reported schizophrenia-like psychoses with temporal epilepsy in cases with no schizophrenic history. Welner and Strömgren (1958) as well as McCabe (1975) reported "psychogenic psychoses," clinically diagnosed, with no prior family history. Obviously, the heterogeneity in the etiology of schizophrenic psychoses is an important problem.

As long as the substrate, or substrates, of the schizophrenic psychoses remain unknown, a careful grouping together of differentiated clinical findings by families and twin pairs is necessary for establishing the genetic etiology of schizophrenia, and the tentative fitting into theoretical genetic models is an important link in isolating the mode of genetic transmission (see Chapter IV).

Twin Studies of Schizophrenia

This section is based on discussion and critiques of twin studies by E. Essen-Möller, I.I. Gottesman, E. Kringlen, S.S. Kety, D. Rosenthal, and F.G. Worden.

Design of Twin Studies

In classical twin studies, differences between MZ (monozygotic) and DZ (dizygotic) twins were attributed to genetic factors on the assumption that, since both members of a twin pair share the same environment, there should be no difference in environmental variance between MZ and DZ twins. It follows that any difference in concordance rates for schizophrenia between MZ and DZ twins would then reflect the fact that MZ twins have an identical genetic endowment while DZ twins share only half their genes on average. However, MZ twins identify with each other, imitate one another, and share virtually all life experiences together much more than do DZ twins (Koch, 1966). If one member of an MZ pair develops a disorder or behavioral pattern that is not genetic, presumably, the chances are that the co-twin will develop the same pattern more often than would the co-twin in a DZ pair. Thus, MZ twins should show a higher concordance rate even for a nongenetic disorder or behavioral pattern. In fact, there is almost never any reason to believe that MZ twins will manifest a lower concordance rate than DZ twins, whether the trait or disorder in question is genetic or not. All findings should go in the same direction; only the magnitude of the difference between the concordance rates in the two types of twins is at issue.

The interpretation of observed differences is therefore complicated not only by the potential methodological weaknesses of the earlier studies but also by questions about the underlying assumption of environmental equivalence between MZ and DZ twin pairs. Of course, the same problems of interpretation apply to any familial trait so long as pairs of relatives are reared together.

Methodological Issues in Twin Studies

Sampling

In the earlier twin studies such as Kallmann's, the index twin (i.e., the one with schizophrenia) was likely to be a severe chronic schizophrenic already hospitalized. Because severity of the illness and sampling directly from a hospital population are associated with high concordance rates, the bias of the earlier samples was toward high concordance rates. If results of twin studies are to be generalized to other than the hospitalized population of schizophrenics, it is necessary to have a systematic sampling procedure that includes nonhospitalized schizophrenics and schizophrenics not in treatment. Failure to meet these sampling criteria undoubtedly contributed to the higher concordance rates found in the earlier studies; however, the results are valid at least for hospitalized, severely ill schizophrenics, and the lower concordance rates found in contemporary studies are more accurate for schizophrenics in general.

Criteria for Concordance

Gottesman stressed the importance of differentiating the three methods of determining concordance (see Allen et al., 1967): (1) the casewise rate refers to the proportion of cases with an affected partner and has the highest value; (2) the pairwise rate refers to the proportion of pairs in which both twins are affected and gives the most conservative value; and (3) the proband method, which gives a value intermediate between the casewise rate and the pairwise rate. This method omits as probands those cases that have not been independently ascertained in a defined manner. The proband method thus calculates concordance as the proportion of probands with an affected partner; it is a casewise rate corrected for mode of ascertainment and is the value most comparable to the calculated risks for other classes of relatives and for the general population (see Gottesman and Shields, 1972).

Zygosity Determination

Zygosity determination, if twin pairs are intact and available for study, is now accurate, but in the earlier studies a small error could be assigned to the difficulty in making judgments of zygosity (see Gottesman and Shields, 1972).

Age of Risk

Some of the variance in age-corrected concordance rates is due to variation between studies in regard to using a shorter or longer age of risk; however, most of the variance comes from whether or not the studies are age-corrected. For example, when Kallmann's study was age-corrected, his MZ concordance rates for "definite schizophrenia" rose from 59% to the much-quoted figure of 86%, and the DZ rate rose from 9% to 15% (see Gottesman and Shields, 1972).

Diagnosis

Diagnosis is not especially difficult for the index twin because doubtful cases can be sequestered or discarded, but diagnosis of the co-twins reported in the literature has been argued at length in different studies. In earlier studies, the investigator usually diagnosed both members of a twin pair, leaving open a serious possibility of bias. A better procedure in contemporary twin studies is to have twins diagnosed by judges who are blind as to whether the twin is a member of an MZ or a DZ pair.

The influence of diagnostic criteria on the discrimination between MZ and DZ twins was studied by Shields and Gottesman (1972). An international panel of seven diagnosticians blindly diagnosed the histories of 114 twins in the Maudsley schizophrenic twin

TABLE 1

Concordance for Judges with the Most Extreme
Criteria of Schizophrenia [Shields and Gottesman, 1972]

Criteria	MZ	DZ	MZ:DZ
Narrowest criteria (Birley)			
Both twins first-choice schizophrenia	3/15 20%	3/22 14%	1.5
Both twins schizophrenia, including			
?? schizophrenia	10/21 48%	3/30 10%	4.8
Consensus diagnosis of 6 judges			
Both twins schizophrenia, including			
? schizophrenia	11/22 50%	3/33 9%	5.5
Broadest criteria (Meehl)			
Both twins chronic or acute schizophrenia	11/22 50%	3/33 9%	5.5
Both twins schizophrenia (including			
borderline schizophrenia) or schizotype	14/24 58%	8/33 24%	2.4

series. It was found that very broad or very strict diagnostic criteria did
not give as reliable a discrimination between MZ and DZ twin
concordance rates as did a middle-of-the-road consensus diagnosis
(Table 1).

Prenatal and Perinatal Factors

Twins are usually born prematurely, have a higher death rate
during the first year than nontwins, and the death rate of MZ twins is
higher than that of DZ twins (Yerushalmy and Sheerar, 1940a,b;
Bulmer, 1970). In a Swedish study (Husén, 1960), twins showed mean
poorer performance than single borns in Swedish, mathematics, and
English. Twins are therefore a deviant sample.

Other possible confounding variables include fusion of the
placenta giving both fetal twins a shared circulation, differences of
intrauterine position between fetal twins, in utero crowding, special
conditions of implantation, and different circumstances during delivery.
Some of these conditions may disadvantage one twin and lead to
increased discordance between the twins, others may increase concordance because of common environmental effects. Comparison of
monochorionic and dichorionic MZ twins would be interesting
(Campion and Tucker, 1973). However, the risk of schizophrenia is not
higher in twins than nontwins and the kinds of schizophrenia observed
in twins do not differ from those in singletons (Rosenthal, 1960).

A Recent Twin Study: E. Kringlen

The largest of the recent twin studies where a personal survey was made of the twins was reported by Kringlen (1967). All twins recorded in the Norwegian birth lists from 1901 to 1930 were checked against the central register of psychoses. This provided a large and, what is more important, a relatively unselected sample of psychotic twins. A final sample of 342 pairs of twins between the ages of 34 and 64 where one or both of the twins had at some time been hospitalized in Norway for functional psychoses was obtained.

Of the 342 pairs, 75 were classified as MZ and 55 of these belonged to the schizophrenic group. The pairwise concordance rate for schizophrenia ranged from 25% to 38% in MZ pairs, and 4% to 12% for DZ pairs, variations depending upon whether the concordance rates were based on registered hospitalized cases or personal investigations and on whether a wide or a strict concept of schizophrenia was employed.

The study showed that the clinical pictures presented by individuals with the same hereditary equipment as a typical schizophrenic (schizophreniform excluded) embraced a graduated series of disorders and personality patterns that ranged from a duplication of the psychosis to neurosis and clinical normalcy. In 31% both twins showed the same psychopathology. In another 9% the co-twins of schizophrenics had either been affected with a reactive psychosis or could be described as borderline cases. In 29% the co-twins were diagnosed as having character disorders, suffering from various neuroses, or being alcoholic. And finally, 31% of the co-twins were considered to be normal.

The investigation showed that clear differences existed in discordant MZ and DZ pairs in premorbid personality traits and nervous symptoms in childhood. Prior to his illness, the schizophrenic displayed a less healthy personality structure than the nonpsychotic twin. Usually, the more introverted, submissive, dependent, and obsessive twin was more prone to develop schizophrenia later on.

In Kringlen's study, no difference between twins and the general population in frequency of functional psychoses was demonstrated, a finding that cast doubt on Jackson's (1960) theory that MZ twins may have a high risk for schizophrenia because of problems of ego formation and confused identity.

A Critical Review of Pairwise and Probandwise Rates:
I.I. Gottesman

Table 2 shows the results of five recent twin studies at two levels—a pairwise range of concordance rates reported by the investigators and a set of probandwise concordance rates using the criterion "affected," which approximates what a consensus panel of seven judges called "S + ?S"; that is, a functional psychosis with schizophrenic-like features not likely to be an affective psychosis. The continued misunderstanding of the different kinds of concordance rates that can calculated from the same twin data pool led to the description of differences between pairwise and probandwise rates above.

TABLE 2

Concordance in Recent Twin Studies
[From Gottesman and Shields, 1976]

	Gottesman and Shields	Kringlen	Fischer	Tienari	Pollin
MZ Pairs					
Pairwise range (%)	40-50	25-38	24-48	0-36	14-27
Number of pairs	22	55	21	17	95
Probandwise concordance (%)	58	45	56	35	43
DZ Pairs					
Pairwise range (%)	9-10	4-10	10-19	5-14	4-5
Number of pairs	33	90	41	20	125
Probandwise concordance (%)	12	15	26	13	9

These data have not been age-corrected.

The studies summarized in Table 2 are presented so as to show how many twins were probands, or index cases, in their own right using each study's criterion. Kringlen (1967) combined the pairs with schizophrenic (45) and schizophreniform (10) diagnoses to reach the sample of 55 MZ pairs. As he used the diagnosis, schizophreniform turned out to be just as "genetic" as schizophrenia. The lower end of the range of pairwise concordance rates, 25%, was obtained by dividing the number of pairs where both twins were hospitalized and registered as schizophrenic or schizophreniform (14) by the total number of pairs (55). The upper limit of 38% was obtained when Kringlen also counted as concordant those pairs where the co-twin, though not on the register, was found by him to be either psychotic (3) or borderline (4). At the level of schizophrenic-like functional psychosis, pairwise concordance is therefore $(14 + 3)/55 = 31\%$. To convert this to a probandwise rate the 14 MZ pairs where both twins appeared on the national psychosis register were added to both the numerator and the denominator to obtain a new fraction, $(14 + 14 + 3)/(14 + 55)$ or $31/69 = 45\%$. This is the percent of independently ascertained (registered) twins with schizophrenia or schizophreniform psychosis (69 probands) who had an affected partner. (If cases that Kringlen diagnosed as borderline on interview were included, the probandwise rate would have gone up to 51%, $35/69$.) The number of concordance rates that can be derived from a study should not be a cause of embarrassment to twin researchers, but rather cause for pause and thoughtful deliberation.

The Maudsley Hospital Twin Study: I.I. Gottesman

The Maudsley-Hospital-based study of Gottesman and Shields was reported late in 1972 and included case histories of both MZ and DZ pairs and blindfolded diagnoses of the 114 twins by a panel of six judges plus a Scandinavian viewpoint from Essen-Möller. Gottesman and Shields's work before and at the conference in 1967 on the transmission of schizophrenia (see Rosenthal and Kety, 1968) made use of four operationally defined categories of disorder/normalcy that they have since abandoned for the consensus diagnosis of a blindfolded panel of international diagnosticians. Their complete reporting of details (Gottesman and Shields, 1972) will permit further analyses and tests of competing or alternative hypotheses by others without the great expenditure of time and energy initially required to collect a sample from sixteen years of consecutive admissions to a regional psychiatric facility. Despite the emphasis of Gottesman and Shields on formal quantitative and population genetics as the framework for evaluating their data, attention was also directed to sociodemographic and hypothesized psychodynamic factors. The condensed summary of their concordance rates in Table 2 shows these studies to be of a piece with the other recent twin studies. The fact that the probands came from consecutive admissions to both inpatient and (mostly) outpatient sources was given as one reason why the MZ concordance rates of Gottesman and Shields were somewhat lower than the earlier twin studies, which had a large proportion of "standing" hospital cases. Extensive psychometric assessments by means of the Minnesota Multiphasic Personality Inventory, the Goldstein-Scheerer Object

Sorting Test, and the Global Psychopathology Rating Scale added new dimensions to this twin study, as did the taped interviews with most of the twins.

By using a genetic criterion, Gottesman and Shields explored a new way for testing the validity of various of the judges' individual and consensus diagnoses of schizophrenia. They asked the judges which concepts of schizophrenia preserved and maximized the difference in concordance rates between MZ and DZ pairs. Aside from the obviously greater reliability obtained for a consensus diagnosis for psychometric reasons, they found that either too narrow or too broad a concept for schizophrenia eroded the MZ/DZ contrasts—too narrow criteria lowered the MZ rate to the value of the DZ rate and too wide criteria raised both the MZ and the DZ rates to dilute an indicator of "biological specificity," the ratio of the MZ/DZ concordance rates (see Table 1). These findings are not unlike those of Carpenter and his collaborators (1973) who showed the effects of too many or too few Schneiderian symptoms (see Schneider, 1971) on the number of false positive and false negative diagnoses of schizophrenia.

Since 1972 Gottesman and Shields have gone on to explore the concepts of schizoidia and the so-called schizophrenia spectrum (Shields, Heston, and Gottesman, 1975) by using the expected and observed rates of various conditions in co-twins as a point of departure. One consequence of their paper with Heston was a revision of the latter's formulation that schizoidia was the basis of most schizophrenias and that schizoidia was caused by a dominant gene with complete penetrance. The revision was occasioned by looking at exactly what conditions were necessary to be included among DZ co-twins of the Maudsley schizophrenic-probands before a DZ rate of 50% affectation was achieved. It was obvious that a concept of schizoidia too wide to be useful outside of family studies was needed to retain the idea of complete penetrance despite the earlier formulation (Heston, 1970) of twin and family data. They agreed to disagree on whether a dominant gene with incomplete penetrance (essentially Slater's theory) was any better or worse than a polygenic threshold theory wherein some genes could have large effects, especially since Gottesman and Shields (1972) had shown that the predictions of the two theories led to indistinguishable differences with the empirically observed risks in relatives of schizophrenics.

One recurring theme in the Gottesman and Shields writings on schizophrenia is that, by construing the disorder as polygenically determined with a threshold effect, a number of heuristic benefits accrue to investigators. Models provided by *Drosophila* genetics (Thoday, 1967), population genetics (Cavalli-Sforza and Bodmer, 1971), mathematical genetics (Falconer, 1965; Smith, 1971; Curnow and Smith, 1975), and leads provided by researchers on such conditions as diabetes and even Huntington's disease become grist for the schizophreniologist's mill. Gottesman and Shields (1967) and Falconer (1965) introduced psychopathologists to the concept of the liability to develop a threshold trait and calculated that the heritability of the liability to develop schizophrenia on present evidence is in the neighborhood of 85%; a naive determinist view of this value is not warranted. Few other schizophrenia researchers have chosen to differentiate between threshold and continuum models, even to support a polygenic view over a monogenic one.

Adoption Studies of Schizophrenia

This section is derived from critiques and discussion of adoption studies by J.A. Clausen, I.I. Gottesman, E. Gruenberg, S.S. Kety, D. Rosenthal, F. Schulsinger, E. Strömgren, and P.H. Wender.

Design of Adoption Studies

In family and twin studies of the transmission of schizophrenia, genetic and environmental variables are confounded because both the genetic endowment and the rearing experience are provided by the same biological parents. The influence of these variables can, however, be more successfully separated in studies of adopted persons because the rearing experience is provided by adoptive parents and the genetic endowment by the biological parents. Exploiting this advantage in a series of studies, Kety, Rosenthal, Wender, Schulsinger, and colleagues have demonstrated the following: (1) The prevalence of schizophrenia is greater among the raised-apart biological relatives of adopted adult schizophrenics than among the raised-apart biological relatives of nonschizophrenics (Kety et al., 1968). (2) The prevalence of schizophrenia, as well as schizophrenia-like disorders, is greater among the adopted-away offspring of schizophrenics than among the adopted-away offspring of nonschizophrenics (Rosenthal et al., 1968, 1971). (3) The adoptive parents of schizophrenics are less disturbed behaviorally and psychologically than the biological parents of schizophrenics (Wender et al., 1968, 1971). (4) Diagnoses of schizophrenia and uncertain schizophrenia are significantly concentrated in the biological relatives of adoptees who become schizophrenic, whereas the biological relatives of controls, adoptive relatives of schizophrenics, and adoptive relatives of controls have no more of these diagnoses than the general population. Furthermore, there was a significant concentration of schizophrenic diagnoses in biological paternal half-siblings of schizophrenic adoptees compared to paternal half-siblings of controls; in utero factors and early mothering experiences are excluded because paternal half-siblings have different mothers. These individuals have therefore shared no environmental influences with the probands.

In a preliminary study, the offspring of normal biological parents, adopted and reared by schizophrenic foster parents, were compared with adopted-away offspring of normal biological parents reared by normal parents and the adopted-away offspring of schizophrenic biological parents reared by normal foster parents. This cross-fostering type of study indicated a greater prevalence of psychopathology among the adopted-away offspring of schizophrenic parents than among either of the other cross-fostered groups. In other words, the tentative conclusion is that rearing by schizophrenic parents does not produce schizophrenia in a child with normal genetic endowment (Wender et al., 1974).

The results of the most recently completed study, unpublished at the time of the conference, are summarized in Table 3. This represents an analysis of blind consensus diagnoses based on psychiatric interviews conducted by Jacobsen with the biological and adoptive relatives of schizophrenic and control adoptees. Of the 512 relatives identified, 119 had died, 26 had emigrated beyond Scandinavia, and 3 had disappeared. More than 90% of those alive and accessible participated in the interviews.

Methodological Issues in Adoption Studies

The ideal method for the separation of genetic and environmental variables would be to study identical twins reared apart from birth. However, there are few such twin pairs with schizophrenia, and there would be severe ascertainment bias if this method were used. For this reason, Kety and his collaborators utilized a sample of nontwin adoptees. The following methodological issues concerning these studies were raised and discussed.

TABLE 3

Summary of Adoption Study Based on Interviews with Relatives
of 33 Schizophrenic Adoptees and Their Matched Controls [Kety et al., 1975]

	Biological relatives		p^*	Adoptive relatives	
	Index	Control		Index	Control
Number identified	173	174		74	91
Died	35	13	.0004	35	36
Alive and residing in Scandinavia	124	149		39	52
Adequate interview obtained	118	140		35	48
Consensus psychiatric diagnosis†					
Normal	30	49		11	11
Organic	7	6		5	6
Neurosis	4	6		3	2
Affective	2	11	.05	1	3
Personality disorder	27	39		8	15
Nonschizophrenia spectrum psychiatric diagnosis	40	62		17	26
Schizophrenia spectrum†					
Definite schizophrenia	11	3	.026	1	2
Chronic	5	0	.03	1	1
Latent	6	3		0	1
Uncertain schizophrenia	13	3	.009	1	3
Total, definite and uncertain schizophrenia	24	6	.0004	2	5
Schizoid or inadequate personality	13	13		2	2
Biological paternal half-siblings only ‡					
Number identified	63	64			
Definite schizophrenia	8	1	.015		
Definite or uncertain schizophrenia	14	2	.001		
Families as units‡					
Number	33	34		33	34
With one or more definite schizophrenia	14	3	.002	1	3

$^*p$ = Fischer's exact probability comparing index and control relatives, where value is .05 or less.

†Diagnoses based on interviews only.

‡Diagnoses based on all information available (interviews and institutional records).

Sampling

　　The cooperation of the Danish government and the quality of Danish records of adoptions, psychiatric illness, and population (Kety et al., 1968) made possible the identification of adoptees in sufficient numbers to permit the research designs that have been employed. Nevertheless, a number of questions about the sample were raised and discussed.

Do the probands really constitute all the adoptees in the area investigated? This question must be answered in the affirmative as a consequence of the complete system of registration of adoptions in Denmark. All legally adopted adults between 25 and 50 years of age where adoption was not by biological relatives in the city and county of Copenhagen have been included in the material. The inclusion of the rest of adoptions in Denmark is in progress.

Are adoptees representative of the general population? Certainly not. For instance, they display considerably higher criminality than the rest of the population of the same age and sex. This does not, however, invalidate comparisons within the group of adoptees. The adoptees are representative of the nonadopted population insofar as the prevalence of schizophrenia in both groups is concerned. In a comprehensive sample of nonadopted individuals matched for the 5483 adoptees in number, age, sex, and socioeconomic class of the rearing family, a search was made for schizophrenic probands using the same techniques of ascertainment and diagnosis employed for the adopted sample. This yielded 31 schizophrenic nonadopted probands as compared with 33 among the adopted group.

Are the schizophrenics found in the adoptee sample representative of schizophrenics in Denmark in general? No. The age distribution of the adoptees does not correspond to that of the general population, as it comprises more young people. As there is a high correlation between age at onset and subtype of schizophrenia, some types may be overrepresented and others underrepresented among the adoptees and their siblings.

Gershon raised the possibility that schizophrenics who do not keep their offspring have a genetically more virulent illness than schizophrenics in general. However, in the adopted-away study of Rosenthal and his co-workers (1971), the modal time of first hospitalization for the biological parents was approximately 11 years after the child was born. So in fact the sample was skewed away from early onset and more severely ill parental schizophrenia.

Are the schizophrenics found in this metropolitan population representative of schizophrenics in Denmark as a whole? Probably not. Kety has reminded us of the possibility that in an urban population there are special environmental conditions that may favor the hospitalization of schizophrenics with the result that known schizophrenia becomes more prevalent in metropolitan areas than in rural areas. Many studies in other countries have supported this observation. The findings are, however, not easy to interpret because the high prevalence of schizophrenia in certain urban districts may be at least partially caused by migration of schizophrenics or schizophrenia-prone individuals to such areas. Careful studies in the United States and England (Goldberg and Morrison, 1963; Turner and Wagenfeld, 1967) seem to show that most, but definitely not all, of the accumulation is caused by migration phenomena. Further evidence for the migration of schizophrenia-prone individuals to disadvantaged urban areas is provided by Wender and his colleagues (1973) in a study of relationships between socioeconomic status and the prevalence of schizophrenia in a population of adoptees. They concluded tentatively that their data support the hypothesis that psychopathology causes people to become ineffectual socially and occupationally and, therefore, to drift downward in the social hierarchy. These data did not, however, support the hypothesis that migration to cities occurred because the subjects were schizophrenic. An equally plausible hypothesis is that, facilities being less available in the country, individuals must be sicker to be admitted to such facilities and thus obtain "official" recognition. There are differences with regard to prevalence of schizophrenia in different parts of Denmark. In this connection, it should be remembered that an area from which people are emigrating will tend to show a high prevalence since the severely disturbed persons tend to stay in that area, whereas a large fraction of the sound population will move to other parts of the country. It has been observed in other countries that in such "residual" populations prevalences of all kinds of incapacitating disorders are high, and this applies to the metropolitan area of Copenhagen as well. In the center of Copenhagen, all kinds of incapacities are more prevalent than in the suburbs to which the more sound and prosperous parts of the population tend to emigrate.

These questions, of course, are not peculiar to adoption studies but are common to family, twin, or any epidemiological study that does not involve an entire country. In the Danish adoption studies, they have little bearing on the conclusions drawn since comparisons are always made against matched controls, the relatives involved are identified, records obtained, and interviews held wherever the family members may have moved in Denmark. Also, the adoptees in the greater Copenhagen sample represented both an urban and suburban population, and thus the sample is already reasonably representative of the Danish population. In any case, these demographic problems will disappear when all adoptees in the total Danish population are included. It is important to remember that, when only offspring of schizophrenics are studied, there is a question of the representiveness in general, since approximately 90% of schizophrenics do not have a schizophrenic parent.

Nongenetic Prenatal, Perinatal, and Neonatal Factors

The expression of genetic factors may be confounded by the action of environmental factors occurring during fetal development, at birth, or in the immediate neonatal period. In the biological relatives of schizophrenics there is a significantly higher death rate than in the biological relatives of controls. Schulsinger and his staff have tracked down the cause of each death from death certificates and other records. The preponderance of deaths in the index biological relatives can be largely accounted for by suicide (5 vs. 0 instances), possible suicide (3 vs. 0), sudden death of unknown cause (3 vs. 0), or homicide (5 vs. 0). Deaths from natural causes are not significantly different between the two groups (19 vs. 15).

Furthermore, the biological mothers of schizophrenics have a higher death rate at an earlier age than the biological mothers of controls. The earlier deaths of the biological mothers suggested to Gruenberg that the biological mothers of the schizophrenic adoptees may live in a harsher physical environment and, consequently, may provide a less favorable intrauterine environment for fetal development. Such environmental factors might influence gene expression so that a schizophrenic genotype that might not manifest itself phenotypically when buffered by a sheltered environment is expressed as schizophrenia. Kety's group was struck by the greater number of deaths among the biological mothers of schizophrenic adoptees than the control biological mothers. There were indeed more deaths among index than among control biological mothers (11 vs. 3), but of these, 4 were suicides, 1 accidental, and 1 of unknown cause. The remaining 5 represented neoplasm (2) or circulatory disease (3). The 3 deaths among the control mothers were from neoplasm, coronary disease, and cirrhosis. An alternative hypothesis would therefore be that the suicides represented unrecognized schizophrenia and that the higher death rate is a genotypic expression, not the result of harsher environmental factors.

At any rate, the operation of prenatal and perinatal factors is ruled out in studies of biological paternal half-siblings of schizophrenics and in studies of the adopted-away offspring of schizophrenic fathers (Rosenthal, 1971) because, in these instances, there is no sharing of uterine or neonatal environment. The data from this group suggest that genetic factors are significant for the transmission of schizophrenia (Kety et al., 1975).

Diagnosis

In the adoptee studies, what is meant by the concept of the schizophrenic spectrum? As a hypothesis to be tested, it proposes that the diagnoses of schizophrenia, uncertain schizophrenia, and schizoid or inadequate personality form a continuum of syndromes related to the schizophrenic genotype (Kety et al., 1968). Although measures of interrater reliability indicate that blind judges agree substantially on the categorization of patients into the schizophrenic spectrum disorders, there is no way of defining how these phenotypic patterns are related to the genotype for schizophrenia. Some evidence suggests that clear-cut psychotic episodes, such as certain acute schizophrenic reactions that occur, for example, in some individuals under severe combat stress, probably have little genetic relationship to true schizophrenia, whereas, conversely, discordant identical twins of "true" schizophrenics who fail to show spectrum disorder manifestations probably have an unexpressed schizophrenic genotype.

A further point is that, in the adoptee studies, blind judges made multiple ratings of a single clinical assessment. Since the manifestations of psychopathology are known to be highly dynamic and variable over time and to interact with changing life circumstances, Clausen suggested that the studies would be strengthened if repeated clinical and social role assessments of the adoptees were obtained. Epidemiological studies entailing repeated measurement suggest substantial turnover between classifications of mild and severe symptoms, especially over a period of years (Srole, 1975).

Also, it is obvious that the precautions taken to secure blindness and lack of bias imply that some error may be introduced by the length of time involved and the number of investigators working on the case history, the personal interview, the case notes, abstracts of case histories, translations from Danish into English, making of diagnoses, and the coding and conclusion. The number of research workers and their helpers participating in the preparation of the material introduces the risk that different diagnostic viewpoints, different opinions of what is important, etc., might have colored the case notes, the abstracts, and the conclusions made on the basis of the written material.

In a study of some of these issues, Kety and his colleagues (1975) investigated the possibility of bias introduced by the person interviewing the subjects and editing the material that was to be submitted to the blind raters. They found that where hunches or other clues had become available during the interview or during the editing of the records, these did not influence the diagnostic judgment, and deletion of all cases where such hunches occurred had no significant influence on the results.

A question remains of whether the different members of the Danish-American team have always understood the viewpoints of the other members. Do they always know what the other members mean by certain expressions in current use within clinical psychiatry? Can they always know what other members regard as abnormal? There are certainly differences between nations and individuals in this respect, not only with regard to viewpoints and evaluations, but also with regard to the way in which they are expressed verbally.

Finally, the real complexity of expression of personality function cannot adequately be communicated in any system of classification or diagnostic labeling. Prose descriptions of individuals and of family units are useful in revealing the nuances of idiosyncratic personalities that might be correlated to the genetic transmission of schizophrenia. Such a correlation might be revealed in the analysis of component symptoms, signs, and behaviors.

Other Issues

Since the schizophrenia risks in the adoptee studies were not age-corrected, it is not yet possible to test genetic models against each other for a best fit. In general, frequencies are expressed as prevalences, which makes comparisons with other frequencies difficult. True expectancies have not been calculated in the adoptee studies, and age corrections have not been carried out to a sufficient degree. Furthermore, separate analysis of first- and second-degree relatives of schizophrenics would improve the studies. It is also important to note that, unless both parents are assessed, we must assume an ignorance of selective processes in matings.

Contributions of Adoption Studies: S.S. Kety

In addressing the methodological problems, one should keep in mind what adoption studies cannot accomplish as well as what they are uniquely qualified to accomplish; in particular, one should consider what hypotheses the adoption studies were designed to test, the validity of the conclusions drawn, and the relevance of the criticism to those issues. The unique value of adoption studies lies in the opportunity they offer to disentangle genetic and environmental variables, which family studies and twin studies, no matter how carefully planned and executed, have not been able to do. They are not especially useful for yielding data pertinent to the mode of genetic transmission or to the "true" prevalence of schizophrenia in a population. Since the prevalence of schizophrenia depends so heavily on factors of ascertainment and diagnoses, Kety and his co-workers decided at the very beginning to control these variables, as well as the possible differences between adopted individuals and their relatives from the rest of the population, by the use of matched controls subjected indiscriminately to the same ascertainment and diagnostic procedures. It is comforting, but not crucial, that what Kety's group calls "definite schizophrenia" is found in approximately 1% of individuals not genetically related to the index cases when the diagnosis is taken from institutional records and in 2% when the diagnosis is based on psychiatric interviews with nearly all of the same population. The compatibility of these figures with those in the literature shows that the incidence of schizophrenia in the relatives of adopted individuals does not differ from the incidence in the general population and that the techniques of ascertainment and diagnosis of Kety's group are not conspicuously idiosyncratic. To age-correct these prevalences or to calculate "true expectancies" seems somewhat pretentious.

Although Kety and his collaborators have reported the diagnoses for the different types of relationships, they have not attempted to make comparisons among them because they are not comparable in terms of ascertainment and other variables. Instead, they have compared biological relatives of index cases with those of control probands where number, relationships, age, and ascertainment are comparable, the only difference being that one group is genetically related to the schizophrenic probands. The consistency with which the biologically related group shows a significantly higher prevalence of

schizophrenia is the most important finding. Many of the methodological problems that have been raised would tend to increase the
variability in the final consensus diagnosis and render a significant
difference less likely to occur by chance. Assortative mating, which
does occur to some extent, would enhance an existing difference
between index and control relatives but would not create a difference.

The interview study has yielded enough new information to
permit examination of the components of the schizophrenia spectrum,
which Kety's group regards as a hypothesis or group of hypotheses that
can be tested for a relationship to classical schizophrenia. Their
diagnosis of chronic schizophrenia (comparable to the classical or
Kraepelinian type) is found by each rater and by the consensus at a
significantly higher rate in the biological index relatives. Their diagnosis
of latent schizophrenia discriminates the two populations less well. On
the other hand, the diagnosis of "uncertain" schizophrenia (by which
each rater signifies that schizophrenia is his best diagnosis, although he
is uncertain because of atypical features, the absence of information, or
of sufficient crucial symptoms) discriminates the two populations
extremely well. Their consensus diagnoses of "schizoid personality" or
"inadequate personality" failed to discriminate these two populations
significantly, although one rater did so with a p value of .001. The
criteria used for their diagnoses have been published, and it would now
seem appropriate to attempt to define these subgroups more explicitly;
this is being done in collaboration with Robert Spitzer and his
colleagues using a computer-based diagnostic system.

X Linkage in Manic-Depressive Psychosis:
W.E. Bunney, Jr., E.S. Gershon, and G. Winokur

The hypothesis of X chromosome transmission of manic-
depressive illness was first advanced by Rosanoff and his colleagues
(1935), but it was Winokur and his co-workers who first presented
evidence using X-chromosome-linked markers to support this hypothesis (Reich et al., 1969; Winokur and Tanna, 1969; Winokur et al.,
1969). A large series of informative families was recently reported by
Mendlewicz and his co-workers (1972, 1975; Mendlewicz and Fleiss,
1974). Their conclusion that a subset of bipolar manic-depressive illness
is linked to marker loci on the X chromosome represents a potentially
crucial breakthrough in our understanding of this disorder.

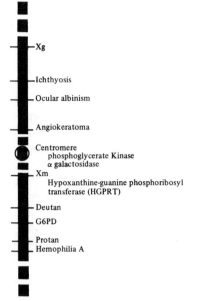

Figure 1. Map of the human X chromosome. Deutan and protan are two forms of color blindness. Xg is a blood-group protein, and Xm is another protein found in the blood. There are at least 93 loci known to belong to the X chromosome, most of which are unmapped, in addition to almost as many others that are believed to be X-linked. Several of the map locations given here are tentative. [From Bodmer and Cavalli-Sforza, 1976]

Sex Chromosome Linkage and Recombination

Chromosomes are transmitted from parent to child either as replicates of one of the original paired chromosomes, or as crossover products (recombinants) of both members of the pair (Cavalli-Sforza and Bodmer, 1971). If the recombination frequency (θ) is 50%, the two markers are said to be unlinked, since this is the expected "recombination" between genes on separate chromosomes. (In fact, genes that are far apart on the same chromosome may often give rise to recombination fractions of 50%.) The human X chromosome is paired in the female but not in the male (where it is associated with the Y chromosome), and it is not transmitted from fathers to sons. Examination of the sons of women heterozygous at two loci therefore allows estimation of the recombination frequency. In the present case, color blindness and the Xg blood group serve as the marker loci whose relationship to bipolar manic-depressive illness is studied. Demonstration of less than 50% recombination between a known X chromosome locus and bipolar illness would prove that a locus on the X chromosome contributes to the risk for manic-depressive illness. Previous studies of linkage between markers on the X chromosome have allowed the chromosome to be mapped (Figure 1), providing reference points for placement of newly discovered loci.

Methodological Problems

In a psychiatric disorder with multiple manifestations and a variable age of onset, the use of analytic methods such as those of Edwards (1971; Morton, 1955)* requiring that each informative person be definitely ill or well does not allow for errors in classification of well persons who have not passed through the age of risk. This problem might be dealt with by introducing an age-of-onset probability density function into the Edwards method (Elston, 1973). An alternative adopted by Mendlewicz and his co-workers (1972, 1975; Mendlewicz and Fleiss, 1974) is to include persons as negative for illness only if they have passed an appreciable portion of the age at risk for the disorder. Clearly, this is only a rough approximation of the probability that a well relative will ever become ill.

The problems of penetrance and the multiple manifestations of affective illness are less easily handled. In order to minimize the number of persons who are genotypically but not phenotypically ill with manic-depressive illness, Mendlewicz and Fleiss (1974) chose families with manifest illness in two generations and interpreted any affective disturbance as a manifestation of the genotype for bipolar illness. Gershon and his co-workers (1976b) noted that this method may select atypical families from among all persons with affective illness but would not be expected to produce a false linkage in the families studied provided that ascertainment is otherwise unbiased.

The presence of multiple forms of the illness (e.g., unipolar and bipolar forms of affective disorder) also presents problems in analyzing for transmission on the X chromosome. Family studies are required to demonstrate that each of the multiple manifestations is indeed related to bipolar illness. Finding that significantly more relatives of bipolar patients than expected have unipolar illness or cycloid personality would demonstrate that some cases of these disorders are related to bipolar illness. The possibility that phenocopies or independent unipolar illness will appear in these pedigrees and produce false linkage findings of illness is not taken into account by the Edwards method, nor is the possibility that nonpenetrance causes a mistaken negative finding of psychiatric normalcy.

Gershon and Bunney concluded that linkage analysis using the Edwards method is not definitive in bipolar manic-depressive illness;

*This method essentially finds the recombination fraction that maximizes the likelihood of the particular distribution pattern of the marker and the trait observed in the sibship.

nevertheless the results are of value for heuristic purposes, and the data may prove suggestive despite the methodological limitations.

Association Between Manic-Depressive Illness and Color Blindness

An assumption of the Edwards method is that the probability of occurrence of coupling and repulsion* is equal in the population from which the subjects are drawn, and that proband selection does not favor either type or family. This assumption does not appear valid in the reported data on color blindness and manic-depressive illness. All male manic-depressive probands studied by Mendlewicz and his co-workers (1972; Mendlewicz and Fleiss, 1974) were color blind, as was the male proband in the Alger family (Reich et al., 1969) included in their analysis. This should, in general, not occur in random sampling of probands, in which half would be expected to be in repulsion. Two possible explanations may be considered: (1) there may have been preferential referral of patients for family investigation if the patient was both color blind and manic-depressive, or (2) there may be an association between color blindness and manic-depressive illness such that, in families of manic-depressive patients, color blind males are more likely to have manic-depressive illness than normal vision males. Preferential referral would not, however, account for coupling being more likely in the families of female probands not deficient in color vision. In the data reviewed in Table 4, a preponderance of coupling is present in the relatives of both male and female probands, suggesting an association between manic-depressive illness and color blindness. Until this association is understood, linkage analysis of color blindness does not appear possible. Note that very close linkage between a "manic-depressive gene" and color blindness could lead to the coupling excess

---

*Coupling and repulsion refer to the alleles present on a single chromosome. In the case of color blindness, a chromosome in repulsion would have a not-manic depressive and a color blindness allele, or the alleles for manic-depressive illness and not-color blindness. In coupling, chromosomes would have alleles for color blindness and manic-depressive illness or alleles for normal vision and psychiatric normalcy. Association must be carefully distinguished from linkage. Association means that two traits are found together in the population. Linkage means that the loci determining the two traits are close to each other on the chromosome. If a mother has a chromosome in the coupling phase, the traits will tend to be associated in her offspring; but if the mother has a chromosome in repulsion, the traits will tend to be negatively associated in her offspring. In the general population, coupling and repulsion are assumed equally likely, so there will be no tendency for association of the traits. For closely linked genes, this assumption may not be correct (see the later discussion on HLA and disease associations).

TABLE 4

Tests for Association Between Trait at
Marker Locus and Manic-Depressive Illness
[Gershon and Bunney]

I. Relatives of male probands*

	CB−	CB+	
MD−	15	1	$x^2 = 27.2, p < .001$
MD+	4	26	

II. Relatives of female probands

	CB−	CB+	
MD−	8	2	$x^2 = 7.15, p < .02$
MD+	2	11	

III. Xg blood group

	Xg−	Xg+	
MD−	15	7	$x^2 = 3.67$, NS
MD+	19	25	

*All informative sons for linkage analysis, and informative maternal uncles or grandfathers for phase determination, included in this tabulation. "Male probands" include one female proband who was found to be demonstrably heterozygous for color blindness on direct examination, using a test that can detect heterozygous persons.

CB = color blindness; MD = manic-depressive illness; NS = not significant.

(linkage disequilibrium*) without any implications of biased sampling or functional association.

In the data on Xg blood group and bipolar illness, there is no preponderance of coupling or repulsion in the informative sons (Table 4).

Review of Pedigrees Informative for Linkage to Xg

Gershon and Bunney reviewed the published pedigrees bearing on the linkage of the Xg blood group to manic-depressive disorder (Winokur and Tanna, 1969; Mendlewicz and Fleiss, 1974; Mendlewicz et al., 1975). In order to maximize the likelihood of finding X linkage,

*Linkage disequilibrium is the nonrandom association of alleles at linked loci due to the effects of natural selection or to the fact that the population has not yet reached equilibrium.

pedigrees were excluded if the father of informative males was not known to be free of affective illness. A uniform criterion of 25 years of age was chosen as the minimum for considering a person to be free of bipolar or unipolar illness. Based on these criteria, some of the reported families were excluded from computation of the recombination fraction.*

Linkage appears to be present, with $\theta \sim 0.2$ (odds favoring linkage 77:1). These data are compatible with the hypothesis of X linkage. Because of the statistical nature of lod scores, the odds should be greater than 1000:1 for linkage to be accepted (Morton, 1955). In view of this and of the methodological and statistical problems described, it would be premature to conclude that linkage is an established finding.

The importance of age of onset as a methodological problem is illustrated by the fact that in eight out of the twenty informative pedigrees, the evidence that the mother is heterozygous for affective disorder is a single well individual between the ages of 26 and 30. Without these families, the linkage would be even further from statistical significance.

Matthysse pointed out the apparent inconsistency of the reported close linkage with known map distances. As determined by Mendlewicz and his collaborators (1975), the linkage of bipolar illness to the protan-deutan and the Xg locus of the X chromosome is quite close (.07 to .10 map units for color blindness, .19 map units for Xg). The distance between Xg and color blindness has been estimated as 0.48 map units (Renwick and Schulze, 1964). This is greater than the sum of maximum-likelihood map distances from protan-deutan to bipolar illness and from Xg to bipolar illness, which is estimated as 0.28 map units from the maximum likelihood values of θ.† Thus there is an apparent incompatibility between the two close linkages (to Xg and color blindness) reported for bipolar illness. This incompatibility would not be present if the apparent linkage between color blindness and bipolar illness were due to an association between the two traits, that is, if color blind people were prone to depression or depressed persons were unable to appreciate color.

*Based on the age criterion, family R was omitted and analysis of family P was modified (Mendlewicz et al., 1975); family W-6 was omitted (Winokur and Tanna, 1969); families RS and E were omitted; and family GR had a modified analysis (Mendlewicz and Fleiss, 1974). Family MO was omitted because of an ill father (Mendlewicz and Fleiss, 1974).

†.01 map unit (one centimorgan) is the distance between two loci on a chromosome that is associated with 1% probability of cross-over occurring between the loci.

Father-Son Transmission in Bipolar Illness

If transmission is through a single locus on the X chromosome, then an ill male proband would always get the allele from his mother, never from his father. His brothers would have a greater probability of illness than the general population. These predictions can be roughly tested in the published family history data. If mothers and daughters of bipolar males are compared with sons and fathers, then there is a statistically significant preponderance of ill mothers and daughters, as predicted by the hypothesis. In a review of 6 published family studies (Gershon et al., 1976b), 10 out of 116 sons and fathers at risk had affective illness, which is higher than reported population prevalences and is not expected if there is X chromosome transmission. The preponderance of illness in mothers and daughters over sons and fathers might, therefore, be due to a general preponderance of females to males with the illness (that is, a sex effect in an autosomally transmitted characteristic). To test this, Gershon and Bunney compared male siblings of bipolar males with male parents-offspring.* This comparison of males with males would not be affected by the greater tendency of women to manifest the disorder. The X chromosome transmission hypothesis predicts a higher probability of illness in male siblings than in male parents-offspring because the trait would have to be transmitted by the mother, but this is not compatible with the observed cases (Table 5). Therefore, the paucity of male-to-male transmissions expected with an X-linked disorder is not generally found in family studies of affective illness, and the observed difference of male and female parents-offspring concordance may be attributable to autosomal or environmental factors. Schulsinger summarized the study by Welner† of 52 male manic probands in which 7 fathers and 11 mothers had affective disorder. This study suggested that significant father-son transmission does occur. Winokur reviewed other family studies in which father-son transmission occurs and proposed a method for calculating the proportion of manic-depressive cases that are X-linked. In the X-linked subpopulation of manic-depressives, the proportion of females should be 67%, assuming that the gene frequency is 1%. This figure is obtained from the Hardy-Weinberg formula. The expected

*Male parents-offspring, or fathers-sons, refers to a group composed of both the fathers of manic-depressive sons and the sons of manic-depressive fathers.
†J. Welner, unpublished data.

TABLE 5

Brothers vs. Fathers-Sons of
Male Bipolar Probands in Five Studies*
[Gershon et al., 1976b]

Relative	Diagnosis†	
	Ill‡	Well
Male siblings	18	129
Male parents and offspring	10	106

*Data of Stendstedt (1952), Winokur (1967), Helzer and Winokur (1974), Goetzl et al. (1974), Gershon et al. (1976a).
†Difference between brothers and fathers-sons is not significant (χ^2 = 0.90, 1df). In a disorder transmitted via the X chromosome, the brothers would have a greater morbid risk than fathers and sons.
‡Major affective illness (unipolar and bipolar).

frequency of a dominant trait in females is $q^2 + 2pq$ = .0199, and the expected frequency in males is q = .01. The proportion of females is therefore (.0199)/(.0199 + .01) = 67%. The gene frequency of 1% is taken from Fremming's (1951) studies of Bornholm Island, where 1% of the male population was found to be manic-depressive. In British first admissions for mania (1965-1966), there were 1500 females out of a total 2556 (Spicer et al., 1973). The percentage of female bipolar patients is not 67%, however; it is about 59%. As there is only 59% females rather than 67%, these data may be interpreted as evidence for heterogeneity in transmission. If x of these cases are of the X-linked form, then .67x + .5 (2556 − x) = 1500, assuming that the non-X-linked form has an equal male/female ratio. Solving for x gives 1306 X-linked cases, or 51% of the total. Winokur thus arrived at an estimate of 51% for the proportion of manic-depressive cases which are X-linked.

In at least one family study in which there was systematic examination of relatives (Winokur et al., 1969), the predicted preponderances of male-to-female transmission and absence of male-to-male transmission were observed. The family study data are therefore compatible with heterogeneity of the disorder in different populations, with some populations or subpopulations showing X-linked transmission.

Conclusions from Contemporary Studies

Twin and adoptee studies of schizophrenia have established the existence of an important genetic element beyond any doubt. They have not, and cannot, explicate the mode of genetic transmission and the specific nature of the genetic disorder, whether it be polygenic or monogenic.

In the adoptee studies, the high prevalence of schizophrenic spectrum disorders in the biological relatives of schizophrenics, even though these relatives do not know of their relationship to a schizophrenic, is strong evidence against the concept that schizophrenia is a myth perpetuated by social and labeling factors.

Twin and adoption methodologies are complementary rather than competitive. Adoption designs can clearly demonstrate the reality of genetic factors. Twin studies can suggest genetic determination but cannot prove it, because identical twins may share a more concordant environment than nonidentical twins. Because monozygotic concordance is always less than 100%, the twin method directly reveals the operation of environmental factors. Adoption studies may indicate an environmental contribution if some of the variance in outcome is accounted for by characteristics of the rearing family; however, the demonstration is less direct, because the adoptees and their biological relatives do not have identical genotypes. As the existence of genetic and environmental factors is no longer subject to doubt, both twin and adoption methodologies have to be put to new uses. On the environmental side, the foremost problem is isolation of specific environmental factors that contribute to the etiology; the mere statement of their existence is no longer sufficient. On the genetic side, the most consequential issue is delineation of the genetically determined phenotype or phenotypes at risk for this illness. Granted that the genotype(s) do not cause the illness with certainty, it should be possible to discover what they do cause. These phenotypic expressions may be defined biochemically, physiologically, or psychologically; it is hoped that when they are defined they will have a higher monozygotic concordance than the illness itself. Now the relative merits of twin and adoption studies are reversed. Twin studies are ideal for revealing phenotypes more directly related to the genotype, because when a co-twin is discordant for the illness, he may still be concordant for a biochemical or psychological trait present in the index twin. Adoption studies are more powerful for revealing specific environmental factors, because when twins are raised together it is difficult to establish differences in their rearing environments with certainty. Consequently, twin and adoption studies are again complementary. The twin design can now be used to clarify the phenotypic component under genetic control, whereas the adoption method can be used to reveal specific environmental factors that contribute to the risk for illness.

So far, the evidence for an X-linked transmission of manic-depressive illness indicates that there may be some subpopulations of manic-depressive patients in which the illness is transmitted on the X chromosome.

It seems clear that new research approaches are needed to clarify the exact nature of the genetic factor in these disorders and the mechanisms operating to produce the genotype-to-phenotype relationships. In the following chapter, opportunities are discussed for the application of new methods in psychiatric genetics.

IV. RESEARCH STRATEGIES FOR PSYCHIATRIC GENETICS

Enzyme Polymorphism: L.L. Cavalli-Sforza

Biochemical analysis is, to some extent, an alternative to twin and adoption studies for isolating the mode of transmission of disease. Physical and chemical differences in a protein are strong evidence of a genetic factor causing a change in one or more of the amino acids in the sequence. If a mutant protein is responsible for a disease, then patients afflicted by this disease should show the variant form of the protein and normal controls should not. But one cannot expect to find such a sharp result all the time. Whenever a disease has multiple etiologies, the group of patients will be heterogeneous and only a fraction of the patients may show a given mutant type. The possibility that a mutant genotype may simply predispose an individual to a disease, which will develop only if some environmental contingencies are also present, is also important. One would then expect only a difference between the frequency of the variant form among controls and patients. If such a variation is found and controls are well chosen and in sufficient number, then the fact that the mutant gene is at least partially responsible for the disease would rest on good presumptive evidence. An alternate explanation that would have to be tested is that the gene responsible is very closely linked (in practice, at 1% to 2% map distance) to the gene controlling the proteins whose variants were found to be associated with the disease. Methods used to search for protein variation include:

1. *Electrophoresis.* This is the best method, but only about one-third of the existing variants can be identified. Also, after electrophoresis, identification of the protein by suitable staining techniques is necessary. A new labeling technique for proteins that involves introducing radioactive ligands (such as, e.g., dopamine or serotonin) as tracers of proteins having an affinity for the ligands, which is followed by electrophoresis and autoradiography, has been developed. Pignatti and Cavalli-Sforza (1975), for example, incubated platelet homogenates with radioactive serotonin and, after electropho-resis and autoradiography, determined which proteins bind the radio-active serotonin. In an application of this technique outside the field of neuroscience, the previously unknown function of an otherwise well-studied Gc protein (group-specific component protein) has been

identified with Vitamin-D-binding protein (Daiger et al., 1975). Radio-active substrates have also been used for "staining" serotonin and dopa decarboxylases after electrophoresis (Cavalli-Sforza et al., 1974). The electrophoretic identity of 5-hydroxytryptophan and dopa decarb-oxylases was thus shown for human liver.* No individual differences were found in the electrophoretic mobility of this enzyme in a sample of about twenty human livers from autopsy.

2. *Heat resistance.* Molecular variants of a protein can be detected by heating them up to a suitable temperature and studying their inactivation in the curves as a function of time. Cavalli-Sforza used this method for the decarboxylases of tryptophan and dopamine.* A temperature of $55°$ gives 90% inactivation in a period of about 3 minutes in some subjects and 20 minutes in others. A simple interpretation in genetic terms was made difficult by the finding of a different behavior of the same enzyme in the same individual in two different organs, the liver and the kidney. Again, there was complete concordance of dopa and 5-hydroxytryptophan decarboxylases.

3. *Relative substrate specificity.* A variant enzyme can have a distinctive pattern of substrate specificity. However, many mutations have no influence on substrate specificity because, unless the variation occurs near the active site, it may not influence substrate specificity.

4. *Inhibitor sensitivity.* This technique is currently used, for example, to detect pseudocholinesterase variants, which are of practical importance as they show different sensitivities to muscle relaxants employed during surgery (see Kalow, 1962).

5. *Immunological reagents.* These reagents can, in principle, be employed to detect genetic differences for given enzymes or proteins.

Harris (1975) has shown that while most such molecular variants, at least those discovered by electrophoresis, occur in fre-quencies of less than 1 per 1000, variants were discovered in frequencies of 2% or more for about 30% of the proteins examined. That is to say that for at least 30% of the gene loci there are relatively common mutants in the population. No doubt when all the techniques outlined above have been brought to bear on this issue a good deal more than 30% of the loci will be shown to be polymorphic. The role of these mutants and why they are so frequent is not yet clear, but if common diseases have any genetic basis, the genes involved must themselves be common. Accordingly, one approach to the elucidation

*L.L. Cavalli-Sforza, unpublished data.

of the genetic origin of schizophrenia might be a study of such relevant enzyme systems as the platelet neurotransmitter pathways to look for variant proteins that might appear in the platelets of schizophrenics and some of their relatives in greater frequency than in the platelets of the general population.

Biochemical Markers in Psychiatry: R.J. Wyatt

Enzymes active in catecholamine synthesis and metabolism have been studied in the major psychiatric disorders. In Table 6, a listing of studies of erythrocyte catechol-O-methyl-transferase (COMT) is presented. In the data of Dunner and his co-workers (1971) and Briggs and

TABLE 6

Erythrocyte Catechol-0-Methyl-Transferase (COMT)
Activity in the Affective Disorders [Wyatt]

Study	Patients	COMT activity compared to controls
Cohn et al., 1970; Dunner et al., 1971	Female unipolar	↓
	Female bipolar	↓
	Male unipolar and bipolar depressed	no change
Briggs and Briggs, 1973	Female depressed	↓
Gershon and Jonas, 1975	Female and male unipolar and bipolar	↑

Briggs (1973), a decrease in activity of this enzyme was found in women with affective disorders. In the study of Gershon and Jonas (1975), however, who used a different substrate for the enzyme assay, there was a tendency for patients with affective disorder to have elevated enzyme activity. Furthermore, elevated enzyme activity distinguished ill from well persons within families. Gershon and Jonas suggested that activity of this enzyme is heritable and that elevated COMT activity may be a genetic marker of vulnerability to affective illness. Uniform differences between unipolar and bipolar illness have not been reported. Study of COMT activity in brain revealed no change in depression (Grote et al., 1974).

Studies of monoamine oxidase (MAO) activity (Murphy and Wyatt, 1972) have revealed a decrease in enzyme activity in platelets of some chronic schizophrenics as compared with controls. In a study of monozygotic twins discordant for schizophrenia (Murphy and Wyatt, 1972; Wyatt et al., 1973a), there was a significant correlation between the members of the twin pair (r = 0.67) (Figure 2), suggesting that monoamine oxidase may be an indicator of genetic vulnerability to schizophrenia. Monozygotic twins discordant for schizophrenia can be used to help separate the genetic contribution from environmental factors such as the use of medications, chronic hospitalization, etc., since the nondisturbed twin has not been exposed to these factors. (Also, a search for common environmental factors between discordant twins may point to a defined nongenetic element, superimposed on the genetic susceptibility.) If low platelet monoamine oxidase were entirely due to events that occurred because the subjects were schizophrenic, then it would be expected that only the schizophrenic twin would have

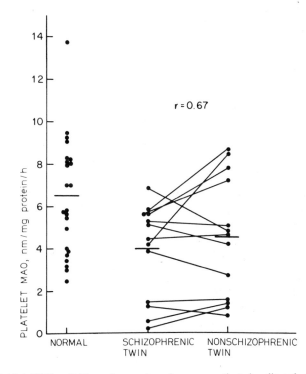

Figure 2. Platelet MAO activities of normals and monozygotic twins discordant for schizophrenia; r = correlation between twin pairs. [Wyatt et al., 1975a]

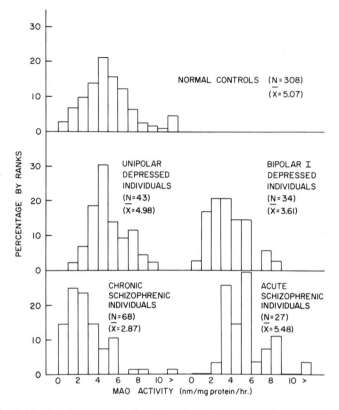

Figure 3. Distribution frequency of platelet MAO activity in normal, chronic schizophrenic, acute schizophrenic, unipolar depressed, and bipolar I depressed individuals. [Wyatt et al., 1975a]

low monoamine oxidase. Such was not the case. Family studies (Wyatt et al., 1975a) of monoamine oxidase in platelets reveal a high correlation between index patients and first-degree relatives (r = 0.73). This correlation is higher than is expected from purely genetic sources of correlation between relatives, suggesting that there may be assortative mating or sampling biases causing the correlation to be spuriously high.* In normal twins, the correlation in MZ twins for platelet MAO is 0.88 and for DZ twins the correlation is 0.45, suggesting that this enzyme activity is heritable (Murphy et al., 1974). As indicated in Figure 3, platelet MAO is decreased in bipolar depressed patients as well as in chronic schizophrenics. No differences were observed in the

*In ten pairs there did appear to be a significant correlation between husband and wife, for both normals and schizophrenics.

Michaelis constant, temperature sensitivity, or substrate specificity of platelet MAO between patients and controls. Cavalli-Sforza observed that the correlation between first-degree relatives may be inflated by selecting a small range or two small ranges widely separated for study.

   Studies of brains of chronic schizophrenics have generally shown decreased activity of enzymes of catecholamine synthesis and metabolism (Wise et al., 1974). The decreases in dopamine-β-hydroxylase activity that have been reported in schizophrenic patients (Wise et al., 1974; Wyatt et al., 1975b) may be related to phenothiazine dosage or to the time between death and storage of the brain. Wyatt and his colleagues found no change in dopamine-specific adenyl cyclase activity in the head of the caudate nucleus (Carenzi et al., 1975). There did not appear to be any differences in brain monoamine oxidase in schizophrenics using tryptamine as the substrate (Schwartz et al., 1974a). After dividing the monoamine oxidases (Schwartz et al., 1974b) into Type A and Type B (according to the preferred substrate), there was still no difference in monoamine oxidase activity between the brains of patients with schizophrenia and controls (Table 7).

TABLE 7

Monoamine Oxidase Activity in Three Areas of
Brain from Mentally Normal and Chronic Schizophrenic
Individuals [Schwartz et al., 1974b]

	Enzyme activity, μmol deaminated (30 min · mg of protein)$^{-1}$ ± SD		Ratio, Mean ± SD
	PEA*	5HT*	5HT/PEA*
Mentally normal			
Temporal cortex	2.4 ± 1.1	6.0 ± 2.1	3.0 ± 1.30
Amygdala	4.4 ± 2.8	8.8 ± 4.4	2.2 ± 0.89
Putamen	2.3 ± 1.9	4.2 ± 2.4	2.3 ± 0.71
Chronic schizophrenics			
Temporal cortex	2.8 ± 1.0	5.9 ± 2.0	2.3 ± 0.86
Amygdala	4.0 ± 1.3	6.2 ± 2.5	1.5 ± 0.52
Putamen	3.3 ± 2.1	5.1 ± 2.6	1.7 ± 0.58

*Brain samples assayed for monoamine oxidase activity in nine normal and eight schizophrenic subjects using β-phenylethylamine (PEA) and serotonin (5HT) as substrates. No statistically significant differences were found when brain samples were compared.

Pharmacogenetics: B.N. La Du

Although the major purpose of pharmacogenetics is under-standing the source of variation in response to drugs and accounting for unusual drug reactions, the subject may also be relevant to psychiatric genetics as a model strategy for studying inherited factors in mental disorders.

Broadly speaking, there are two kinds of reactions that drugs can undergo in the body: (1) direct chemical attack on functional groups—oxidations, reductions, dealkylations and other changes (these reactions generally lead to pharmacologically less active or inactive products, but some drugs are metabolically transformed in the body to their active forms), and (2) conjugation of the drug or its metabolites, e.g., with glucuronic acid or sulfate.

Both types of reactions are enzymatically catalyzed and subject to genetic variability; individual differences in drug metabolism tend to be rather large, and tenfold differences are not uncommon. Genetic rather than environmental factors are primarily responsible, and twin studies of drug metabolism have shown that monozygotic twin pairs agree more closely than dizygotic twin pairs (Vesell, 1973). Most of the variation in the rate of isoniazid acetylation, for example, is genetic (Bönicke and Lisboa, 1957).

Various types of adverse drug reactions may be inherited. Acute drug toxicity is exemplified by prolonged apnea during anesthesia resulting from a diminished rate of succinylcholine metabolism (Kalow, 1962). Genetically determined slow metabolism (acetylation) of isoniazid can result in cumulative toxicity as residual amounts of the drug gradually accumulate from repeated doses (Hughes et al., 1954). The same genetic trait can also cause untoward drug interactions: isoniazid inhibits the metabolism of diphenylhydantoin in the liver, so that slow acetylators of isoniazid tend to accumulate diphenylhydan-toin and are subject to toxic effects when both drugs are given (Brennan et al., 1970). Side reactions to drugs can also occur in particular individuals; for example, primaquine produces hemolysis in patients having certain types of glucose 6-phosphate dehydrogenase deficiencies (Beutler, 1972). Drug resistance or ineffectiveness can be caused by a deficiency of an enzyme needed to convert a drug to its active form. For example, a deficiency of hypoxanthine-guanine phosphoribosyltransferase prevents the transformation of allopurinol and a number of purine antimetabolite drugs to their active nucleotide forms (Kelley et al., 1969).

Another kind of drug resistance can be genetically traced in selected family pedigrees. Two large pedigrees are known in which certain members carry a dominant gene causing them to require about twenty times as much coumarin anticoagulant as the average patient needs to produce prolongation of prothrombin time (O'Reilly, 1970). Resistant individuals are also unusually sensitive to the anticoagulant antidote, vitamin K. A further example of a familial condition inherited as a dominant trait is hyperthermia and rigidity, induced by anesthetic agents such as halothane and succinylcholine (Kalow, 1972). This is a serious condition since affected members have a 50% probability of a fatal outcome (Britt and Kalow, 1968).

Although some pharmacogenetic conditions are easily detected, others lack suitable analytical methods. Satisfactory methods for studying individual variations in drug metabolism can be illustrated by using serum pseudocholinesterase, the enzyme that hydrolyzes succinylcholine. The levels of serum esterase activity follow a normal distribution in the general population; however, drug-sensitive individuals are not primarily at the low end of the population. Instead, their enzyme is active in a modified form that gives it very low affinity for succinylcholine (Kalow, 1962). There is also a "missing enzyme" type of succinylcholine sensitivity, but people with no serum pseudocholinesterase are very rare. An "inhibition index" in vitro test using serum with dibucaine as the inhibitor has been developed to identify atypical pseudocholinesterase. The rate of benzoylcholine hydrolysis, with and without dibucaine and under standard conditions, shows that normal pseudocholinesterase is inhibited 80% and the atypical esterase is inhibited 20% (Kalow and Genest, 1957). In fact, the population distribution of esterase inhibition is trimodal rather than normal, with modes at 20%, 60%, and 80%, corresponding to atypical homozygous, heterozygous, and normal, or usual, individuals. The dibucaine inhibition test is useful in family studies for detecting carriers of the drug sensitivity trait, and it also permits us to identify which people will be sensitive to succinylcholine without directly exposing them to the drug.

The time course of drug metabolism is an important factor to be considered in establishing genetic differences. Roughly half of the population acetylates isoniazid slowly and half rapidly, the rate being controlled by two allelic genes at a single locus, slow acetylators being homozygous for the recessive gene (Evans et al., 1960). The phenotypic classification (rapid or slow) of individuals can be made by measuring the plasma concentration of isoniazid six hours after giving a test dose of the drug. The bimodal distribution of plasma levels of isoniazid at six hours is used; earlier time points are influenced by absorption and distribution of the drug, rather than metabolism, and at later times, the acetylation reaction rate is no longer rate-limiting.

The *pattern* of drug metabolism as well as the rate may account for some pharmacogenetic conditions. Minor pathways of metabolism can be exaggerated by genetic traits and lead to unusual drug effects. Acetophenetidin is ordinarily metabolized in the liver by O-dealkylation to N-acetyl-p-aminophenol, which is then conjugated as the sulfate or glucuronide and excreted. Some individuals apparently are deficient in the O-dealkylation enzyme and metabolize aceto-phenetidin by another route, leading to 2-hydroxyphenetidin and 2-hydroxyphenacetin. The latter metabolites account for the extensive degree of hemolysis and methemoglobinemia that these people develop when given standard amounts of the drug (Shahidi, 1968).

Brief mention should be made of the application of pharmaco-genetic principles in studies of the metabolism of environmental chemicals. The latter compounds are handled by the same biochemical reactions in the body as employed for therapeutic agents, and genetic traits can affect both types of substrates. Thus, it is of interest that aryl hydrocarbon (benzo(a)pyrene) hydroxylase of human lymphocytes can be induced by 3-methylcholanthrene, and the degree of inducibility of this enzyme system is variable and under genetic control (Kellerman et al., 1973a). The conversion of environmental aromatic compounds to reactive chemicals, possibly toxic agents, is thought to influence their biological activity, and genetic traits presumably account for individual differences in susceptibility to these agents.

How does pharmacogenetics relate to further studies on genetic factors in mental disorders? It seems reasonable to suggest that drugs can be used as indicators of unusual metabolic reactions in patients with mental diseases. Studies of the rate and pattern of drug metabolism and metabolites might reveal differences not apparent from measurements of endogenous compounds and their metabolites. Drugs represent a wide spectrum of potential substrates for probing metabolic reactions, and drug metabolism reflects numerous internal conditions of the tissues (transport systems, cofactor levels, inhibitors, special receptors, etc.). Furthermore, the response to drugs (pharmacological effects) and the influence of drugs on the metabolism of endogenous compounds might also provide clues to genetic differences in mental disorders.

In the discussion it was noted that some differences in the effects of exogenous substances have already been reported in schizophrenia. In 1923 Whitehorn observed a smaller wheel-and-flare reaction (a skin reaction to intradermal application of histamine) in schizophrenia than in normal subjects. This difference has been replicated in a number of studies. Schizophrenics also appear to have a reduced blood pressure and blood sugar response to norepinephrine. Sensitivity to the physiological effects of chlorpromazine has been found to be markedly reduced in schizophrenics, and the insensitivity does not appear to be attributable to hyperactivity, emotional turmoil, or tolerance because it occurs both when the patient is in remission and when the drug is first administered. However, it is not known if this insensitivity to the effects of chlorpromazine in schizophrenics is caused by a difference in the way the drug is metabolized or if it represents a true difference in responsiveness to the drug. Chlorpromazine has about sixty metabolites, some of which have pharmacological activity, and is thus a difficult drug to study. La Du suggested that it might be worth studying analogues of chlorpromazine that have less complicated metabolic patterns to see if the differences are still found. Such studies might show if the differences are caused by the pharmocokinetics of the drug (and drug metabolism) or by responses to the drug.

Another drug having idiosyncratic effects is reserpine, which causes depression in some patients. It might be valuable to compare the pattern of reserpine metabolism in patients with and without depressive reactions. There might be qualitative or quantitative differences, which could best be revealed by careful study of metabolite patterns in a few patients using techniques such as gas chromatography–mass spectrometry.

However, finding a difference in drug response by patients with schizophrenia is but the first step; many explanations for the difference can be imagined, such as differences in drug metabolism, drug metabolites, cellular receptors, interactions with endogenous constituents, and altered affinity of tissue enzymes. Unfortunately, there is no simple formula for determining the basis of the difference observed. It is like establishing the biochemical basis of a new inborn error of metabolism, with each problem requiring a unique approach. Nevertheless, using drugs as probes for genetic traits associated with mental disorders is an approach for further investigation that merits imaginative consideration and discussion.

The HLA System and Linkage Analysis in Cell Culture: W.F. Bodmer

Much progress has been made in the assignment of genes to specific human chromosomes and in the detection of their spatial relationships, one to another. The knowledge of such chromosome markers may be helpful in human genetics in two ways: (1) they may be used in establishing the genetic origin of a phenotype whose distribution in families indicates its close association with the marker, and (2) a known linkage may help to establish the presence in a particular genotype of a gene that is not manifest or that may not express itself until later in development. An account of the use of the HLA leukocyte blood group system as such a marker and of progress in gene assignment by cell culture techniques follows.

The HLA system was initially detected as a white blood cell system and is now known to be likely to contain at least a few hundred if not a thousand or more genes. (It is usually observed as an antigenic polymorphism on lymphocytes, or platelets, and seems to be the major human histocompatibility system.) The HLA system has proved to be important in immune response and organ transplantation rejection and also contributes significantly to disease susceptibility (Bodmer, 1972, 1973, 1975). The existence of genes that control susceptibility to infection illustrates the complete intertwining of genetic and environmental factors. HLA has two major series of antigens present on most types of cells, each series representing a family of alleles at one locus: the A (formerly LA) and B (formerly 4) loci. These two loci, though closely linked, may encompass hundreds to many thousand loci between them. Some of these intervening loci are known to control cell surface antigens, which have a more restricted tissue distribution than those of the A and B loci. The two main loci are highly polymorphic; 75% of the Caucasian population will, on the average, have four different HLA-A and HLA-B locus antigens and less than 2% will have only two antigens. The equivalent of HLA in the mouse is the H-2 system. Genes in the H-2 region are known to control immune response, complement functions, and graft rejection, as in the HLA region (see, e.g., Klein, 1975).

The HLA system is associated with a number of diseases (Table 8), as was expected because in the mouse H-2 region there are genes known to control the ability to make antibodies to various antigens as well as genes affecting susceptibility to virally induced leukemias (Lilly, 1970). Ankylosing spondylitis is the most striking example of an HLA association to disease. The antigen B27 of the B locus occurs in about 90% of patients as compared to only 7% of controls (see, e.g., Brewerton, 1975). The frequency of the disease is about one in a thousand in males and some four times lower in females; thus 1% to 2% of males and about 0.25% of females who have B27 get the disease, at least in its severest forms. The association is not specific for this diagnosis, however, because Reiter's disease and acute anterior uveitis, which are often associated with ankylosing spondylitis, are also associated significantly with B27. The HLA association is more than just a genetic marker; it indicates an immunological cause of the disease.

If immune response genes are the basis for at least some of the HLA and disease associations, then these genes will have a much greater association with the relevant disease than that detected by alleles of the A and B loci. The association with the alleles of the A and B loci then only occurs because of the existence of linkage disequilibrium. In the case of multiple sclerosis, for example, there is a weak association with HLA-A and HLA-B locus alleles *A3* and *B7*, but a strong association with an allele at the HLA-D locus controlling the mixed lymphocyte culture response determinant DW2 (formerly LD7A). Diabetes is now also known to be associated with HLA. In this case the association may be mediated by an immune response gene affecting the response to coxsackie or another virus, or perhaps by the production of auto-antibodies to insulin-producing cells of the pancreas. Studies of HLA association in schizophrenia might be worthwhile if there were thought to be any possibility of either autoantibodies or slow virus infections being involved in the etiology of the disease.

The genetics of biochemical characters can now be studied in tissue culture using human-mouse and other cell hybrids produced by fusion with Sendai virus (see, e.g., Bodmer, 1971; Ephrussi, 1972, 1975; Bengtsson and Bodmer, 1975; van Heyningen et al., 1975). When the nuclei fuse, hybrid cells are formed that contain genetic material

TABLE 8

HLA and Disease Associations [McDevitt and Bodmer, 1974]

Disease	Number of studies	Antigen	Frequency in patients (%)	Frequency in controls (%)	Average relative risk
Ankylosing spondylitis	5	B27	90	7	141.0
Reiter's disease	3	B27	76	6	46.6
Acute anterior uveitis	2	B27	55	8	16.7
	6 }	B13	18	4	5.0
Psoriasis	6 }	BW17	29	8	5.0
	4	BW16	15	5	2.9
Graves' disease	1	B8	47	21	3.3
Coeliac disease	6	B8	78	24	10.4
Dermatitis herpetiformis	3	B8	62	27	4.5
Myasthenia gravis	5	B8	52	24	4.6
Chronic hepatitis	3	B8	55	25	3.6
Juvenile diabetes	4 }	B8	48	25	2.4
		BW15	27	15	2.3
Systemic lupus erethymatosus	2	BW15	33	8	5.1
	4 }	A3	36	25	1.7
Multiple sclerosis		B7	36	25	1.5
		DW2	70	16	12.2
Acute lymphatic leukemia	7 }	A2	63	37	1.7
	8	BW35	25	16	1.6
Hodgkin's disease	7 }	A1	39	32	1.3
	7	B8	26	22	1.3
Ragweed hayfever, Ra5 sensitivity	1	B7	50	19	4.0
Streptococcal antigen response	1	B5	31	7	6.0

from both parental cell lines. Selection conditions can be imposed that favor the survival of hybrids containing specific human chromosomes. Any marker detectable at the cellular level (including, for example, inborn errors of metabolism, drug idiosyncracies such as response to phenothiazines in the case of schizophrenia, and possibly abnormal receptors to dopamine) can be analyzed genetically by using the techniques of somatic cell genetics and, thus, the relevant genes can be assigned to their specific chromosome. In some cases, two forms of an enzyme can be distinguished solely by genetic assignment to different chromosomes, without observation of differentiating biochemical properties.

Differences in Incidence Rates Predicted by the Single Major Locus and Multifactorial Models: S. Matthysse

Matthysse and Kidd* have shown that the frequencies of illness among some classes of relatives of affected individuals, as predicted by simple forms of the single major locus and multifactorial models, differ substantially. If first-degree relatives alone are considered, their predictions are indistinguishable, at least for traits with one threshold (Reich et al., 1972).

The single major locus (monogenic) model requires four parameters: q, f_0, f_1, f_2, where q is the gene frequency; f_0, the probability of contracting the illness in the absence of the gene (the frequency of phenocopies); f_2, the probability of illness in the homozygote; and f_1, the probability of illness in the heterozygote. $f_1 = f_0$ for recessive traits, $f_1 = f_2$ for dominants (James, 1971). The multifactorial (polygenic) model has three independent parameters: V_A, V_D, T. It is assumed that genetic vulnerability for the disease is normally distributed, with additive and dominance variances V_A and V_D. An independent, normally distributed environmental variable is superimposed with the stipulation that the sum of the genetic and environmental contributions has variance one (Cavalli-Sforza and Bodmer, 1971). An individual is affected if his sum exceeds the threshold T. This formulation is equivalent to assuming a cumulative normal risk function (Curnow, 1972).

*Unpublished data.

For the single major locus model, it can be shown that

$$IMZ = 4(ISS) - 2(IPO) - GI$$

where IMZ is the predicted incidence of the illness in monozygotic twins of affected individuals; ISS, the incidence in sibs; IPO, the incidence in offspring; and GI, the incidence in the general population.* When ISS = IPO, the predicted incidence in offspring of dual matings, I(S × S), can be shown to be equal to IMZ.*

The multifactorial case is less tractable, but an approximate formula for IMZ in terms of ISS, IPO, and GI could be derived, using an approximation devised by Smith (1970). Define the following symbols:

$$s = \log \ ISS/\log GI$$

$$p = \log \ IPO/\log GI$$

$$m = \log \ IMZ/\log GI$$

$$\text{then } m \approx \frac{2w - (1-w^2)}{2w + (1-w^2)}$$

$$\text{where } w = \frac{2s - p(1-s^2)}{1 - s^2 + 2sp}$$

An explicit formula for I(S × S) could not be found, but for the case ISS = IPO, values based on Monte Carlo computations are available (Kidd and Cavalli-Sforza, 1973).

Application of these formulas to the frequency data on schizophrenia shows that the models make strikingly different predictions. For schizophrenia, we may take GI = .87%, ISS = IPO = 10.4%. These figures were derived from Slater's (1968) review of the published literature. The values for ISS and IPO given in Slater's tabulation differ slightly (8.7% and 12.0%, respectively), but they have been averaged and equated for this analysis. For monozygotic concordance, the single major locus model predicts 19.9%, and the multifactorial model predicts approximately 60.7%, a major difference. The actual figure is in the vicinity of 47% (average of five recent studies reported in Gottesman and Shields, 1972). Because of common environment, the actual monozygotic concordance rate would be expected to be higher than the prediction, but it is unlikely that a discrepancy as large as the

---

*Deviations will be published in a forthcoming paper by S. Matthysse and K.K. Kidd.

difference from the single major locus estimate can be explained in that way. For incidence in offspring of dual matings, the single major locus model predicts 19.9% (same as IMZ), and the Monte Carlo multifactorial prediction is approximately 42% to 45%. The actual figure is between 35% and 44% (Erlenmeyer-Kimling, 1968), in between the two predictions but somewhat closer to the polygenic.

Matthysse suggested that a two-gene model might fit the data on schizophrenia better than the single major locus model because gene interaction effects (epistatic variance) can increase monozygotic concordance relative to sibling and offspring incidences. Such a model would be heuristically preferable to the multifactorial theory, because traits or biochemical markers associated with the individual genes might be sought.

Discussion

Childs suggested that the differentiation between monogenic and polygenic models has not been, and will probably not be, helpful for progress in understanding the specific actions of individual genes. He suggested that schizophrenia will probably be found to be caused by mutants at a single locus in some individuals and by the combined effects of two or more, and perhaps many genes, in others. These possibilities can be explicated only by appropriate laboratory research.

Edwards stated that the use of mathematical models is not the way progress has usually been made in biological sciences where genetic models have been built on the basis of demonstrable structure. The use of mathematical models in multidimensional space is an attempt to short-circuit the necessary investigation of physical structural characteristics associated with the disorders in question and is unlikely to be fruitful. For example, one can consider the data on intelligence as it would have appeared in relation to phenylketonuria before the metabolic basis of retardation in this disorder was known. If one looks at fair-hairedness and intelligence as two characteristics that may be correlated with each other, this could be explained as a polygenic or multifactorial trait, although when one is able to measure the levels of phenylalanine in the blood, it is unmistakably clear that this is a single trait for which there is no overlap between persons with severe retardation resulting from phenylketonuria and members of the normal population. Therefore, when looking at the distribution of two traits that may be related genetically, with overlapping characteristics in relatives, the use of segregation analysis may not be effective for behavioral characteristics.

Pedigree Analysis: J.H. Edwards

Another research strategy is pedigree analysis, but one needs very penetrant loci to study with this method. If at one locus there are several alleles, but one predominates, then even though this appears to show continuous variation, it is indistinguishable from a single major locus situation. Even in such a case, if there is a wide variability of expression associated with each genotype, as well as overlap among the genotypes, then what seems to be a normal distribution of the characteristic will appear in the population, and one would be tempted to use, erroneously, a polygenic model. The two so-called models, multifactorial and single major locus, do not appear to be distinct at all, and it is a source of confusion to attempt to distinguish them from each other.

Pedigree analysis is valuable only if the relationship of the illness to a chromosomal linkage marker is evident upon drawing the pedigree. There may be little point in applying mathematical analysis to large family pedigrees in which the linkage is doubtfully present.

Kety suggested that there is no point in further studying schizophrenia in the families of schizophrenics, but that it is worth studying the biological characteristics of the families of schizophrenics.

With any model, an observed correlation between relatives and a population prevalence that presumably reflects zero correlation in the absence of inbreeding can be demonstrated. This observed correlation is related to the true genetic correlation, but there are other components in it. The observed phenotypic correlation between relatives reflects the genetic correlation only to the extent that the environmental correlation between relatives is zero. The genetic correlation is defined at conception, and as time proceeds the genetic correlation is a relatively smaller part of the phenotypic correlation unless the environmental correlation is zero. Only if the environmental correlation is zero can heritability be a meaningful concept. In fact, this does not happen in man. So the usefulness of the approach of studies of correlations between relatives is limited and has low resolving power compared to laboratory methods.

Behavioral Pattern Analysis: A.H. Leighton

Leighton suggested that in order to find more orderly genetic relationships in mental illness we must reconsider our methods for identifying mental illness phenotypes. Most behavior comes in the form of patterns that occur over and over again. What we recognize clinically as schizophrenia, depression, and personality disorder are gross aggregates made up of component patterns. Efforts to relate genotype to phenotype might be more successful if the phenotypic units consisted of the component subpatterns rather than the gross aggregates.

Concepts and methods for identifying component subpatterns of the psychoses have begun to emerge in recent years in psychiatric epidemiology as a result of efforts to explore environmental influences. It seems likely that subpatterns of behavior would be equally relevant for studying genotypic influences. Furthermore, it has been found advisable to identify and classify adaptive as well as maladaptive behavior patterns in order to distinguish better the existence of relationships to environmental influences (Beiser et al., 1972). This is in line with comments above about the desirability of studying the distribution of capabilities in persons manifesting psychopathology.

Such mapping and codification of behavior patterns is found in one form or another across all the behavioral sciences, and it is possible that psychiatric genetics can profit from an acquaintance with these experiences. In the study of brain function, for example, von Holst and St. Paul (1962) demonstrated the importance of detailed codification of children's behavior as a prerequisite to determining the effect of localized brain stimulation. Ethologists such as Dilger have evolved highly discriminating descriptive categories in order to identify inherited, species-specific behavior patterns in birds. Similar methods were developed by Bales (1970) for studying small group behavior among humans. Many other illustrations could be added to suggest that these methods and concepts could help in designing models for classifying human behavior patterns that enter into the composition of the schizophrenic phenotype.

These suggestions do not mean that Leighton has rejected the clinical syndromes as unsuitable for investigation. On the contrary, they are still fruitful for many purposes; but they do not, since they are gross aggregates of patterns, provide the best classification for the purpose of uncovering the etiology of psychiatric disorders. Total patterns of behavior, such as that of schizophrenia, may not be amenable to genetic analysis, but, as Childs has already suggested in reference to coronary risk factors, components may prove useful. Components that look like reasonable possibilities are anxiety, recurrent patterns of concentration difficulty, insomnia, and low thresholds for arousal of fear or suspicion.

Animal Behavior Patterns: W.C. Dilger and D. Ploog

Dilger is working with a genus of African parrot (love birds) that has a short generation time (Dilger, 1960). He has developed a list of normal behaviors of these parrots and the variability characteristic of each particular species. These birds have behavior patterns with heavy genetic loading, some so rigid that almost no experience can change them. Experimentally, it is possible to distort the experiences presumed to be important for normal development of the bird or, conversely, to distort the genotype by hybridization, allowing the hybrids to develop under normal environmental conditions.

Dilger described a particular behavior pattern of nest building: these parrots carry materials such as strips of grass by stuffing them into the feathers of their rump. Analysis of this grass-stuffing behavior reveals that it can be broken down into components. The first step consists of three simultaneous actions: the head is turned back, the feathers on the rump are extended, and the wing is lowered to get it out of the way. The second step has two components: holding the grass in its beak, the parrot makes a shoving movement and, simultaneously, very small movements of the beak called "hooking" that result in stuffing the grass material between the feathers. In the third step, the strip of grass is released from the beak. The fourth step reverses the first—the head is put back up, the feathers are put down, and the wing is brought up.

In normal animals, this sequence occurs in a precise, finely tuned straight line over time. When such an animal is crossed with a species that does not carry material by stuffing it into its feathers, the hybrid offspring show a nonfunctional behavior pattern that consists of all the normal steps except the second, which is omitted. That is, they do not shove or hook with the beak. As a result, these animals cannot carry materials in their feathers and sooner or later learn with great difficulty to carry materials in their beak instead; but it may take two years for this learning to occur.

In another experiment, the rump feathers of a normal animal are shaved before any grass stuffing has occurred. As a result, the animal fails in attempts to stuff the grass into the rump feathers; there is a complete breakdown in this behavior pattern as soon as the bird tries one variant after another of the four different normal behavior components. Eventually, this breakdown leads to stereotyped behavior idiosyncratic for each animal. That is, each animal ends up with his own peculiar way of doing things.

Ploog observed that the basic ethological concepts developed from the behavior of birds and fish have been found to be true, or at least stimulating, when applied to mammals (Ploog, 1972). However, analysis of social behavior in squirrel monkeys has shown that the elements are never as predetermined as in the rather fixed sequence of birds and fish; rather, the combination of elements is, at the present state of our knowledge, unpredictable and may only be analyzed by stochastic mathematics. On the other hand, there are examples of rigidly performed, prewired behavior, such as vocalization patterns that, in squirrel monkeys, are certainly innate and only modifiable by learning within limits. From investigations of squirrel monkeys with different karyograms, Ploog and his colleagues (1976) have shown that certain karyograms can be correlated with certain dialects of vocal patterns.

Human Behavior Patterns: R.C. Benfari, A.H. Leighton, and J.M. Murphy

Leighton and his associates have been concerned with counting the frequency of mental illnesses in geographically defined populations. For this purpose they used a representative sample of each population and gathered data pertaining to all the individuals in the sample. The focus was on behavior relevant to mental health and mental illness that was obtained by (1) responses to a standard questionnaire, (2) description of the behavior during the interview in which the questionnaire data were obtained, and (3) reports from general practitioners in the community about the subjects.

Classification and analysis of the data posed several difficulties. For example, it was necessary from the outset to avoid the bias that the use of clinical terms already infused with interpretive meaning might introduce. Diagnostic concepts such as reactive and endogenous were avoided in order to let the behavior patterns stand on their own.

Benfari used computerized multivariate analysis of the questionnaire data to develop the components of behavior patterns across populations of sample members. One advantage of this computerized approach is that it eliminates the problem of "rater drift" (i.e., change over time in behavioral ratings by human judges). Through these procedures, clusters of patterns similar to the clinical categories have emerged; however, other types not included in the clinical categories have also emerged. The latter may correspond to risk factors or components of larger syndromes. For example, Benfari and his colleagues (1974) developed five dimensions of psychological disorder: (1) physical anxiety (e.g., shortness of breath, trembling), (2) topically oriented depression (worries about external realities), (3) physiological process disturbance (e.g., insomnia, loss of appetite), (4) noncognitive depression, and (5) alienation or withdrawal.

Based upon a cluster analysis of the five dimensions, six types were developed for the sample of 530 respondents. The types were given numerical designations to avoid premature classification. Type 1 (24% of the total sample) scored low on symptomatology and high on involvement. This type had the lowest scores on the psychoneurotic factors and, conversely, high scores on involvement. Type 2 (12% of the sample) scored low on symptomatology and high on alienation. This type was similar to type 1 with the exception of the high score on alienation. Type 3 (23% of the sample) received average scores on symptomatology and high scores on involvement. This type had either an average score on the five dimensions or one slightly lower than average. There was nothing distinctly prominent in this group. Type 4 (15% of the sample) scored moderately high on somatic depression and moderately high on alienation. Type 5 (11% of the sample) contained topical depressives with physiological concomitants and scored high on involvement. Type 6 (8% of the sample) contained anxious types with all manifestations of depression-alienation. And finally, residuals (7% of the sample) were similar to type 6, but showed greater variability on all the dimensions. No coherent pattern emerged from this group although they had extreme scores on some of the dimensions.

These types were found to correlate with various diseases. For example, type 4 was high in skin disorders and gastrointestinal disturbances, type 5 frequently had gastrointestinal disturbances and allergic reactions, and type 6 often had symptomatology associated with the greatest impairment of functional capacity (Benfari et al., 1974).

Murphy discussed similar problems regarding the classification of social behaviors and interpersonal environments. Among the behavioral science concepts designed to measure differences in the patterns of social environment, cultural diversity and social class are undoubtedly the most pervasive in influence. This influence long ago reached into psychiatric research.

Culture is the pattern, or "way of life," of a group of people who share language, philosophy, religion, and other attributes based on heritage. The difference in such patterns that has been thought relevant to schizophrenia is referred to by dichotomies such as Western and non-Western or primitive and civilized. For many years schizophrenia has been thought of as a disease of civilization. However, the expanding body of systematic data from non-Western areas has, to a large extent, disproved this hypothesis (see Edgerton, 1968; Murphy, 1971, 1976).

Class or socioeconomic status (SES) is also a pattern of social environment. It refers to the "way of life" of groups who share a similar position in a hierarchy based mainly on economic resources and prestige. There are now innumerable indications that in modern industrial societies some kind of a relationship exists between social class and psychiatric illness, including schizophrenia (Faris and Dunham, 1939; Hollingshead and Redlich, 1958; Dohrenwend and Dohrenwend, 1969).

In prevalence studies of large urban agglomerates, it is common to find high rates in the lower SES categories. Clausen and Kohn (1959) and Turner and Wagenfeld (1967) have suggested that the relationship is complex and equivocal. Such investigations raise questions about the hypothesis that prevalence correlations mean that the stress of a low SES environment has causative influence for the emergence of schizophrenia. Nevertheless, environmental measures, including improved techniques for assessing social class, are needed before the interaction between social and genetic factors can be understood.

The early studies of social class made use of multiple indicators (see Warner, 1963). Then it became customary to use an index based on area of residence, occupation, and years of schooling (Clausen and Kohn, 1959). At the present time the Hollingshead two-factor index,* consisting of occupation and education, is the most commonly used, although social class ratings are frequently based solely on occupation. It is time to ask again if occupation or occupation with education do, in

*A.B. Hollingshead (1957): Two factor index of social position. (Mimeo.) New Haven, 1965 Yale Station.

fact, index the behavior pattern meant by the concept of social class, and if they function in the same way in all contemporary social systems. National differences in welfare policies may profoundly influence the subculture of groups in certain occupational categories. Historical changes also need to be taken into account. In the postindustrial societies of North America, Europe, and Scandinavia, there is marked increase in the number of people engaged in service occupations. In the existing occupational rating schemes, the service occupations are at a higher position than primary industries. Thus, the secular drift of an occupational rating system is upward (Lebergott, 1968). If a group of schizophrenic males, for example, are at the same location on the occupational scale as were their fathers, this represents a downward shift relative to the general trend.

In the same study described above (Benfari et al., 1974), Murphy found that patterns of social behavior, like those of psychological functioning, were clarified by the use of multivariate analysis using a large pool of individual items.* Six patterns were discovered that markedly distinguished between environments chosen a priori from census data and first-hand observation as advantaged and disadvantaged in a global sense. The principal component factor that accounted for the greatest amount of variance in this analysis was one relevant to social class. In rank order of the strength of correlation, this factor included education, education relative to that of parents, income, certain leisure activities, certain material possessions, and, finally, occupation. Other factors referred to the quality of neighbor behavior, features of contact with friends and relatives, subjective evaluation of the environment as a locale in which to live, involvement in religious activities, and ethnic homogeneity.

Environmental measures such as these have been useful for studying large populations in a systematic way and may prove useful for selecting limited numbers of cases for deeper inspection into the more proximate interpersonal settings in which patients and controls live. At this proximal level, most of the existing research regarding schizophrenic patients concerns intrafamilial measures, with special attention given in recent years to patterns of communication within families (Bateson et al., 1956; Lidz et al., 1965; Mishler and Waxler, 1968). Two other measures that may prove useful are social network and behavioral setting.

*J.M. Murphy, R.C. Benfari, and A.H. Leighton: "Urban locales and mental illness," manuscript in preparation.

A considerable methodology has been developed by British behavioral scientists for assessing the range, activation, and meaning of the networks of social relationships in which individuals are enmeshed (see Bott, 1971; Mitchell, 1969). Similar attention has been given in the United States to measuring behavioral settings (Barker and Gump, 1964; Barker and Schoggen, 1973). Behavioral setting refers to reliably distinguishable patterns involving the coalescence of three environmental attributes: (1) the physical environment, (2) recurring patterns of interaction, and (3) regular participants as occupants of settings. An attractive aspect of behavioral setting research is that it has already been demonstrated that settings vary in terms of pressure for participation and, alternatively, in the lack of pressure and accommodation of individuals who are essentially supernumerary. A measure of the degree to which a setting allowed individuals to be understimulated, underused, and essentially redundant could prove to be important for assessing the contribution of environmental patterns in the etiology of schizophrenia.

THE NEW RESEARCH STRATEGIES–A CRITIQUE

S. Matthysse

The consensus of this meeting was clearly that we must work out a strategy for discovering the single gene effects that contribute to the predisposition to mental disorders. As Childs suggested, even if the major mental illnesses are etiologically complex with several risk factors, each of these may be traceable to a single gene. The question is: What are the best strategies for finding these single gene effects? A number of possible directions for research were discussed, including the measurement of enzymes in peripheral tissues such as platelets, the separation of isoenzymes, and the analysis of linkage. Since each of these programs involves substantial expense and effort, it is worthwhile to estimate their power in advance. "Power" is meant in the statistician's sense: Given a real effect, what is the probability that the test will detect this effect? In this section, the power of each of the new tools that have been discussed (enzyme polymorphisms, biochemical markers, pharmacogenetics, HLA association, mathematical models, and behavioral pattern analysis) will be estimated informally, rather than in the exact sense in which the statistician uses the term.

The power of biochemical screening depends upon the plausibility of the hypotheses guiding it. It is reasonable to expect that there is genetic variability in the enzymes and other proteins involved in neurotransmitter function; there could be a qualitative or quantitative alteration in some circulating biochemical factor. On the other hand, the change might be confined to the brain; it might be morphological rather than enzymatic (genes make proteins, to be sure, but not all proteins are enzymes), or a biochemical alteration might have been manifest only in utero or during early postnatal development. The morphological consequences of single gene mutations can be profound even without any obvious accompanying enzymatic error; for example, in agenesis of the corpus callosum in mice, the corpus callosum is absent, but compensatory changes, such as formation of a longitudinal callosal bundle, take place (Sidman et al., 1965). Wyatt's measurements of monoamines and their enzymes in brain and in platelets are promising because these substances are related to neurotransmitter function. Cavalli-Sforza's studies of variant forms of transmitter-related enzymes have the same advantage over general screening programs.

Pharmacogenetic research may well yield valuable knowledge concerning either unusual drug reactions specific to particular mental illnesses or pharmacologically defined genetic subtypes. For example, the discovery that there are subgroups of depressives that differ from each other in therapeutic responsiveness to classes of antidepressants would be a step toward an understanding of the etiology of the disorders. The informal observation that schizophrenics react less strongly to the peripheral effects (e.g., hypotension) of phenothiazines is an intriguing clue. It would also be interesting to study the responses of schizophrenics to drugs that affect dopamine receptors, since we already have reason to believe that they may be abnormal in schizophrenia (Kety, 1974). For example, the threshold for emesis induced by apomorphine, a dopamine-receptor stimulant, might be abnormally low.

The power of all these biochemical methods would be increased if there were a way to select homozygotes rather than heterozygotes or phenocopies* for biochemical study. On a single major locus model, some affected individuals are phenocopies, some are heterozygotes, and some are homozygotes. Most schizophrenics, according to this model, are phenocopies or heterozygotes rather than homozygotes (Matthysse and Kidd, 1976). It may be that only the homozygote will manifest a biochemical deviation (deficient or variant enzyme, or abnormal drug response) even though the phenocopies and heterozygotes under study also have the symptomatic illness. The biochemical error could be limited to the brain or to a particular developmental period. In the homozygote, however, the error might also be found in peripheral tissues and in maturity. In a mixed sample containing all three genetic types, a few deviant values might represent the homozygotes, but there would be no way to identify them as homozygotes. And statistical analysis of the whole sample might show no significant difference from normal. Although we cannot identify homozygotes with certainty, selection procedures exist that might increase the proportion of homozygous individuals in the sample. The best of these is selection of offspring of dual matings, especially individuals who developed the illness and who were reared apart from their biological parents (Matthysse and Kidd, 1976).

For revealing the mode of transmission, the power of mathematical analysis of the frequency of illness among relatives of affected individuals is limited. Simple models do not fit the data, and if the

*On a single major locus model, phenocopies are affected individuals who are genetically normal.

models incorporate features such as assortative mating, gene interaction, common environment, cultural transmission, and hetero-geneity, discrimination of single major locus from multifactorial models is probably not possible.

Linkage analysis is potentially more powerful. Consider, for example, a disease caused by a single autosomal dominant gene with high penetrance, such as Huntington's chorea. A marker is likely to be useful for linkage analysis only if its distance is less than about 20 recombination units from the trait locus; otherwise the number of sibships required is too large (Morton, 1955). To be informative, markers must be highly polymorphic. Elston and Lange (1975) calculated the probability of at least one of thirty markers lying within twenty recombination units of an arbitrary trait locus to be approxi-mately 30%. This encouraging result has to be tempered by the less favorable circumstances that prevail in psychiatry, such as uncertainty regarding mode of transmission and incomplete penetrance. It would be worthwhile to estimate the power of linkage analysis more exactly, given the factors mentioned and also considering that any one family is informative for only a few marker loci.

If an effect such as differential response to phenothiazines could be demonstrated in cell culture, then the assignment to a specific chromosome could, in principle, be worked out by using somatic cell genetic techniques. As more and more polymorphic markers are discovered and located on the human gene map, the probability that a suitable marker will be close to one detected in cell culture increases. Such a polymorphic marker could then be used as a basis for pedigree linkage studies to ascertain whether the effect detected in cell culture bore any relationship to schizophrenia as diagnosed clinically.

HLA association and linkage studies are potentially very powerful because, if associations or linkages exist between mental diseases and HLA alleles (or loci), they could easily be demonstrated because these loci are highly polymorphic. HLA studies are, however, a "long shot" because the HLA system, from this point of view, represents just another position on the genetic map. The expectation of success would, of course, be increased if we had a theory implicating immune response genes in schizophrenic or manic-depressive psychoses. The "autoimmunity theory" of Heath does indeed make such an implication, but its empirical status is dubious (Matthysse and Lipinski, 1975).

Edwards observed that it is not very efficient to confine linkage analysis to two-generation families; more can be learned from larger pedigrees with three generations. It is also possible to search for linkage to a large number of markers at once. It is very inefficient to do linkage analysis without planning it, and especially inefficient on non-Mendelian diseases. But if one can work with large three-generation families and freeze cells and serum, the effort is justified. The study on the markers themselves would be informative even if no strong locus influencing schizophrenia, should one exist, were near the locus of a marker.

Behavioral pattern analysis could, in principle, have considerable power because there might be behavioral patterns, or constellations of such patterns, with much higher concordance rates in monozygotic twins than either the schizophrenia syndrome or the syndromes of affective disorders. Leighton and Benfari made two suggestions in this connection: (1) to develop identification of the behavioral pattern subunits from empirical data derived from the malfunctional aspects of the psychotic syndromes and (2) to develop behavioral pattern subunits based on the surviving capabilities of persons who suffer from these syndromes. Both call for major effort directed at the development of methods for detecting and categorizing behavioral patterns along the lines initiated in psychiatric epidemiology (see Leighton, 1959; Benfari et al., 1972, 1974; Wing et al., 1974).

Matthysse and his associates have been interested in patterns whose presence might indicate increased risk of the psychotic syndromes. Thus, they have focused on a pattern of "disattention defect." "Disattention," as defined by the psychologist Cromwell, is "the adaptive ability of an organism to withdraw his attention from a stimulus after having attended to it" (Cromwell and Dokecki, 1968). Difficulty in disattending might be the mental equivalent of stereotyped behavior in animals and, therefore, might be related to hyperdopaminergic function. Some aspects of antipsychotic drug action can perhaps be understood in terms of disattention. Insofar as these drugs block norepinephrine, they have been thought to exert a calming and sedative effect. Insofar as they block dopamine, they may counteract the rigidity of attention of the schizophrenic patient, decreasing his perseverative rumination on delusional ideas and freeing him for more constructive thinking. It is interesting that in the twin series of Pollin and his colleagues (1966), five of the seven discordant twins were described as "obsessive."

Schulsinger described the method of studying risk groups as a useful extension of the more "classical" studies in psychiatric genetics. Since 1962, he and Mednick have followed a group of 207 children of severely schizophrenic parents and a control group of 104 children of "nonpsychiatric" parents (Mednick and Schulsinger, 1974). The group is now between 20 and 30 years old; 15 of the high-risk and 1 of the low-risk subjects have become schizophrenic. Some have signs of schizophrenic thought disorder or show paranoid tendencies but are far from ill or maladjusted. The clinical follow-up assessment has been very detailed (Schulsinger, 1976).

Schulsinger pointed out that the special value of the high-risk design is that it permits us to study the influence of defined environmental factors on a specific genetic disposition and the influence of a single environmental factor on genetic high-risk versus genetic low-risk subjects. For example, the mental health scores of children with a high degree of parental separation were compared to the scores of children without such separation. Low-risk children who had a low degree of parental separation had high mental health scores, whereas a high degree of parental separation was correlated with lower mental health scores. If the children also had a severely schizophrenic mother (i.e., were high-risk), the mental health score became even lower. It was also possible to demonstrate additive or interactive effects between genetic and environmental factors, such as parental separation and perinatal complications for psychophysiological parameters.

Mednick and his colleagues (1974a*) have recently demonstrated that in 10- to 12-year-old children matched for the exact course of pregnancy and delivery, perinatal complications resulted in much more frequent neurological abnormalities in children whose mother was a schizophrenic (high-risk) than in children whose mother was normal (low-risk). The largest neurological differences were spontaneous nystagmus, reciprocal coordination difficulties, associated movements, and certain posture and gait abnormalities. Most of these abnormalities in the 10- to 12-year-olds would not be abnormalities if found in 5- or 6-year-olds. In other words, there might have been some kind of retardation of maturation of the central nervous system. An extensive review of methodological issues and ongoing studies using the high-risk method may be found in Garmezy (1974) and Garmezy and Streitman (1974).

Winokur noted that, in the past, we have not been at all certain of having a homogeneous group of patients in which to look for a genetic factor. Pedigree methodology offers an additional option for achieving homogeneity; in addition to the clinical picture, course of the

*Also, unpublished data.

illness, age, and sex, the specific family constellation can help define homogeneous subgroups.

Childs emphasized that heterogeneity has been either explicit or implicit in almost everything that the geneticists have said. In other words, schizophrenia is too broad a phenotype to continue to study as such. Studies like those of Wyatt and Murphy in which the biochemical abnormalities in schizophrenia are explored should be given high priority, but rewards will also accrue to studies in which children at risk for schizophrenia, especially in families with heavy concentrations of cases, are carefully examined. Childs also asked whether some of the subjective criteria for the diagnosis of schizophrenia could not be articulated so as to score them quantitatively. This might lead to subcategories analogous to the risk factors of coronary artery disease. Family studies and segregation analysis of such subtypes could then be carried out. Studies of this kind might yield some characteristics that could be studied in persons who are not (yet) overtly schizophrenic and that might also make the biochemical approach easier. The important point is the rigor of the classification system.

With respect to the biochemical aspects, Schmitt pointed out that genes do more than specify enzymes. In one mutant mouse there are no granule cells in the cerebellum. Another mutant has no Bergmann glia. In searching for biochemical abnormalities in the brain of schizophrenics, we might look not only for changes in neurotransmitters but also for defects in receptors and neuromodulators. The latter are proteins thought to modulate the postsynaptic polarization by intervening, in ways still unknown, somewhere in the chain that includes receptor, adenylate cyclase, and protein kinase. Schmitt wondered if we could postulate that whole parts of the nervous system are normal in schizophrenia, for example, the sensory-motor systems composed of Golgi type I neurons. This would focus attention on the Golgi type II, or local circuit neurons, thought by many to underlie higher brain function (see Rakic, 1975).

Ploog recalled that at an earlier Work Session on schizophrenia, Teuber (1972) reviewed brain lesions that mimic schizophrenia and pointed out that, in general, a number of different systems have to be involved to give a picture similar to schizophrenia. The lesion most frequently misdiagnosed as schizophrenia is damage to the temporal lobe. Basal frontal lobe lesions are also frequently misdiagnosed as schizophrenia. Certain cases of brain atrophy cannot be differentiated on the basis of psychopathology from chronic schizophrenia. If one considers that the brain has so many different jobs to do, it makes sense to imagine that to produce the full schizophrenic syndrome it is necessary that several different domains of brain activity be disturbed or impaired. Conversely, in view of the fact that one can make a large lesion in the brain without producing any behavioral disturbance, it is not surprising that gross abnormalities are not found in the schizophrenic brain.

In pharmacogenetic studies, it might be possible to study the comparative pharmacokinetics of particular brain systems. Differences in neurotransmitter agents (norepinephine, serotonin, and dopamine) might be recognized or accentuated by drugs known to affect the synthesis, turnover, and metabolism of these endogenous compounds. Risk research could also be used to point toward specific brain systems. For example, in Schulsinger's children, the greatest disturbance seems to be in spontaneous nystagmus, posture, gait, and coordinated movements, and the systems that are responsible for these symptoms could be studied.

In summary, although one can never be certain of success, the new tools have sufficient power to justify applying them vigorously to the genetics of mental disorders.

BIBLIOGRAPHY

This bibliography contains two types of entries: (1) citations given or work alluded to in the report, and (2) additional references to pertinent literature by conference participants and others. Citations in group (1) may be found in the text on the pages listed in the right-hand column.

Page

Allen, G., Harvald, B., and Shields, J. (1967): Measures of twin concordance. *Acta Genet. Stat. Med.* 17:475-481.   30

Bales, R.F. (1970): *Personality and Interpersonal Behavior.* New York: Holt, Rinehart and Winston.   73

Barker, R.G. and Gump, P. (1964): *Big School, Small School.* Stanford: Stanford University Press.   79

Barker, R.G. and Schoggen, P. (1973): *Qualities of Community Life.* San Francisco: Jossey Bass Publishers.   79

Bateson, G., Jackson, D.D., Haley, J., and Weakland, J. (1956): Toward a theory of schizophrenia. *Behav. Sci.* 1:251-264.   78

Beiser, M., Feldman, J.J., and Egelhoff, C.J. (1972): Assets and affects. A study of positive mental health. *Arch. Gen. Psychiatry* 27:545-549.   73

Belmaker, R., Beckmann, H., Goodwin, F., Murphy, D., Pollin, W., Buchsbaum, M., Wyatt, R., Ciaranello, R., and Lamprecht, F. (1975): Relationships between platelet and plasma monoamine oxidase, plasma dopamine-β-hydroxylase, and urinary 3-methoxy-4-hydroxy phenylglycol. *Life Sci.* 16:273-279.

Belmaker, R.H., Murphy, D.L., Wyatt, R.J., and Loriaux, D.L. (1974): Human platelet monoamine oxidase changes during the menstrual cycle. *Arch. Gen. Psychiatry* 31:553-556.

Belmaker, R., Pollin, W., Wyatt, R.J., and Cohen, S. (1974): A follow-up of monozygotic twins discordant for schizophrenia. *Arch. Gen. Psychiatry* 30:219-222.

Belmaker, R.H. and Wyatt, R.J. (1975): Possible X-linkage in a family with varied psychoses. *Israel Med. J.* (In press)

Benfari, R.C., Beiser, M., Leighton, A.H., and Mertens, C. (1972): Some dimensions of psychoneurotic behavior in an urban sample. *J. Nerv. Ment. Dis.* 155:77-90.   83

Benfari, R.C., Beiser, M., Leighton, A., Murphy, J., and Mertens, C. (1974): The manifestation of types of psychological states in an urban sample. *J. Clin. Psychol.* 30:471-483.   76,78, 83

Benfari, R.C. and Leighton, A.H. (1970): PROBE: A computer instrument for field surveys of psychiatric disorder. *Arch. Gen. Psychiatry* 23:352-358.

Benfari, R.C., Leighton, A.H., Beiser, M., and Coen, K. (1972): CASE: Computer assigned symptom evaluation. *J. Nerv. Ment. Dis.* 154:115-124.

Bengtsson, B. and Bodmer, W.F. (1975): The strategy of gene assignment using hybrids: the number of lines needed to exclude chance associations. *Second International Workshop on Human Gene Mapping, Birth Defects: Original Article Series XI/3.* New York: The National Foundation, pp. 62-66.   67

Benzer, S. (1971): From the gene to behavior. *J. Am. Med. Assoc.* 218:1015-1022.   25

Benzer, S. (1973): Genetic dissection of behavior. *Sci. Am.* 229:24-37.   25

Berg, K. and Bearn, A.G. (1968): Human serum protein polymorphisms. *Annu. Rev. Genet.* 2:341-362.

Beutler, E. (1972): Glucose 6-phosphate dehydrogenase deficiency. *In: The Metabolic Basis of Inherited Disease.* (3rd Ed.) Stanbury, J.B., Wyngaarden, J.B., and Frederickson, D.S., eds. New York: McGraw-Hill, pp. 1358-1388.   15,62

Bleuler, E. (1911): *Dementia Praecox or the Group of Schizophrenias.* Zinkin, J., trans. New York: International Universities Press, 1950.   11,12

Bodmer, W.F. (1971): Linkage analysis using human-mouse hybrid cells. *In: Human Genetics.* (Proceedings of the Fourth International Congress of Human Genetics, Paris, 6-11 September 1971.) Amsterdam: Excerpta Medica, pp. 365-373.   67

Bodmer, W.F. (1972): Evolutionary significance of the HL-A system. *Nature* 237:139-145.   66

Bodmer, W.F. (1973): The genetics of the HLA and H-2 major histocompatibility systems. *In: Defence and Recognition.* Porter, R.R., ed. London: Butterworth, Inc., pp. 295-328.   66

Bodmer, W.F. (1975): *In: Histocompatibility Testing.* Kissmeyer-Nielsen, F., ed. Baltimore, Md.: Williams and Wilkins.   66

Bodmer, W.F. and Cavalli-Sforza, L.L. (1976): *Genetics, Evolution, and Man.* San Francisco: W.H. Freeman. (In press)   47

Bönicke, R. and Lisboa, B.P. (1957): Über die Erbbedingtheit der intraindividuellen Konstanz der Isoniazidausscheidung beim Menschen (Untersuchungen an eineiligen und zweieligen Zwillingen). *Naturwissenschaften* 44:314.   62

Bott, E. (1971): *Family and Social Network.* (2nd Ed.) New York: The Free Press.   79

Brennan, R.W., Dehejia, H., Kutt, H., Verebely, K., and McDowell, P. (1970): Diphenylhydantoin intoxication attendant to slow inactivation of isoniazid. *Neurology* 20:687-693.   62

Brewerton, D.A., ed. (1975): Symposium on histocompatibility and rheumatic disease. *Ann. Rheum. Dis.* 34, Suppl. 1.   67

Neurosciences Res. Prog. Bull., Vol. 14, No. 1   **89**

Page

Briggs, M.H. and Briggs, M. (1973): Hormonal influences on erythrocyte catechol-O-methyl transferase activity in humans. *Experientia* 29:278-280.

58

Britt, B.A. and Kalow, W. (1968): Hyperrigidity and hyperthermia associated with anesthesia. *Ann. N.Y. Acad. Sci.* 151:947-958.

63

Brugger, P. (1929): Zur Frage einer Belastungsstatistik der Durchschnitts-bevölkerung. *Z. ges. Neurol. Psychiatr.* 118:459-488.

26

Bulmer, M.G. (1970): *Biology of Twinning in Man.* New York: Oxford University Press.

32

Cadoret, R.J. and Winokur, G. (1972): Genetic principles in the classification of affective illnesses. *Int. J. Ment. Health* 1:159-175.

Campion, E. and Tucker, G. (1973): A note on twin studies, schizophrenia and neurological impairment. *Arch. Gen. Psychiatry* 29:460-464.

32

Carenzi, A., Gillin, J.C., Guidotti, A., Schwartz, M.A., Trabucchi, M., and Wyatt, R.J. (1975): Dopamine-sensitive adenylyl cyclase in human caudate nucleus. *Arch. Gen. Psychiatry* 32:1056-1059.

61

Carpenter, W.T., Jr., Strauss, J.S., and Bartko, J.J. (1973): Flexible system for the diagnosis of schizophrenia: Report from the WHO International Pilot Study on Schizophrenia. *Science* 182:1275-1277.

36

Cavalli-Sforza, L.L. (1973): Analytic review: Some current problems of human population genetics. *Am. J. Hum. Genet.* 25:82-104.

Cavalli-Sforza, L.L. (1974): Letter: Controversial issues in human population genetics. *Am. J. Hum. Genet.* 26:266-271.

Cavalli-Sforza, L.L. and Bodmer, W.F. (1971): *The Genetics of Human Populations.* San Francisco: W.H. Freeman.

37,47, 69

Cavalli-Sforza, L.L. and Feldman, M.W. (1973): Cultural versus biological inheritance: Phenotypic transmission from parents to children (a theory of the effect of parental phenotypes on children's phenotypes). *Am. J. Hum. Genet.* 25:618-637.

Cavalli-Sforza, L.L. and Kidd, K.K. (1972): Genetic models for schizophrenia. *Neurosciences Res. Prog. Bull.* 10:406-419. Also *In: Neurosciences Research Symposium Summaries, Vol. 7.* Cambridge, Mass.: M.I.T. Press, 1973, pp. 406-419.

Cavalli-Sforza, L.L., Santachiara, S.A., Wang, L., Erdelyi, E., and Barchas, J. (1974): Electrophoretic study of 5-hydroxytryptophan decarboxylase from brain and liver in several species. *J. Neurochem.* 23:629-634.

57

Chapman, L.J. and Chapman, J.P. (1974): *Disordered Thought in Schizophrenia.* Englewood Cliffs, N.J.: Prentice Hall.

12

Childs, B. (1972): Genetic analysis of human behavior. *Annu. Rev. Med.* 23:373-406.

Childs, B. (1974): The William Allen Memorial Award Lecture. A place for genetics in health education, and vice versa. *Am. J. Hum. Genet.* 26:120-135.

Clark, S.W., Glaubiger, G.A., and La Du, B.N. (1968): Properties of plasma cholinesterase variants. *Ann. N.Y. Acad. Sci.* 151:710-722.

Clausen, J.A. and Kohn, M.L. (1959): Relation of schizophrenia to the social   77
structure of a small city. *In: Epidemiology of Mental Disorder.* Pasamanick, B., ed. Washington, D.C.: American Association for the Advancement of Science, pp. 69-94.

Clausen, J.A. and Kohn, M.L. (1960): Social relations and schizophrenia: A research report and a perspective. *In: The Etiology of Schizophrenia.* Jackson, D.D., ed. New York: Basic Books, pp. 295-320.

Clayton, P.J., Pitts, F.N., Jr., and Winokur, G. (1965): Affective disorder: IV. Mania. *Compr. Psychiatry* 6:313-322.

Cohn, C.K., Dunner, D.L., and Axelrod, J. (1970): Reduced catechol-O-methyl-   58
transferase activity in red blood cells of women with primary affective disorder. *Science* 170:1323-1324.

Cromwell, R.L. and Dokecki, P.R. (1968): Schizophrenic language: a disattention   83
interpretation. *In: Developments in Applied Psycholinguistics Research.* Rosenberg, S. and Koplin, J.H., eds. New York: MacMillan, pp. 209-260.

Curnow, R.N. (1972): The multifactorial model for the inheritance of liability to   69
disease and its implications for relatives at risk. *Biometrics* 28:931-946.

Curnow, R.N. and Smith, C. (1975): Multifactorial models for familial diseases in   37
man. *J.R. Stat. Soc. A.* (In press)

Daiger, S.P., Schanfield, M.S. and Cavalli-Sforza, L.L. (1975): Group-specific   57
component (Gc) proteins bind vitamin D and 25-hydroxyvitamin D. *Proc. Nat. Acad. Sci.* 72:2076-2080.

Dilger, W.C. (1960): The comparative ethology of the African parrot genus   74
Agapornis. Z. Tierpsychol. 17:649-685.

Dohrenwend, B.P. and Dohrenwend, B.S. (1969): *Social Status and Psychological*   77
Disorder. New York: Wiley-Interscience.

Dunner, D.L., Cohn, C.K., Gershon, E.S., and Goodwin, F.K. (1971): Differential   58
catechol-O-methyltransferase activity in unipolar and bipolar affective illness. *Arch. Gen. Psychiatry* 25:348-353.

Ebaugh, I.A., Freiman, M., Woolf, R.B., Sherman, A.I., and Winokur, G. (1968): Chromosome studies in patients with affective disorder (manic depressive illness). *Arch. Gen. Psychiatry* 19:751-752.

Neurosciences Res. Prog. Bull., Vol. 14, No. 1

91

Page

Edgerton, R. (1968): Conceptions of psychosis in four East African societies. *Am. Anthropol.* 68:408-425.　　　77

Edwards, J.H. (1969): Familial predisposition in man. *Brit. Med. Bull.* 25:58-64.

Edwards, J.H. (1971): The analysis of X-linkage. *Ann. Hum. Genet.* 34:229-250.　　　48

Edwards, J.H. (1972): The genetical basis of schizophrenia. *In: Genetic Factors in "Schizophrenia."* Kaplan, A.R., ed. Springfield, Ill.: C.C Thomas, pp. 310-314.

Elston, R.C. (1973): Ascertainment and age of onset in pedigree analysis. *Hum. Hered.* 23:105-112.　　　48

Elston, R.C., Kringlen, E., and Namboodiri, K.K. (1973): Possible linkage relationships between certain blood groups and schizophrenia or other psychoses. *Behav. Genet.* 3:101-106.

Elston, R.C. and Lange, K. (1975): The prior probability of autosomal linkage. *Ann. Hum. Genet.* (In press)　　　82

Elston, R.C. and Stewart, J. (1971): A general model for the genetic analysis of pedigree data. *Hum. Hered.* 21:523-542.

Ephrussi, B. (1972): *Hybridization of Somatic Cells.* Princeton, N.J.: Princeton University Press.　　　67

Ephrussi, B. (1975): *In: Second International Workshop on Human Gene Mapping, Birth Defects: Original Article Series XI/3.* New York: The National Foundation.　　　67

Erlenmeyer-Kimling, L. (1968): Studies on the offspring of two schizophrenic parents. *In: The Transmission of Schizophrenia.* Rosenthal, D. and Kety, S.S., eds. Oxford: Pergamon Press, pp. 65-83.　　　71

Essen-Möller, E. (1935): Untersuchungen über die Fruchtbarkeit gewisser Gruppen von Geisteskranken (Schizophrenen, Manischdepressiven und Epileptikern). *Acta Psychiatr. Neurol.* Suppl. 8:1-314.

Essen-Möller, E. (1936): Die Heiratshäufigkeit der Geschwister von Schizophrenen. *Arch. Rass. u. Gesellechaftsbiol.* 30:367-379.

Essen-Möller, E. (1941): Psychiatrische Untersuchungen an einer Serie von Zwillingen. *Acta Psychiatr. Neurol.* Suppl. 23:1-200.　　　26

Essen-Möller, E. (1946): The concept of schizoidia. *Monatsschr. Psychiatr. Neurol.* 112:258-271.

Essen-Möller, E. (1955): The calculation of morbid risk in parents of index cases, as applied to a family sample of schizophrenics. *Acta Genet. Stat. Med.* 5:334-342.

Essen-Möller, E. (1959): Mating and fertility patterns in families with schizophrenia. *Eugen. Q.* 6:142-147.

Essen-Möller, E. (1963): Uber die Schizophreniehäufigkeit bei Müttern von Schizophrenen. *Schweiz. Arch. Neurol. Neurochir. Psychiatr.* 91:260-266.

Essen-Möller, E. (1965): Twin research and psychiatry. *Int. J. Psychiatry* 1:466-475.

Essen-Möller, E. (1970): Twenty-one psychiatric cases and their MZ co-twins: a thirty years' follow-up. *Acta Genet. Med. Gemellol.* 19:315-317.

Essen-Möller, E. (1975): Aspects of continuity, including reference to the psychiatry of H. Sjöbring. *Psychiatry* (In press)

Essen-Möller, E., Larsson, H., Uddenberg, C.-E., and White, G. (1956): Individual traits and morbidity in a Swedish rural population. *Acta Psychiatr. Neurol. Scand.* Suppl. 100:1-160.

Evans, D.A.P., Manley, K.A., and McKusick, V.A. (1960): Genetic control of   64
isoniazid metabolism in man. *Brit. Med. J.* 2:485-491.

Falconer, D.S. (1965): The inheritance of liability to certain diseases, estimated   37
from the incidence among relatives. *Ann. Hum. Genet.* 29:51-76.

Faris, R.E.L. and Dunham, H.W. (1939): *Mental Disorders in Urban Areas: An*   77
Ecological Study of Schizophrenia and Other Psychoses. Chicago: Chicago University Press.

Fieve, R.R., Mendlewicz, J., and Fleiss, J.L. (1973): Manic depressive illness: Linkage with the Xg blood group. *Am. J. Psychiatry* 130:1355-1359.

Fischer, M. (1973): Genetic and environmental factors in schizophrenia: A study of   28
schizophrenic twins and their families. *Acta Psychiatr. Scand.* 238(Suppl.):9-142.

Fremming, K. (1951): *The Expectation of Mental Infirmity in a Sample of the*   26,53
Danish Population. (Occasional papers on eugenics, No. 7.) London: Cassell and Co.

Garmezy, N. (1974): Children at risk: The search for the antecedents of   84
schizophrenia. Part II. Ongoing research programs, issues, and intervention. *Schizophrenia Bull.* 9:55-125.

Garmezy, N. and Streitman, S. (1974): Children at risk: The search for the   84
antecedents of schizophrenia. Part I. Conceptual models and research methods. *Schizophrenia Bull.* 8:14-90.

Geist, V. (1975): *Mountain Sheep and Man in the Northern Wilds.* Ithaca, N.Y.: Cornell University Press.

Gershon, E.S., Baron, M., and Leckman, J. (1976a): Genetic models of the transmission of affective disorders. *J. Psychiatr. Res.* (In press)

Page

Gershon, E.S., Bunney, W.E., Jr., Leckman, J.F., Van Eerdewegh, M., and   48,52,
DeBauche, B.A. (1976b): The inheritance of affective disorders: A review of   53
data and of hypotheses. *Behav. Genet.* (In press)

Gershon, E.S. and Jonas, W.Z. (1975): Erythrocyte soluble catechol-O-methyl   58
transferase activity in primary affective disorder: A clinical and genetic study.
Arch. Gen. Psychiatry 32:1351-1356.

Gershon, E.S., Mark, A., Cohen, N., Belizon, N., Baron, M., and Knobe, K.E.
(1976c): Transmitted factor in the morbid risk of affective disorders: A
controlled study. *J. Psychiatr. Res.* (In press)

Goetzl, U., Green, R., Whybrow, P., and Jackson, R. (1974): X linkage revisited: A
further family study of manic-depressive illness. *Arch. Gen. Psychiatry*
31:665-672.

Goldberg, E.M. and Morrison, S.L. (1963): Schizophrenia and social class. *Brit. J.*   41
Psychiatry 109:785-802.

Goldstein, J.L. and Brown, M.S. (1975): Hyperlipidemia in coronary heart disease: 16
a biochemical genetic approach. *J. Lab. Clin. Med.* 85:15-25.

Gottesman, I.I. (1968): Severity/concordance and diagnostic refinement in the
Maudsley-Bethlem schizophrenic twin study. *In: The Transmission of Schizophrenia.* Rosenthal, D. and Kety, S.S., eds. New York: Pergamon Press,
pp. 37-48.

Gottesman, I.I. (1974): Developmental genetics and ontogenetic psychology:
overdue detente and propositions from a matchmaker. *In: Minnesota Symposia
on Child Psychology.* Pick, A., ed. Minneapolis: University of Minnesota Press,
pp. 55-80.

Gottesman, I.I. and Heston, L.L. (1972): Human behavioral adaptations. Speculations on their genesis. *In: Genetics, Environment and Behavior.* Ehrman, L.,
Omenn, G.S., and Caspari, E., eds. New York: Academic Press, pp. 105-122.

Gottesman, I.I. and Shields, J. (1966): Schizophrenia in twins: 16 years'
consecutive admissions to a psychiatric clinic. *Brit. J. Psychiatry* 112:809-818.

Gottesman, I.I. and Shields, J. (1967): A polygenic theory of schizophrenia. *Proc.*   37
Nat. Acad. Sci. 58:199-205.

Gottesman, I.I. and Shields, J. (1972): *Schizophrenia and Genetics: A Twin Study*   28,31,32,
Vantage Point. New York: Academic Press.   35,36,70

Gottesman, I.I. and Shields, J. (1973): Genetic theorizing and schizophrenia. *Brit.*
J. Psychiatry 122:15-30.

Gottesman, I.I. and Shields, J. (1976): A critical review of adoption, twin, and   34
family genetic studies of schizophrenia. *Schizophrenia Bull.* (In press)

Gottesman, I.I., Shields, J., and Heston, L.L. (1976): Characteristics of the twins of schizophrenics as fallible indicators of schizoidia. *In: First International Congress of Twin Studies, Rome, October 30, 1974.* Rome: G. Mendel Institute. (In press)

Grote, S.S., Moses, S.G., Robins, E., Hudgens, R.W., and Croninger, A.B. (1974): A   58
study of selected catecholamine metabolizing enzymes: A comparison of depressive suicides and alcoholic suicides with controls. *J. Neurochem.* 23:791-802.

Gruenberg, E.M. (1966): Epidemiology of mental retardation. *Int. J. Psychiatry* 2:78-134.

Gruenberg, E.M. (1968): Epidemiology and medical care statistics. *In: The Role and Methodology of Classification in Psychiatry and Psychopathology.* Katz, M.H., Cole, J.O., and Barton, W.E., eds. Washington, D.C.: U.S. Government Printing Office, pp. 76-99.

Gruenberg, E.M. (1968): Foreword to *Diagnostic and Statistical Manual of Mental Disorders, Second Edition.* American Psychiatric Association, Committee on Nomenclature and Statistics. Washington, D.C.: American Psychiatric Association, pp. vii-x.

Gruenberg, E.M. (1974): Benefits of short-term hospitalization. *In: Strategic Intervention in Schizophrenia: Current Developments in Treatment.* Cancro, R., Fox, N., and Shapiro, L.E., eds. New York: Behavioral Publications, pp. 251-259.

Gruenberg, E.M. (1974): The epidemiology of schizophrenia. *In: American Handbook of Psychiatry, Second Edition, Vol. II. Child and Adolescent Psychiatry, Sociocultural and Community Psychiatry.* Caplan, G., ed. New York: Basic Books, pp. 448-463.

Gruenberg, E.M. (1974): The social breakdown syndrome and its prevention. *In: American Handbook of Psychiatry, Second Edition, Vol. II. Child and Adolescent Psychiatry, Sociocultural and Community Psychiatry.* Caplan, G., ed. New York: Basic Books, pp. 697-710.

Hanson, D., Gottesman, I., and Heston, L. (1976): Some possible childhood indicators of adult schizophrenia inferred from children of schizophrenics. *Br. J. Psychiatry* (In press)

Harris, H. (1975): *The Principles of Human Biochemical Genetics, 2nd Ed.* New   57
York: American Elsevier.

Helzer, J.E. and Winokur, G. (1974): A family interview study of male manic depressives. *Arch. Gen. Psychiatry* 31:73-77.

Heston, L.L. (1966): Psychiatric disorders in foster home reared children of   28
schizophrenic mothers. *Brit. J. Psychiatry* 112:819-825.

Heston, L.L. (1970): The genetics of schizophrenic and schizoid disease. *Science*   36
167:249-256.

Neurosciences Res. Prog. Bull., Vol. 14, No. 1   **95**

Page

Heyningen, V. van, Bobrow, M., Bodmer, W.F., Gardiner, S.E., Povey, S., and   67
Hopkinson, D.A. (1975): Chromosome assignment of some human enzyme loci:
mitochondrial malate dehydrogenase 7, mannosephosphate isomerase and
pyruvate kinase to 15 and, probably, esterase D to 13. *Ann. Hum. Gen.*
38:295-303.

Hollingshead, A.B. and Redlich, F.C. (1958): *Social Class and Mental Illness.* New   77
York: John Wiley and Sons, Inc.

Holst, E. von and St. Paul, U. von (1962): Electrically controlled behavior. *Sci. Am.*   73
206:50-59.

Hughes, H.B., Biehl, J.P., Jones, A.P., and Schmidt, L.H. (1954): Metabolism of   62
isoniazid in man as related to the occurrence of peripheral neuritis. *Am. Rev.
Tuberculosis* 70:266-273.

Husén, T. (1960): Abilities of twins. *Scand. J. Psychol.* 1:125-135.   32

Jackson, D.D. (1960): A critique of the literature on the genetics of schizophrenia.   27,33
In: The Etiology of Schizophrenia. Jackson, D.D., ed. New York: Basic Books,
pp. 37-87.

James, J.W. (1971): Frequency in relatives for an all-or-none trait. *Ann. Hum.*   69
Genet. 35:47-49.

Kallmann, F.J. (1938): *The Genetics of Schizophrenia.* New York: Augustin.   26

Kallmann, F.J. (1946): The genetic theory of schizophrenia. An analysis of 691   26
schizophrenic twin index families. *Am. J. Psychiatry* 103:309-322.

Kallmann, F.J. (1950): The genetics of psychoses: An analysis of 1,232 twin index   26
families. *Congrès International de Psychiatrie, Paris,* 6:1-40.

Kalow, W. (1962): *Pharmacogenetics: Heredity and the Response to Drugs.*   57,62,63
Philadelphia: W.B. Saunders Co.

Kalow, W. (1972): Succinylcholine and malignant hyperthermia. *Fed. Proc.*   63
31:1270-1275.

Kalow, W. and Genest, K. (1957): A method for the detection of atypical forms of   63
human serum cholinesterase. Determination of dibucaine numbers. *Canad. J.
Biochem. Physiol.* 35:339-346.

Kaplan, A.R., ed. (1972): *Genetic Factors in "Schizophrenia."* Springfield, Ill.: C.C
Thomas.

Karlsson, J.L. (1966): *The Biologic Basis of Schizophrenia.* Springfield, Ill.: C.C   28
Thomas.

Kellermann, G., Luyten-Kellermann, M., and Shaw, C.R. (1973a): Genetic variation   64
of aryl hydrocarbon hydroxylase in human lymphocytes. *Am. J. Hum. Genet.*
25:327-331.

Kellermann, G., Shaw, C.R., and Luyten-Kellermann, M. (1973b): Aryl hydro- 16
carbon hydroxylase inducibility and bronchogenic carcinoma. *New Engl. J. Med.*
289:934-937.

Kelley, W.N., Green, M.L., Rosenbloom, F.M., Henderson, J.F., and Seegmiller, J.E. 63
(1969): Hypoxanthine-guanine phosphoribosyltransferase deficiency in gout.
Ann. Int. Med. 70:155-206.

Kety, S.S. (1959): Biochemical theories of schizophrenia. Part I of a two-part
critical review of current theories and of the evidence used to support them.
Science 129:1528-1532.

Kety, S.S. (1959): Biochemical theories of schizophrenia. Part II of a two-part
critical review of current theories and of the evidence used to support them.
Science 129:1590-1596.

Kety, S.S. (1967): Current biochemical approaches to schizophrenia. *New Engl. J.
Med.* 276:325-331.

Kety, S.S. (1974): From rationalization to reason. *Am. Psychiatry* 131:957-963.

Kety, S.S., editor-in-chief (1974): Symposium on catecholamines and their 81
enzymes in the neuropathology of schizophrenia. May 18-21, 1973, Strasbourg,
France. *J. Psychiatr. Res.* 11:1-364.

Kety, S.S. and Matthysse, S. (1972): Prospects for research on schizophrenia.
Neurosciences Res. Prog. Bull. 10:369-507. Also *In: Neurosciences Research
Symposium Summaries, Vol. 7.* Schmitt, F.O. et al., eds. Cambridge, Mass.:
M.I.T. Press, 1973, pp. 369-507.

Kety, S.S., Rosenthal, D., Wender, P.H., and Schulsinger, F. (1968): The types and 37,39,43
prevalence of mental illness in the biological and adoptive families of adopted
schizophrenics. *J. Psychiatr. Res.* 6(Suppl. 1):345-362.

Kety, S.S., Rosenthal, D., Wender, P.H., Schulsinger, F., and Jacobsen, B. (1975): 39,43,44
Mental illness in the biological and adoptive families of adopted individuals who
have become schizophrenic: A preliminary report based on psychiatric interviews. *In: Genetic Research in Psychiatry.* Fieve, R.R., Rosenthal, D., and Brill,
H., eds. Baltimore, Md.: The Johns Hopkins University Press, pp. 147-165.

Kidd, K.K. and Cavalli-Sforza, L.L. (1973): An analysis of the genetics of 70
schizophrenia. *Soc. Biol.* 20:254-265.

Klein, J. (1975): *Biology of the Mouse Histocompatibility-2 Complex: Principles of* 67
Immunogenetics Applied to a Single System. Berlin: Springer-Verlag.

Klemperer, J. (1933): Zur Belastungsstatistik der Durchschnittsbevölkerung: 26
Psychosenhäufigkeit unter 1000 stichprobenmässig aus den Geburtsgegistern der
Stadt München (Jahrgang 1881-1890) ausgelesen Probanden. *Z. ges. Neurol.
Psychiatr.* 146:277-316.

Neurosciences Res. Prog. Bull., Vol. 14, No. 1   97

Page

Koch, H.L. (1966): *Twins and Twin Relations*. Chicago: University of Chicago   30
Press.

Kohn, M.L. and Clausen, J.A. (1955): Social isolation and schizophrenia. *Am.
Sociol. Rev.* 20:265-273.

Kohn, M.L. and Clausen, J.A. (1956): Parental authority behavior and schizophrenia. *Am. J. Orthopsychiatry* 26:297-313.

Kraepelin, E. (1919): *Dementia Praecox and Paraphrenia*. Edinburgh: Livingstone.   12

Kringlen, E. (1964a): Discordance with respect to schizophrenia in monozygotic
male twins: Some genetic aspects. *J. Nerv. Ment. Dis.* 138:26-31.

Kringlen, E. (1964b): *Schizophrenia in Male Monozygotic Twins*. Oslo: University   27
Press. Also *In: Acta Psychiatr. Scand.* 40(Suppl. 178):1-76.

Kringlen, E. (1966): Schizophrenia in twins. An epidemiological-clinical study.
Psychiatry 29:172-184.

Kringlen, E. (1967): *Heredity and Environment in the Functional Psychoses. An*   28,33,34
Epidemiological-Clinical Twin Study. Oslo: University Press.

Kringlen, E. (1968): An epidemiological-clinical twin study on schizophrenia. *In:
The Transmission of Schizophrenia*. Rosenthal, D. and Kety, S.S., eds. Oxford:
Pergamon Press, pp. 49-63.

Kringlen, E. (1970): New studies on the genetics of schizophrenia. *In: The World
Biennial of Psychiatry and Psychotherapy, Vol. 1*. Arieti, S., ed. New York:
Basic Books, pp. 476-504.

La Du, B.N. (1972): Isoniazid and pseudocholinesterase polymorphisms. *Fed. Proc.*
31:1276-1285.

La Du, B.N. (1972): Pharmacogenetics: Defective enzymes in relation to reactions
to drugs. *Annu. Rev. Med.* 23:453-468.

La Du, B.N. (1973): Biochemical studies of metabolic disorders associated with
mental retardation. *In: Inborn Errors of Metabolism*. Hommes, F.A. and Van
Den Berg, C.J., eds. New York: Academic Press, pp. 1-13.

La Du, B.N. (1974): Pharmacogenetics: Single gene effects. *In: Pharmacology and
Pharmacokinetics*. Teorell, T., Dedrick, R.L., and Condliffe, P.G., eds. New
York: Plenum Press, pp. 253-260.

La Du, B.N. and Dewald, B. (1971): Genetic regulation of plasma cholinesterase in
man. *Adv. Enzyme Reg.* 9:317-332.

La Du, B.N. and Zannoni, V.G. (1971): Basic biochemical disturbance in aromatic
amino acid metabolism in phenylketonuria. *In: Phenylketonuria and Some
Other Inborn Errors of Amino Acid Metabolism*. Bickel, H., Hudson, F.P., and
Woolf, L.I., eds. Stuttgart: Georg Thieme Verlag, pp. 6-14.

Lamprecht, F., Wyatt, R.J., Belmaker, R., Murphy, D.L., and Pollin, W. (1973): Plasma dopamine-beta-hydroxylase in identical twins discordant for schizophrenia. *In: Frontiers in Catecholamine Research.* New York: Pergamon Press, pp. 1123-1126.

Lebergott, S. (1968): Labor force and employment trends. *In: Indicators of Social Change.* Sheldon, E.B. and Moore, W.E., eds. New York: Russell Sage Foundation, pp. 97-143.   78

Leighton, A.H. (1959): *My Name is Legion. Foundation for a Theory of Man in Relation to Culture, Vol. I.* New York: Basic Books.   83

Leighton, A. (1967): Is social environment a cause of psychiatric disorder? *In: Psychiatric Research Report 22, American Psychiatric Association, April, 1967,* pp. 337-345.

Leighton, A.H. and Hughes, J.M. (1961): Cultures as causative of mental disorder. *Milbank Mem. Fund Q.* 39:446-488.

Leighton, A.H., Leighton, D.C., and Danley, R.A. (1966): Validity in mental health surveys. *Canad. Psychiatr. Assoc. J.* 11:167-178.

Leighton, A.H. and Murphy, J.M. (1965): The problem of cultural distortion. *Milbank Mem. Fund Q.* 43:189-198.

Leonard, C.O., Chase, G.A., and Childs, B. (1972): Genetic counseling: A consumers' view. *New Engl. J. Med.* 287:433-439.

Lidz, T., Fleck, S., and Cornelius, A. (1965): *Schizophrenia and the Family.* New   78
York: International Universities Press.

Lilly, F. (1970): Fv-2: Identification and location of a second gene governing the   67
spleen focus response to Friend leukemia virus in mice. *J. Nat. Cancer Inst.* 45:163-169.

Luxenburger, H. (1928a): Demographische und psychiatrische Untersuchungen in   26
der engeren biologischen Familie von Parelytikerehegetten. *Z. ges. Neurol. Psychiatr.* 112:331-491.

Luxenburger, H. (1928b): Vorläufiger Bericht über psychiatrische Serienunter-   26
suchungen an Zwillingen. *Z. ges. Neurol. Psychiatr.* 116:297-326.

Luxenburger, H. (1934): Die Manifestations wahrscheinlichkeit der Schizophrenie   26
im Lichte der Zwillingsforschung. *Z. psych. Hygiene* 7:174-184.

McCabe, M.S. (1975): Reactive psychoses, a clinical and genetic investigation. *Acta*   29
Psychiatr. Scand. Suppl. 259:1-133.

McDevitt, H.O. and Bodmer, W.F. (1974): HL-A, immune-response genes, and   68
disease. *Lancet* I:1269-1275.

Neurosciences Res. Prog. Bull., Vol. 14, No. 1   99

Page

Marten, S.A., Cadoret, R.J., Winokur, G., and Ora, E. (1972): Unipolar depression: A family history study. *Biol. Psychiatry* 4:205-213.

Matthysse, S. and Haber, S. (1975): Animal models of schizophrenia. *In: Model Systems in Biological Psychiatry.* Ingle, D.J. and Schein, H.M., eds. Cambridge, Mass.: M.I.T. Press, pp. 4-25.   24

Matthysse, S. and Kidd, S.S. (1976): Estimating the genetic contribution to schizophrenia. *Am. J. Psychiatry* (In press)   81

Matthysse, S. and Lipinski, J. (1975): Biochemical aspects of schizophrenia. *Annu. Rev. Med.* 26:551-565.   82

Mednick, S.A., Mura, E., Schulsinger, F., and Mednick, B. (1974a): Perinatal conditions and infant development in children with schizophrenic parents. *In: Genetics, Environment and Psychopathology.* Mednick, S.A., Schulsinger, F., Higgins, J., and Bell, B., eds. New York: American Elsevier, pp. 231-248.   84

Mednick, S.A. and Schulsinger, F. (1965): Children of schizophrenic mothers. *Bull. Int. Assoc. Appl. Psychol.* 14:11-27.

Mednick, S.A. and Schulsinger, F. (1965): A longitudinal study of children with a high risk for schizophrenia: A preliminary report. *In: Methods and Goals in Human Behavior Genetics.* Vandenberg, S.G., ed. New York: Academic Press, pp. 255-295.

Mednick, S.A. and Schulsinger, F. (1974): Studies of children at high risk for schizophrenia. *In: Genetics, Environment and Psychopathology.* Mednick, S.A., Schulsinger, F., Higgins, J., and Bell, B., eds. New York: American Elsevier, pp. 103-116.   84

Mednick, S.A., Schulsinger, F., Higgins, J., and Bell, B., eds. (1974b): *Genetics, Environment and Psychopathology.* New York: American Elsevier.

Meehl, P.E. (1972): Classical symptoms of schizophrenia. *Neurosciences Res. Prog. Bull.* 10:377-380. Also *In: Neurosciences Research Symposium Summaries, Vol. 7.* Schmitt, F.O. et al., eds. Cambridge, Mass.: M.I.T. Press, 1973, pp. 377-380.   21

Mendlewicz, J. and Fleiss, J.L. (1974): Linkage studies with X-chromosome markers in bipolar (manic-depressive) and unipolar (depressive) illnesses. *Biol. Psychiatry* 9:261-294.   46,48,49, 50,51

Mendlewicz, J., Fleiss, J.L., and Fieve, R.R. (1972): Evidence for X-linkage in the transmission of manic-depressive illness. *J. Am. Med. Assoc.* 222:1624-1627.   46,48,49

Mendlewicz, J., Fleiss, J.L., and Fieve, R.R. (1975): Linkage studies in affective disorders: The Xg blood group and manic-depressive illness. *In: Genetic Research in Psychiatry.* Fieve, R.R., Rosenthal, D., and Brill, H., eds. Baltimore, Md.: The Johns Hopkins University Press, pp. 219-232.   46,48,50, 51

Nichol, S., Seal, U.S., and Gottesman, I.I. (1973): Serum from schizophrenic patients. *Arch. Gen. Psychiatry* 29:744-751.

O'Reilly, R.A. (1970): The second reported kindred with hereditary resistance to oral anticoagulant drugs. *New Engl. J. Med.* 282:1448-1451.   63

Pignatti, P.F. and Cavalli-Sforza, L.L. (1975): Serotonin binding proteins from human blood platelets. An experimental model system for studies on properties of synaptic vesicles. *Neurobiology* 5:65-74.   56

Ploog, D.W. (1967): The behavior of squirrel monkeys (*Saimiri sciureus*) as revealed by sociometry, bioacoustics, and brain stimulation. *In: Social Communication among Primates.* Altmann, S.A., ed. Chicago: University of Chicago Press, pp. 149-184.

Ploog, D. (1972): Breakdown of the social communication system: A key process in the development of schizophrenia? *Neurosciences Res. Prog. Bull.* 10:394-396. Also *In: Neurosciences Research Symposium Summaries, Vol. 7.* Schmitt, F.O. et al., eds. Cambridge, Mass.: M.I.T. Press, 1973, pp. 394-396.   75

Ploog, D., Hupfer, K., Jürgens, U., and Newman, J.D. (1976): Neuroethological studies of vocalization in squirrel monkeys with special reference to genetic differences of calling in two subspecies. *In: Growth and Development of the Brain: Nutritional, Genetic, and Environmental Factors (IBRO Monograph Series).* Brazier, M.A.B., ed. New York: Raven Press. (In press)   75

Ploog, D. and Maurus, M. (1973): Social communication among squirrel monkeys: analysis by sociometry, bioacoustics and cerebral radio-stimulation. *In: Comparative Ecology and Behaviour of Primates.* Michael, R.P. and Crook, J.H., eds. New York: Academic Press, pp. 211-233.

Polani, P.E. (1969): Abnormal sex chromosomes and mental disorder. *Nature* 223:680-686.   18

Pollin, W., Allen, M.G., Hoffer, A., Stabenau, J.R., and Hrubec, Z. (1969): Psychopathology in 15,909 pairs of veteran twins: Evidence for a genetic factor in the pathogenesis of schizophrenia and its relative absence in psychoneurosis. *Am. J. Psychiatry* 126:597-610.   27

Pollin, W., Stabenau, J.R., Mosher, L., and Tupin, J. (1966): Life history differences in identical twins discordant for schizophrenia. *Am. J. Orthopsychiatry* 36:492-509.   28,83

Rakic, P. (1975): Local circuit neurons. *Neurosciences Res. Prog. Bull.* 13:289-446.   85

Reich, T., Clayton, P.J., and Winokur, G. (1969): Family history studies: V. The genetics of mania. *Am. J. Psychiatry* 125:1358-1368.   46,49

Reich, T., James, J.W., and Morris, C.A. (1972): The use of multiple thresholds in determining the mode of transmission of semi-continuous traits. *Ann. Hum. Genet.* 36:163-184.   69

Renwick, J.H. and Schulze, J. (1964): An analysis of some data on the linkage   51
between Xg and colorblindness in man. *Am. J. Hum. Genet.* 16:410-418.

Rosanoff, A.J., Handy, L.M., and Plesset, I.R. (1935): The etiology of manic-   46
depressive syndromes with special reference to their occurrence in twins. *Am. J.
Psychiatry* 91:725-762.

Rosanoff, A.J., Handy, L.M., Plesset, I.R., and Brush, S. (1934): The etiology of   26
so-called schizophrenic psychoses with special reference to their occurrence in
twins. *Am. J. Psychiatry* 91:247-286.

Rosenthal, D. (1959): Some factors associated with concordance and discordance
with respect to schizophrenia in monozygotic twins. *J. Nerv. Ment. Dis.*
129:1-10.

Rosenthal, D. (1960): Confusion of identity and the frequency of schizophrenia in   32
twins. *Arch. Gen. Psychiatry* 3:297-304.

Rosenthal, D. (1961): Sex distribution and the severity of illness among samples of
schizophrenic twins. *J. Psychiatr. Res.* 1:26-36.

Rosenthal, D. (1962a): Familial concordance by sex with respect to schizophrenia.
Psychol. Bull. 59:401-421.

Rosenthal, D. (1962b): Problems of sampling and diagnosis in the major twin   27
studies of schizophrenia. *J. Psychiatr. Res.* 1:116-134.

Rosenthal, D., ed. (1963): *The Genain Quadruplets.* New York: Basic Books.

Rosenthal, D. (1966): The offspring of schizophrenic couples. *J. Psychiatr. Res.*
4:169-188.

Rosenthal, D. (1971): A program of research on heredity in schizophrenia. *Behav.
Sci.* 16:191-201.

Rosenthal, D. (1973): Evidence for a spectrum of schizophrenic disorders. Paper
presented at the Annual Meeting of the American Psychological Association,
Montreal, Canada, August 30, 1973.

Rosenthal, D. and Kety, S.S., eds. (1968): *The Transmission of Schizophrenia.* New   35
York: Pergamon Press.

Rosenthal, D., Wender, P.H., Kety, S.S., Schulsinger, F., Welner, J., and Østergaard,   37
L. (1968): Schizophrenics' offspring reared in adoptive homes. *In: The
Transmission of Schizophrenia.* Rosenthal, D. and Kety, S.S., eds. New York:
Pergamon Press, pp. 377-391.

Rosenthal, D., Wender, P.H., Kety, S.S., Welner, J., and Schulsinger, F. (1971): The   37,40
adopted-away offspring of schizophrenics. *Am. J. Psychiatry* 128:307-311.

Rüdin, E. (1916a): *Studien über Vererbung und Enstehung Geistiger Störungen.*
Berlin: Springer-Verlag.

Neurosciences Res. Prog. Bull., Vol. 14, No. 1   103

Page

Rüdin, E. (1916b): *Zur Vererbung und Neuentstehung der Dementia Praecox.*   26
Berlin: Springer-Verlag.

Schneider, K. (1971): *Klinisches Psychopathologie.* (9th Ed.) Stuttgart: Thieme.   36

Schulsinger, H. (1976): A ten years follow-up of children of schizophrenic mothers: 84
The clinical assessment. *Acta Psychiatr. Scand.* (In press)

Schulz, B. (1927): Zur Frage einer Belastungsstatistik der Durchschnitts-   26
bevölkerung. Geschwisterschaften und Elternschaften von 100 Hirnarterio-
sklerotiker-Ehegatten. *Z. ges. Neurol. Psychiatr.* 109:15-48.

Schulz, B. (1932): Zur Erbpathologie der Schizophrenie. *Z. ges. Neurol. Psychiatr.*   29
143:175-293.

Schulz, B. (1934): Versuch einer genealogisch-statistischen Überprüfung eines   29
Schizophreniemateriales auf biologische Einheitlichkeit. *Z. ges. Neurol.
Psychiatr.* 151:145-170.

Schwartz, M.A., Aikens, A.M., and Wyatt, R.J. (1974a): Monoamine oxidase   61
activity in brains from schizophrenic and mentally normal individuals. *Psychopharmacologia* 38:319-328.

Schwartz, M.A., Wyatt, R.J., Yang, H.Y., and Neff, N.H. (1974b): Multiple forms   61
of brain monoamine oxidase in schizophrenic and normal individuals. *Arch. Gen.
Psychiatry* 31:557-560.

Shahidi, N.T. (1968): Acetophenetidin-induced methemoglobinemia. *Ann. N.Y.*   64
Acad. Sci. 151:822-832.

Shields, J. and Gottesman, I.I. (1972): Cross-national diagnosis of schizophrenia in
twins. *Arch. Gen. Psychiatry* 27:725-730.

Shields, J. and Gottesman, I.I. (1973): Genetic studies of schizophrenia as signposts
to biochemistry. *Biochem. Soc. Spec. Publ.* 1:165-174.

Shields, J., Gottesman, I.I., and Slater, E. (1967): Kallmann's 1946 schizophrenia
twin study in the light of new information. *Acta Psychiatr. Scand.* 43:385-396.

Shields, J., Heston, L.L., and Gottesman, I.I. (1975): Schizophrenia and the   36
schizoid: The problem for genetic analysis. *In: Genetic Research in Psychiatry.*
Fieve, R.R., Rosenthal, D., and Brill, H., eds. Baltimore, Md.: The Johns
Hopkins University Press, pp. 167-197.

Sidman, R.L., Green, M.C., and Appel, S.H. (1965): *Catalog of the Neurological*   80
Mutants of the Mouse. Cambridge, Mass.: Harvard University Press.

Siemens, H.W. (1924): *Die Zwillingspathologie. Ihre Bedeutung—Ihre Methodik—
Ihre Bisherigen Ergebnisse.* Berlin: Springer-Verlag.

Sjögren, T. (1935): Investigations of the heredity of psychoses and mental   26
deficiency in two North Swedish parishes. *Ann. Eugen., Camb.* 6:253-318.

Slater, E. (1953): Psychotic and neurotic illnesses in twins. *In: Medical Research*   26
Council Special Report Series No. 278. London: Her Majesty's Stationery
Office.

Slater, E. (1968): A review of earlier evidence on genetic factors in schizophrenia.   70
In: The Transmission of Schizophrenia. Rosenthal, D. and Kety, S.S., eds.
Oxford: Pergamon Press, pp. 15-26.

Slater, E., Beard, A.W., and Glithero, E. (1963): The schizophrenia-like psychoses   29
of epilepsy. *Brit. J. Psychiatry* 109:95-150.

Smith, C. (1970): Heritability of liability and concordance in monozygous twins.   70
Ann. Hum. Genet. 34:85-91.

Smith, C. (1971): Recurrence risks for multifactorial inheritance. *Am. J. Hum.*   37
Genet. 23:578-588.

Spicer, C.C., Hare, E.H., and Slater, E. (1973): Neurotic and psychotic forms of   53
depressive illness: evidence from age-incidence in a national sample. *Brit. J.*
Psychiatry 123:535-541.

Srole, L. (1975): Measurement and classification in sociopsychiatric epidemiology: 43
Midtown Manhattan study (1954) and midtown Manhattan restudy (1974). *J.*
Health Soc. Behav. (In press)

Stenstedt, A. (1952): A study in manic depressive psychoses. Clinical, social, and
genetic investigations. *Acta Psychiatr. Neurol. Scand. Suppl.* 79:1-111.

Strömgren, E. (1935): Zum Ersatz des Weinbergschen abgekürzten Verfahrens,
Zugleich ein Beitrag zur Frage von der Erblichkeit des Erkrankungsalters bei der
Schizophrenie. *Z. ges. Neurol. Psychiatr.* 153:784-797.

Strömgren, E. (1938): Beiträge zur psychiatrischen Erblehre. Auf Grund von   26
Untersuchungen an einer Inselbevölkerung. *Acta Psychiatr. Suppl.* 19:1-259.

Strömgren, E. (1950): Statistical and genetical population studies within
psychiatry. *Congrés Int. Psychiatr.* 6:155-192.

Strömgren, E. (1961): Recent studies of prognosis and outcome in the mental
disorders. *In: Comparative Epidemiology of the Mental Disorders*. Hoch, P.H.,
and Zubin, J., eds. New York: Grune and Stratton, pp. 120-131.

Strömgren, E. (1962): Trends in psychiatric genetics in Scandinavia. *In: Expanding*
Goals of Genetics in Psychiatry. Kallmann, F.J., ed. New York: Grune and
Stratton, pp. 228-234.

Strömgren, E. (1965): "Schizophreniform psychoses." *Acta Psychiatr. Scand.*
41:483-489.

Strömgren, E. (1967): Nachtrag 1964 zur Psychiatrischen Genetik. *In: Psychiatrie*
der Gegenwart: Forschung und Praxis, Band I/1. Grundlagenforschung zur
Psychiatrie, Teil A. Gruhle, H.W., Jung, R., Mayer-Gross, W., and Müller, M., eds.
New York: Springer-Verlag, pp. 60-69.

Neurosciences Res. Prog. Bull., Vol. 14, No. 1

105

Page

Strömgren, E. (1967): Neurosen und Psychopathien. *In: Humangenetik: Ein kurzes Handbuch in fünf Bänden. Band V/2.* Becker, P.E., ed. Stuttgart: Georg Thieme Verlag, pp. 578-598.

Strömgren, E. (1967): Psychiatrische Genetik. *In: Psychiatrie der Gegenwart: Forschung und Praxis, Band I/1. Grundlagenforschung zur Psychiatrie, Teil A.* Gruhle, H.W., Jung, R., Mayer-Gross, W., and Müller, M., eds. New York: Springer-Verlag, pp. 1-59.

Strömgren, E. (1968): *Contributions to Psychiatric Epidemiology and Genetics. Acta Jutlandica.* Vol. 40, No. 4.

Strömgren, E. (1969): Uses and abuses of concepts in psychiatry. *Am. J. Psychiatry* 126:777-788.

Talamo, R.C. (1975): Basic and clinical aspects of the alpha$_1$-antitrypsin. *Pediatrics* 56:91-99.   16

Tanna, V.L. and Winokur, G. (1968): A study of association and linkage of ABO blood types and primary affective disorder. *Brit. J. Psychiatry* 114:1175-1181.

Teuber, H.-L. (1972): Effects of focal brain lesions. *Neurosciences Res. Prog. Bull.*   85
10:381-384. Also *In: Neurosciences Research Symposium Summaries, Vol. 7.* Schmitt, F.O. et al., eds. Cambridge, Mass.: M.I.T. Press, 1973, pp. 381-384.

Thoday, J.M. (1967): New insights into continuous variation. *In: Proceedings of*   37
the Third International Congress of Human Genetics. Crow, J.F. and Neel, J.V., eds. Baltimore, Md.: The Johns Hopkins University Press, pp. 339-350.

Tienari, P. (1963): Psychiatric illnesses in identical twins. *Acta Psychiatr. Scand.*   27
Suppl. 171.

Turner, R.J. and Wagenfeld, M.O. (1967): Occupational mobility and schizo-   41,77
phrenia: An assessment of the social causation and social selection hypotheses. *Am. Sociol. Rev.* 32:104-113.

Vesell, E.S. (1973): Advances in pharmacogenetics. *Prog. Med. Genet.* 9:291-367.   62

Warner, L., ed. (1963): *Yankee City.* New Haven: Yale University Press.   77

Welner, J. and Strömgren, E. (1958): Clinical and genetic studies on benign   29
schizophreniform psychoses based on a follow-up. *Acta Psychiatr. Neurol. Scand.* 33:377-399.

Wender, P.H. (1972): Adopted children and their families in the evaluation of nature-nurture interactions in the schizophrenic disorders. *Annu. Rev. Med.* 23:355-372.

Wender, P.H., Rosenthal, D., and Kety, S.S. (1968): A psychiatric assessment of the   38
adoptive parents of schizophrenics. *In: The Transmission of Schizophrenia.* Rosenthal, D. and Kety, S.S., eds. Oxford: Pergamon Press, pp. 235-250.

Page

Wender, P.H., Rosenthal, D., Kety, S.S., Schulsinger, F., and Welner, J. (1973):   41
Social class and psychopathology in adoptees. A natural experimental method
for separating the roles of genetic and experiential factors. *Arch. Gen. Psychiatry*
28:318-325.

Wender, P.H., Rosenthal, D., Kety, S.S., Schulsinger, R., and Welner, J. (1974):   68
Crossfostering. A research strategy for clarifying the role of genetic and
experiential factors in the etiology of schizophrenia. *Arch. Gen. Psychiatry*
30:121-128.

Wender, P.H., Rosenthal, D., Zahn, T.P., and Kety, S.S. (1971): The psychiatric   38
adjustment of the adopting parents of schizophrenics. *Am. J. Psychiatry*
127:1013-1018.

Whitehorn, J.C. (1923): Aporrhegma reactions in psychoses. *Am. J. Psychiatry*   65
2:421-426.

Wing, J.K., Cooper, J.E., and Sartorius, N. (1974): *The Measurement and*   83
Classification of Psychiatric Symptoms. Cambridge: Cambridge University Press.

Winokur, G. (1967): X-borne recessive genes in alcoholism. *Lancet* II:466.

Winokur, G. (1969): Genetic principles in the clarification of clinical issues in
affective disorder. *In: Psychochemical Research in Man.* Mandell, A.J. and
Mandell, M.P., eds. New York: Academic Press, pp. 329-342.

Winokur, G. (1970): Genetic findings and methodological considerations in manic
depressive disease. *Brit. J. Psychiatry* 117:267-274.

Winokur, G. (1972): Depression spectrum disease: Description and family study.
Compr. Psychiatry 13:3-8.

Winokur, G. (1972): Types of depressive illness. *Brit. J. Psychiatry* 120:265-266.

Winokur, G. (1973a): Genetic aspects of depression. *In: Separation and Depression.*
Washington, D.C.: American Association for the Advancement of Science,
pp. 125-137.

Winokur, G. (1973): The types of affective disorders. *J. Nerv. Ment. Dis.*
156:82-97.

Winokur, G. (1974): The division of depressive illness into depression spectrum
disease and pure depressive disease. *Int. Pharmacopsychiatry* 9:5-13.

Winokur, G., Cadoret, R., Dorzab, J., and Baker, M. (1971): Depressive disease: A
genetic study. *Arch. Gen. Psychiatry* 24:135-144.

Winokur, G. and Clayton, P. (1967): Family history studies: 1. Two types of
affective disorder separated according to genetic and clinical factors. *In: Recent
Advances in Biological Psychiatry, Vol. IX.* Wortis, J., ed. New York: Plenum
Press, pp. 35-50.

Neurosciences Res. Prog. Bull., Vol. 14, No. 1   **107**

Page

Winokur, G., Clayton, P.J., and Reich, T. (1969): *Manic Depressive Illness*. St.   46,53
Louis: C.V. Mosby.

Winokur, G., Morrison, J., Clancy, J., and Crowe, R. (1973): The Iowa 500:
Familial and clinical findings favor two kinds of depressive illness. *Compr.
Psychiatry* 14:99-106.

Winokur, G. and Pitts, F.N., Jr. (1965): Affective disorder: VI. A family history
study of prevalences, sex-differences and possible genetic factors. *J. Psychiatr.
Res.* 3:113-123.

Winokur, G. and Reich, T. (1970): Two genetic factors in manic-depressive disease.
Compr. Psychiatry 11:93-99.

Winokur, G. and Tanna, V.L. (1969): Possible role of X-linked dominant factor in   46,50,51
manic depressive disease. *Dis. Nerv. Syst.* 30:89-94.

Wise, C.D., Baden, M.M., and Stein, L. (1974): Post-mortem measurement of   61
enzymes in human brain: evidence of a central noradrenergic deficit in
schizophrenia. *J. Psychiatr. Res.* 11:185-199.

Wyatt, R.J., Belmaker, R., and Murphy, D. (1975a): Low platelet monoamine   59,60
oxidase and vulnerability to schizophrenia. *In: Modern Problems of Pharmacopsychiatry, Vol. 10. Genetics and Psychopharmacology.* Mendlewicz, E.J., ed.
Basel: S. Karger, pp. 38-57.

Wyatt, R.J., Murphy, D.L., Belmaker, R., Cohen, S., Donnelly, C.H., and Pollin, W.   59
(1973a): Reduced monoamine oxidase activity in platelets: A possible genetic
marker for vulnerability to schizophrenia. *Science* 179:916-918.

Wyatt, R.J., Saavedra, J.M., Belmaker, R., Cohen S., and Pollin, W. (1973b): The
dimethyltryptamine-forming enzyme in blood platelets: A study in monozygotic
twins discordant for schizophrenia. *Am. J. Psychiatry* 130:1359-1361.

Wyatt, R.J., Schwartz, M.A., Erdelyi, E., and Barchas, J.D. (1975b): Dopamine   61
β-hydroxylase activity in brains of chronic schizophrenic patients. *Science*
187:368-370.

Yerulshalmy, J. and Sheerar, S.E. (1940a): Studies on twins. I. The relation of   32
order of birth and age of parents to the frequency of like-sexed and unlike-sexed
twin deliveries. *Hum. Biol.* 12:95-113.

Yerulshalmy, J. and Sheerar, S.E. (1940b): Studies on twins. II. On the early   32
mortality of like-sexed and unlike-sexed twins. *Hum. Biol.* 12:247-263.

Zerbin-Rudin, E. (1967): Endogen psychosen. *In: Humangenetik: Ein kurzes
Handbuch in fünf Bänden. Band V/2.* Becker, P.E., ed. Stuttgart: Georg Thieme
Verlag, pp. 446-577.

THE NEUROBIOLOGY OF LITHIUM

Based on an NRP Work Session
held November 3-5, 1974 and updated by participants

by

William E. Bunney, Jr.

and

Dennis L. Murphy

National Institute of Mental Health
Bethesda, Maryland

Ava B. Nash
NRP Writer-Editor

CONTENTS

PARTICIPANTS

Floyd E. Bloom
Arthur V. Davis Center for
    Behavioral Neurobiology
Salk Institute
P.O. Box 1809
San Diego, CA 92112

Elkan R. Blout
Department of Biological Chemistry
Harvard Medical School
25 Shattuck Street
Boston, MA 02115

William E. Bunney, Jr.
Adult Psychiatry Branch, DCBR
    IRP, NIMH
Bldg. 10, Rm. 3N-212
9000 Rockville Pike
Bethesda, MD 20014

Jonathan L. Costa
National Institute of Neurological
    and Communicative Disorders and
    Stroke
Bldg. 10, Rm. 3S-229
National Institutes of Health
Bethesda, MD 20014

Mac V. Edds, Jr.*
Neurosciences Research Program
165 Allandale Street
Jamaica Plain, MA 02130

Manfred Eigen
Karl-Friedrich-Bonhoeffer-Institut
Max-Planck-Institut für
    biophysikalische Chemie
D-3400 Göttingen-Nikolausberg
Federal Republic of Germany

George Eisenman
Department of Physiology
Center for the Health Sciences
University of California
Los Angeles, CA 90024

Bertil Hille
Department of Physiology and Biophysics
SJ-40, Health Sciences Building
University of Washington
Seattle, WA 98195

Seymour S. Kety
Psychiatric Research Laboratories
Massachusetts General Hospital
Boston, MA 02114

Alexander Leaf
Massachusetts General Hospital
Boston, MA 02114

Jean-Marie Lehn
Institut de Chimie
Université Louis Pasteur
1, rue Blaise Pascal
B.P. 296/R8
67008 Strasbourg Cedex, France

Robert B. Livingston
Department of Neurosciences
University of California, San Diego
    School of Medicine
La Jolla, CA 92037

Arnold J. Mandell
Department of Psychiatry
University of California, San Diego
    School of Medicine
P.O. Box 109
La Jolla, CA 92093

*Dr. Edds died November 29, 1975.

Dennis L. Murphy
Laboratory of Clinical Sciences
Section on Clinical Neuropharmacology
National Institute of Mental Health
Bldg. 10, Rm. 3S-229
Bethesda, MD 20014

Lars Onsager
Center for Theoretical Studies
University of Miami
Coral Gables, FL 33124

Gardner C. Quarton
Mental Health Research Institute
University of Michigan
Ann Arbor, MI 48104

Virginia Ross
Massachusetts Institute of
    Technology—Rm. 6-123
Cambridge, MA 02139

George Sakalosky
Nuclear Engineering Department
Boston Edison Company
800 Boylston Street
Boston, MA 02199

Francis O. Schmitt
Neurosciences Research Program
165 Allandale Street
Jamaica Plain, MA 02130

Mogens Schou
Psychopharmacology Research Unit
Department of Psychiatry
Psychiatric Hospital
Aarhus University
DK-8240 Risskov, Denmark

Irwin Singer
Department of Medicine
University of Pennsylvania
    School of Medicine
Philadelphia, PA 19104

C.H. Suelter
Department of Biochemistry
Michigan State University
East Lansing, MI 48824

R.J.P. Williams
Department of Chemistry
Wadham College
Oxford OX1 3PN, England

Ruthild Winkler
Karl-Friedrich-Bonhoeffer-Institut
Max-Planck-Institut für
    biophysicalische Chemie
D-3400 Göttingen-Nikolausberg
Federal Republic of Germany

Jan Wolff
National Institute of Arthritis, Metabolism,
    and Digestive Diseases
Bldg. 10, Rm. 8N-315
National Institutes of Health
Bethesda, MD 20014

Frederic G. Worden
Neurosciences Research Program
165 Allandale Street
Jamaica Plain, MA 02130

Note: NRP Work Session reports are reviewed and revised by participants prior to publication.

I. INTRODUCTION

The finding that lithium carbonate is unusually effective as a psychoactive agent in the treatment of manic-depressive disorders has, over the last two decades, stimulated many studies of biological effects of lithium. Early studies of various lithium salts clearly revealed that it was the lithium ion itself that was responsible for the therapeutic effects of lithium that are observed in mania and in the prophylaxis of manic-depressive cycles. The fact that a single, naturally abundant metal affects complex human behavior has led to speculations that understanding how lithium works might further the understanding of the postulated neurochemical origin of manic-depressive cycles.

Lithium is an alkali metal found in many minerals in the earth's crust, in sea water in concentrations of approximately 0.014 mM, and in some mineral water from springs in concentrations as high as 0.8 mM. Very small quantities are found in animal tissues and plants, but no necessary physiologic function subserved by the trace amounts of this metal is known.

Lithium is the lightest of all solid elements, with an atomic weight of 6.94. It has the smallest crystal radius of all the alkali metals (Table 1). Upon hydration, lithium's radius is increased out of

TABLE 1

Some Properties of the Group I Alkali Metals and
the Group II Alkaline Earth Metals

	Atomic Number	Atomic Weight	Ionic Radius (A)	Charge Density*
I. Lithium	3	6.94	0.78	0.22
Sodium	11	22.99	0.95	0.088
Potassium	19	39.10	1.33	0.045
Rubidium	37	85.47	1.48	0.036
Cesium	55	132.91	1.67	0.029
II. Beryllium	4	9.01	0.31	1.660
Magnesium	12	24.31	0.65	0.380
Calcium	20	40.08	0.99	0.160
Strontium	38	87.62	1.13	0.120
Barium	56	137.34	1.35	0.088
Radium	88	226.05	1.43	0.078

*Coulombs/A^2, calculated as charge on ion divided by $4 \pi A^2$.

proportion to those of sodium, potassium, rubidium, and cesium, such that in physiologic situations lithium has the lowest diffusion coefficient and is the least lipid-soluble of the alkali metals. Its dissimilarity to rubidium and cesium in many biochemical properties and even in its behavioral effects may represent manifestations of such differences in physical properties.

Lithium's electron affinity is higher than that of the other alkali metals and hence is closer to that of the alkaline earth elements. Williams (1973) and others have noted that charge and size considerations suggest that lithium may interact in biological situations not only with sodium and potassium but also with magnesium and calcium; for example, lithium seems to behave in some chemical and biological situations as a "weak" sodium and in others to act antagonistically with magnesium or calcium.

This NRP Work Session on the neurobiology of lithium brought together physical chemists, neurophysiologists, biologists, and psychiatrists with a common interest in the way lithium and other metals act at the molecular and cellular level, with the hope that the interdisciplinary meeting would throw more light on results obtained clinically with lithium administration. The summary presented here is not a moment-to-moment account of the meeting but rather is an edited, comprehensive synthesis of its main points incorporating additional data from the literature. It is presented as a timely comment on some of the major research areas that might contribute to the understanding of the mechanisms of action of lithium.

II. CLINICAL BEHAVIORAL EFFECTS OF LITHIUM

Clinical Prophylactic Effects and Clinical Pharmacology of Lithium: M. Schou

Prophylactic Effects of Lithium

Lithium was first used clinically for the treatment of mania (Cade, 1949), but its most important clinical effect today is the prophylactic action: its ability to attenuate or prevent recurrences of manic and depressive episodes in bipolar and unipolar depressive patients. At least eight double-blind studies document this finding along with hundreds of nonblind studies (reviews: Schou, 1973d; Schou and Thomsen, 1975). Figure 1 illustrates the first observation of a prophylactic effect on both manic and depressive recurrences. Figure 2 shows in diagrammatic form the outcome of the first systematic nonblind study on lithium prophylaxis.

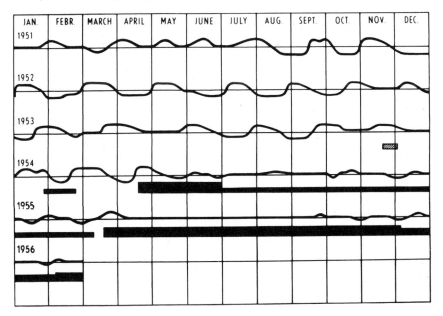

Figure 1. Graphic presentation of the disease history of a patient with bipolar manic-depressive disorder. Lithium treatment (cross-hatched bar, lithium citrate; black bars, lithium carbonate) led to attenuation of the manic and depressive symptoms. Observations shown until March 1, 1956. [Schou, 1956]

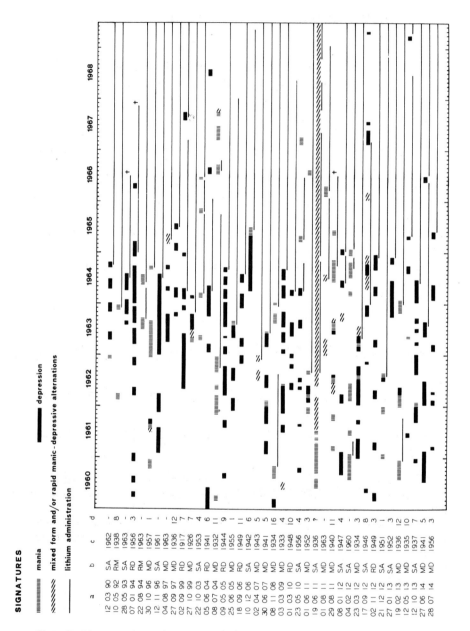

Figure 2. Diagrammatic case histories of patients first described by Baastrup and Schou (1967), here up-dated to July 1, 1969. Column a, the case number with day, month, and year of patient's birth. Column b, the diagnosis: MD = manic-depressive disorder, bipolar type; RM =

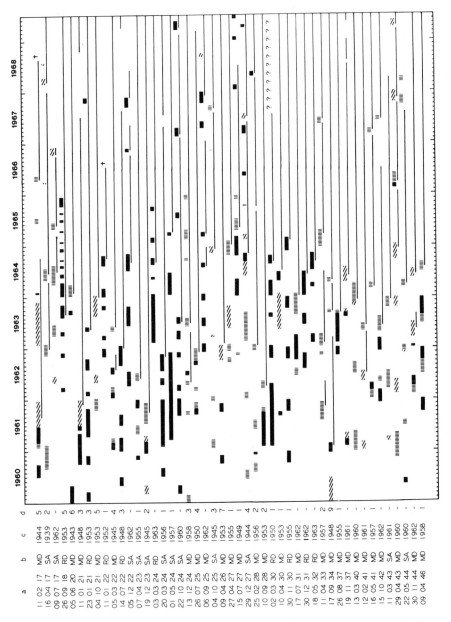

recurrent manias; RD = recurrent endogenous depressions; SA = recurrent schizo-affective psychosis. Column c, year of first manic or depressive episode. Column d, number of episodes before January 1, 1960. [Schou, 1973d]

In the double-blind studies, two general methods have been used: (1) selecting patients who respond to lithium and splitting the sample into a group that continues on lithium and another group in which placebo is substituted for lithium (Melia, 1970; Baastrup et al., 1970; Hullin et al., 1972; Cundall et al., 1972; Prien et al., 1973a,b); and (2) assigning manic-depressive patients either to lithium treatment or to treatment with placebo or other compounds (Coppen et al., 1971; Stallone et al., 1973). Table 2 summarizes the eight double-blind

TABLE 2

Two-Group Double-Blind Trials. (Adapted from Schou and Thomsen, 1975)

Author	Diagnostic group	Medication	Total no.	Relapsed during trial period[†]	p[‡]
Melia (1970)	Bipolar + monopolar	Lithium	9	5	
		Placebo	9	7	n.s.
Baastrup et al.	Bipolar	Lithium	28	0	
(1970)		Placebo	22	12	p < 0.001
	Monopolar	Lithium	17	0	
		Placebo	17	9	p = 0.001
	Bipolar + monopolar	Lithium	45	0	
		Placebo	39	21	p < 0.001
Coppen et al.	Bipolar	Lithium	16	3	
(1971)		Placebo	22	21	p < 0.001
	Monopolar	Lithium	11	2	
		Placebo	14	11	p = 0.01
	Bipolar + monopolar	Lithium	27	5	
		Placebo	36	32	p < 0.001
Hullin et al.	Bipolar + monopolar	Lithium	18	1	
(1971)		Placebo	18	6	p = 0.05
Cundall et al.	Bipolar	Lithium	12	4	
(1972)		Placebo	12	10	p < 0.05
	Monopolar	Lithium	4	3	
		Placebo	4	2	n.s.
	Bipolar + monopolar	Lithium	16	7	
		Placebo	16	12	n.s.
Stallone et al.	Bipolar	Lithium	19	5	
(1973)		Placebo	23	21	p < 0.001
Prien et al.	Bipolar	Lithium	85	36	
(1973a)		Placebo	86	75	p < 0.001
Prien et al.	Bipolar	Lithium	14	5	
(1973b)		Placebo	10	9	p < 0.05
	Monopolar	Lithium	23	13	
		Placebo	21	19	p < 0.05
	Bipolar + monopolar	Lithium	37	18	
		Placebo	31	28	p < 0.001

*Excluding patients who dropped out of the study for irrelevant reasons.
†Including patients who dropped out of the study because they relapsed.
‡One-tailed four-fold table test for significance (Diem and Lentner, 1970) for $N \leqslant 60$; χ^2-test for $N > 60$.

studies. They show convincingly (1) that lithium exerts a prophylactic action that is significantly superior to that of placebo; (2) that it protects against depressions as well as against manias; and (3) that lithium is prophylactically as effective in the unipolar cases, those with depressions only, as in the bipolar cases, those with both manias and depressions.

Because lithium has this double effect against both manias and depressions, the current, rather simple, up-or-down amine hypotheses of affective disorders cannot be readily applied to this drug. We must look for a stabilizing action on the (hypothetical) neurophysiological or neurochemical processes that underlie "endogenous mood swings." By this term Schou means such pathological changes in the general level of mood and mental energy that occur without, or with only slight, enviromental cause and which, if untreated, continue for many months until they disappear, again without any obvious external reason.

Effects on Normal Mental Functions

When administered in prophylactic doses, lithium has very little effect on normal mood and only slight effects on other mental functions (Schou, 1968; Small et al., 1972). Some patients and healthy human volunteers describe tiredness and mild difficulty in concentrating early in the drug trial. Later, there are no effects. Occasionally patients may complain of a slight decrease in reaction speed, for example, in certain kinds of athletics, or they may complain that they have suffered a loss in creative power, at least temporarily. The latter effect may be due to removal of slight manic features (Marshall et al., 1970; Polatin and Fieve, 1971; Schou and Baastrup, 1973).

Distribution and Concentrations

The concentrations of lithium attained in blood and tissues during administration of clinically effective doses are of importance for the planning and the evaluation of experiments. So are concentrations met with during lithium poisoning. Table 3 shows the lithium concentrations during treatment and poisoning as well as extracellular and tissue sodium concentrations.

Lithium is not distributed evenly among the organs. In some tissue, for example liver, the intracellular:extracellular concentration ratio is below unity. In others, such as kidney, thyroid, and bone, it is above. The concentration in whole brain is approximately the same as

TABLE 3

Concentrations of Lithium and Sodium in Extracellular
Fluids and in Tissues [Schou]

	Lithium		Sodium
	Therapy and prophylaxis	Poisoning	
Extracellular fluids	0.5 - 1.2 mmol/l	2 - 10 mmol/l	ca 140 mmol/l
Tissues	0.3 - 5 mmol/kg w.w.	1 - 15 mmol/kg w.w.	10 - 40 mmol/kg w.w.

in the extracellular fluid. Lowest concentrations are found in the spinal cord and pons, highest in the basal ganglia, but no one area of the brain accumulates lithium in excessive concentration.

Excretion of Lithium

Lithium elimination takes place almost exclusively through the kidneys. After filtration through the glomerular membrane, lithium is reabsorbed with sodium and water in the proximal kidney tubules; little or no lithium is reabsorbed in the distal parts of the nephron (Thomsen and Schou, 1968). The renal lithium clearance is therefore identical with the proximal clearance of sodium, about 20% of the glomerular filtration rate. It increases slightly with increasing sodium clearance but is unaffected by procedures that influence only distal sodium reabsorption.

Sodium balance plays a major, although not a solitary role in renal lithium clearance. The latter falls under conditions of severe sodium deficiency resulting from, for example, administration of a low-sodium diet or long-term administration of thiazides (Thomsen and Schou, 1973; Petersen et al., 1974). This fall may to a large extent be accounted for by an increase of the fractional proximal reabsorption of sodium and hence of lithium.

Lithium administration may in itself lower the capacity of the kidneys for conserving sodium (Thomsen et al., 1974), presumably by decreasing the response of the kidneys to mineralocorticoids (Thomsen et al., 1976a). The lowered capacity for conserving sodium leads to a rise in the minimum requirement for sodium. If the requirement exceeds the intake, sodium deficiency develops. This leads to a fall of the renal lithium clearance, resulting in further rise of the serum lithium concentration and additional increase of the minimum sodium requirement, so that a vicious cycle may be started (Thomsen et al., 1976b).

Side Effects and Poisoning

The most common side effects of lithium treatment are slight hand tremor (which may yield to treatment with β-receptor blocking agents), polyuria with secondary polydipsia (which may be caused by lowered response of the kidney to antidiuretic hormone), goiter or myxedema (caused primarily by inhibition of release of thyroglobulin from the thyroid gland), and weight gain.

Gradually developing lithium poisoning is heralded by a coarse tremor of the hands, neuromuscular incoordination, sluggishness, and dysarthria. A fully developed intoxication resembles the clinical picture of cerebral hemorrhage. If untreated, it may lead to death during prolonged coma, anuria, or circulatory failure.

Time Factors Involved

When lithium is used therapeutically, full antimanic action develops in the course of 6 to 10 days. When lithium is used prophylactically, it may take longer (weeks or months) before full protection against relapses is achieved. From a clinical point of view, one is therefore less interested in acute biological experiments in which the effects of a single or a few lithium doses are studied. Of much more interest are studies in which lithium is administered over days, weeks, or months. That acute and chronic lithium administration may produce entirely different effects has been seen in studies on brain amine concentration and turnover (Corrodi et al., 1967; Corrodi et al., 1969; Genefke, 1972), liver glycogen concentration (Plenge et al., 1970; Olesen and Thomsen, 1974), thyroid iodide transport and metabolism (Berens and Wolff, 1975), and thirst and urine flow (Thomsen, 1970).

Certain biological effects of lithium may persist not only after lithium administration has been stopped but also after complete disappearance of lithium from the organism. Such independence of the actual presence and concentration of the lithium ion has been observed in studies on lithium-induced polyuria, renal adenyl cyclase activity, synaptosome transport systems, and choline transport in red blood cells (Baldessarini and Yorke, 1970; Thomsen, 1970; Geisler et al., 1972; Wraae et al., 1972; Harris and Jenner, 1972; Lee et al., 1974). The observations indicate that some lithium effects may be indirect, produced by changes that persist after disappearance of the lithium ion.

Mode of Administration of Lithium

It should be noted that entirely different results may be obtained from experiments in which lithium is given as intraperitoneal injections once or twice during the day and experiments in which it is administered with the food. Under the former circumstances, the serum lithium concentration shows very large fluctuations, with high concentration peaks shortly after the administration and very low concentrations before the next administration. When lithium is administered with the food, the serum lithium concentration shows little variation around the clock and may be maintained at the same levels as those achieved in patients receiving lithium salt tablets. These differences should be kept in mind both when experiments are planned and when experimental data are assessed.

Conclusion

The introduction of lithium treatment and prophylaxis into psychiatry has meant that we can now combat a distressing and dangerous mental disorder with considerable efficiency. The question of the biochemical mode of action of lithium is a challenge to those of us who do research in biological psychiatry. The very simplicity of this drug is apt to lead us into believing that elucidation of its mode of action will be simple. Schou is afraid the opposite is the case.

Acute Behavioral Effects of Lithium Carbonate:
W.E. Bunney, Jr.

Lithium has a number of acute behavioral effects in man. A major medical use is the result of its ability to reverse severe manic symptomatology and, at times, depressive symptomatology in manic-depressive illness. This effect was first discovered in 1949 by John Cade. In order to understand the acute effects of lithium on manic-depressive illness, it is important to review behavioral characteristics of this illness and recent findings concerning it.

Symptomatology in Manic-Depressive Illness

The manic-depressive disorders are characterized by a chronic course lasting over many years during which manic phases alternate with depressive phases. These may occur as infrequently as every three to five years and as frequently as every other day. The manic phase is characterized by increased motor and verbal activity, grandiose thoughts, intrusiveness, bizarre behavior, and, at times, psychotic thinking and euphoria. The depressive phase is characterized by depressive affect, retardation of speech and movement, thoughts of death and dying, loss of interest in life, decreased libido, and difficulty in concentrating.

Hypothesized Biological Defect in Manic-Depressive Illness

Strong evidence now exists that there are genetic factors in manic-depressive illness (Gershon et al., 1971). There is an increased incidence of manic-depressive illness in family members when compared to the general population. The concordance rate for this illness in dizygotic twins is about 15% while the concordance rate in monozygotic twins ranges between 60% and 80% (Gershon et al., 1976). Evidence suggests that a genetic marker, red-green color blindness, is located on the short arm of the X-chromosome and may be linked to the loci for manic-depressive illness (Bunney et al., 1976; Mendlewicz and Fleiss, 1974). In some family studies, both red-green color blindness and manic-depressive illness occur together in patients. Genetic factors in an illness suggest that there may be an enzyme or protein defect and that the drugs that can activate or reverse the illness may be activating or reversing the defect. All of the drugs that activate or reverse manic-depressive illness alter amine neurotransmission in brain (Bunney et al., 1972a,b) and so the chemistry and physiology of neurotransmitters has come to be a major area in which to search for a biological dysfunction in this illness. Lithium's effect in manic-depressive illness is to normalize manic mood, manic activity, and psychotic thinking.

Diagnostic Considerations in Characterizing Affective Illness

Two major diagnostic subtypes are currently proposed for affective illness. These are unipolar depressions, which include patients with a history of recurrent depressive illness and no history of mania, and bipolar depressions, which include patients with a history of recurrence of both manic and depressive episodes. Unipolar patients have an age of onset that peaks at about 45 years and a low incidence of mania in relatives, as revealed by extensive family studies. Bipolar patients have a peak age of onset at 25 years and a much higher incidence of mania in relatives.

One other important characteristic of manic-depressive illness is the suddenness of the change: patients may continue for many months in a retarded, depressed, dozing, nonverbal condition and then, over the course of a few hours, may switch to a hyperactive, talkative, bizarre, and psychotic state. There is probably no change in human behavior as dramatic as the switch from retarded depression to mania, with its completely altered mood, cognition, and behavior. Patients have been studied who switched every 24 hours between mania and depression for up to ten years. In these patients, the switch into mania often occurred between 1 A.M. and 2 A.M. (Bunney and Hartmann, 1965).

Acute Effects of Lithium in Mania and Depression

Lithium carbonate has been administered to patients during acute manic episodes in many double-blind studies carried on all over the world. Within five to eight days, it can produce a complete normalization of the manic condition.

Figure 3 records a patient who was extremely manic, as noted on the daily nurses' ratings, and who showed a rapid response to

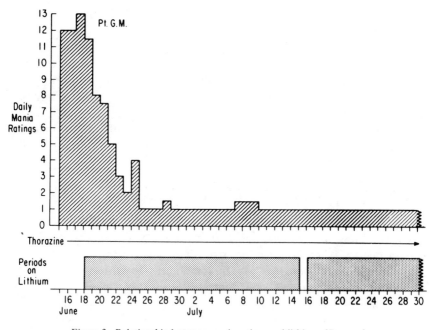

Figure 3. Relationship between mania ratings and lithium. [Bunney]

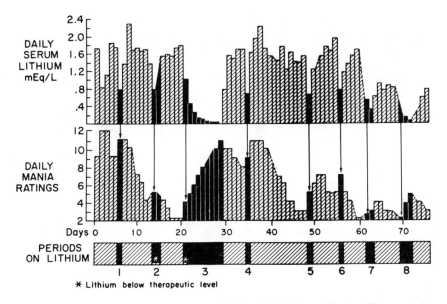

Figure 4. Sensitivity of mania to temporary withdrawal of lithium medication. [Bunney et al., 1968]

lithium carbonate. Figure 4 shows that there is a sensitivity of mania to temporary withdrawal of lithium medication when placebo is substituted. The black bars represent placebo substitution under double-blind conditions. As can be seen in the upper part of the figure, the daily serum lithium levels drop each time placebo is substituted, and the daily mania ratings increase each time placebo is substituted.

Figure 5 illustrates placebo period 3 from Figure 4. This patient was rated "blindly" by a physician and the quotes were documented "blindly" by the nursing staff. This figure illustrates the behavioral characteristics of a period of increasing mania when placebo is substituted. On lithium, the patient is described as calm, logical, insightful, reasonable; the patient states: "I'm just back to the good old Jane, and she's quiet." On the first day of placebo substitution, the patient is described as humming, singing occasionally, talking a bit faster. The patient says, "If things had continued, I would have been as high as a kite. I felt on the spot like a caged animal." The mania progresses to a point where she is described as "some increase in push of speech and paranoia, psychotic thinking, preoccupied." She states, "My brain is going so fast I feel exhausted." Finally, at the peak of mania, during the placebo substitution period, the patient is described

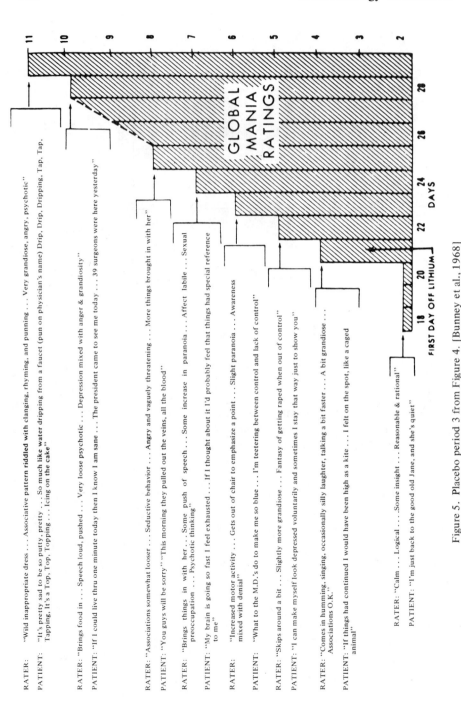

RATER: "Wild inappropriate dress . . . Associative pattern riddled with clanging, rhyming, and punning . . . Very grandiose, angry, psychotic"

PATIENT: "It's pretty sad to be so putty, pretty . . . So much like water dripping from a faucet (pun on physician's name) Drip, Drip, Dripping, Tap, Tap, Tapping, It's a Top, Top, Topping . . . Icing on the cake"

RATER: "Brings food in . . . Speech loud, pushed . . . Very loose psychotic . . . Depression mixed with anger & grandiosity"

PATIENT: "If I could live thru one minute today then I know I am sane . . . The president came to see me today . . . 39 surgeons were here yesterday"

RATER: "Associations somewhat looser . . . Seductive behavior . . . Angry and vaguely threatening . . . More things brought in with her"

PATIENT: "You guys will be sorry" "This morning they pulled out the veins, all the blood"

RATER: "Brings things in with her . . . Some push of speech . . . Some increase in paranoia . . . Affect labile . . . Sexual preoccupation . . . Psychotic thinking"

PATIENT: "My brain is going so fast I feel exhausted . . . If I thought about it I'd probably feel that things had special reference to me"

RATER: "Increased motor activity . . . Gets out of chair to emphasize a point . . . Slight paranoia . . . Awareness mixed with denial"

PATIENT: "What to the M.D.'s do to make me so blue . . . I'm teetering between control and lack of control"

RATER: "Skips around a bit . . . Slightly more grandiose . . . Fantasy of getting raped when out of control"

PATIENT: "I can make myself look depressed voluntarily and sometimes I stay that way just to show you"

RATER: "Comes in humming, singing, occasionally silly laughter, talking a bit faster . . . A bit grandiose . . . Associations O.K."

PATIENT: "If things had continued I would have been high as a kite . . . I felt on the spot, like a caged animal"

RATER: "Calm . . . Logical . . . Some insight . . . Reasonable & rational"

PATIENT: "I'm just back to the good old Jane, and she's quiet"

Figure 5. Placebo period 3 from Figure 4. [Bunney et al., 1968]

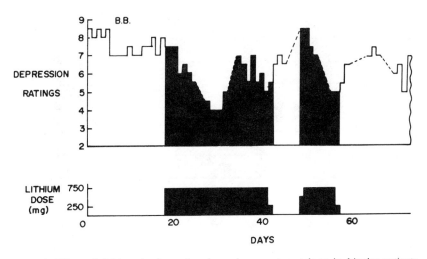

Figure 6. Effect of lithium in decreasing depressive symptomatology in bipolar patients. [Goodwin et al., 1972]

as "wild with inappropriate dress, associative speech pattern riddled with clanging, rhyming and punning, very grandiose, angry and psychotic." The patient is almost talking in word salad: "drip, drip, dripping, tap, tap, tapping, on its top, top, topping, icing on the cake." The patient states, "The President came to see me today; 39 surgeons were here yesterday." In most patients, lithium carbonate reverses these psychotic symptoms.

A number of investigators have observed that lithium is moderately effective in decreasing depressive symptomatology in bipolar patients, as illustrated in one patient in Figure 6 (Goodwin et al., 1972).

One of the major challenges in the field of psychobiology today is the development of a theoretical model to explain the mode of action of lithium carbonate in terms of its capacity to acutely reverse manic symptomatology, partially reverse acute depressive symptomatology, and to prevent the recurrence of both manic and depressive episodes.

Drug Studies Relevant to the Mode of Action of Lithium in Manic Illness

Psychopharmacological studies in man have produced various clues regarding the mode of action of lithium carbonate. Three types of compounds are known to "activate" mania and hypomania in bipolar

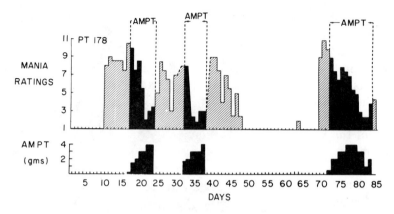

Figure 7. Clinical response of mania to α-methyl-*p*-tyrosine (AMPT). [Brodie et al., 1971]

manic-depressive illness. These include tricyclic compounds, monoamine oxidase inhibitors, and L-dopa, the metabolic precursor of
dopamine and norepinephrine. All of these compounds effectively
increase functional brain neurotransmitter amines. Three compounds,
in addition to lithium, can reverse manic symptomatology: alpha-
methyl-para-tyrosine (AMPT), which blocks the synthesis of dopamine
and norepinephrine at the rate-limiting step, the phenothiazines, and
the butyrophenones. Figure 7 illustrates one patient on AMPT, where
the black shaded areas indicate the periods on AMPT and the white
areas those of placebo substitution (Brodie et al., 1971). There is
additional evidence for the involvement of neurotransmitters derived
from the mode of action of phenothiazines and butyrophenones, which
specifically block dopamine receptors and which can often decrease
acute manic symptomatology. All of these compounds affect functional
brain amines at the synaptic cleft (Table 4).

TABLE 4

Pharmacological Agents Associated with Triggering
or Decreasing Manic Symptomatology [Bunney]

Drugs	Effect on mania	Effect on brain neurotransmitter amines
Tricyclic antidepressants	Increase mania	↑
Monoamine oxidase inhibitors	Increase mania	↑
L-Dopa	Increase mania	↑
Lithium	Decrease mania	↓
Phenothiazines	Decrease mania	↓
Butyrophenones	Decrease mania	↓
α-Methyl-*p*-tyrosine	Decrease mania	↓

Acute Clinical Uses of Lithium

Accepted clinical application of lithium in acute situations includes its use in mania, hypomania, depression, some schizo-affective disorders, and thyrotoxicosis. Additional suggested possible applications include its use in the treatment of Meniere's syndrome and in blocking the "high" of drugs of abuse. This last use is of interest in terms of the acute effects of lithium. One of the components of mania is euphoria, which is also usually associated with drugs of abuse, including amphetamines, marijuana, alcohol, cocaine, and heroin. Lithium may have an effect in blocking the "high" of amphetamines (van Kammen and Murphy, 1975), and there are a number of current studies in animals (Sinclair, 1974; Ho and Tsai, 1975) and man (Kline et al., 1974) investigating its use in decreasing alcohol ingestion.

Any clues concerning the mode of action of lithium carbonate may increase our understanding of manic-depressive illness and, in a larger sense, of mood, cognition, behavior, and the functioning of the human brain.

III. PHYSICAL CHEMISTRY AND TRANSPORT

Introduction

In any study of how Li^+ may affect mammalian cells, it is useful to compare the properties of Li^+ with those of the four cations most abundant in cells: Na^+, K^+, Ca^{2+}, and Mg^{2+}. The physiochemical properties of Li^+—its size, charge, charge density, and energy of hydration—group it with these four cations, and the properties of all five cations overlap to such an extent that in several model systems most of them can mimic and/or compete with one another. Evidence discussed here indicates that Li^+ interacts with a number of cellular systems recognizing Ca^{2+}, Na^+, Mg^{2+}, or K^+. In addition, Li^+ may be capable of affecting cellular systems that normally interact with functional ammonium groups of the biogenic amines and related compounds.

This section focuses specifically on the variety of molecular systems that Li^+ may influence as well as on the manner in which Li^+ may produce its effects. There are several cellular sites where Li^+-cation interactions may take place: (1) Li^+ may affect cellular carriers or receptors (protein or otherwise) that normally bind other Group I and II cations. In order to understand the nature of the interaction between cations and receptors or carriers, the most important factor must be the balance between a cation's energy of hydration and the energy of the complex when the cation binds to the receptor/carrier. (2) Li^+ may affect cellular proteins, whether enzymatic, structural, or regulatory. Because many protein functions are sensitive to, or dependent on, local variations in Na^+, K^+, Ca^{2+}, or Mg^{2+} concentrations, it seems likely that Li^+ may also alter protein function. In this case, the most likely mode of action is by an alteration in a protein's conformational state. (3) Li^+ may occupy sites normally sensitive to changes in concentration of some other cation. By competing effectively for Ca^{2+}-binding sites, for example, Li^+ might enhance or suppress calcium-dependent cyclic adenosine monophosphate (cAMP) generation or exocytotic release of stored compounds. (4) Li^+ may affect the ion-carrying channels of cell membranes. Here the size of the channel's pore and the nature of its cation-binding groups seem to be most critical in determining how Li^+ may act to alter cellular function.

Design of Synthetic Receptor and Carrier Molecules
for the Li$^+$ Cation: J.-M. Lehn

One approach to examining the binding and/or transport of various cations is to design different chemical structures that behave as cation receptors or carriers. A receptor for a given cation is a molecule that specifically binds that cation with high stability, high selectivity, and slow exchange rates. A cation carrier may be defined as a molecule that can transport cations between two aqueous phases separated by a barrier (usually lipid or a hydrophobic solvent) through which the cations will normally not pass. A carrier should display high selectivity for a given cation but also fast enough exchange rates (fast release of the cation) while retaining sufficient stability (sufficient extraction of the cation into the membrane). The design of a specific cation carrier thus requires a compromise between thermodynamics (stability) and kinetics of complexation as well as sufficient lipophilicity to ensure solubility in the membrane phase. A series of molecules that can serve as cation receptors or carriers can be constructed as macropolycyclic polyethers containing oxygen and nitrogen binding sites arranged in a 2- or 3-dimensional array (Lehn, 1973). Such molecules are able to form inclusion complexes in which the cation is contained in the central molecular cavity (i.e., cryptate complexes: Lehn et al., 1970; Cheney and Lehn, 1972; Cheney et al., 1972; Dietrich et al., 1973b,c; Lehn, 1973; Lehn et al., 1973a,b). By studying the selectivity and affinity of such ethers for Li$^+$ and other Group I and II cations, we can obtain some clues about how these cations may interact with structures serving as receptors and/or carriers for cells.

Characteristics of a Lithium Receptor

Ideally a selective Li$^+$ receptor should have a cavity approximately 0.8 A in radius in which the ion could fit, surrounded by binding sites that could form strong bonds with Li$^+$ (and thus substitute themselves for the cation's water of hydration). A cavity of this size would be able to contain Li$^+$ but would exclude all other alkali and alkaline earth cations except Mg^{2+}.

In order to make the receptor favor Li$^+$ over Mg^{2+}, the binding sites should be electrically neutral. Charged binding sites would bind divalent cations more strongly than monovalent ones, because the divalents have a higher charge density (i.e., the same ionic radius but a higher charge, so that the charge distributed over the surface of the ion produces a higher average charge per unit area). Electrically neutral ether oxygens (or nitrogens), for example those present in the compounds described here, provide neutral, dipolar cation-binding sites with the appropriate selectivity to favor binding Li^+ over Mg^{2+}.

In a general way, when one actually attempts to synthesize compounds that will favor monovalent over divalent cations, or that will specifically favor Li^+ over other cations, one encounters the problem of constructing a molecule with a high degree of selective bonding of monovalents in the presence of appreciable concentrations of divalent cations. Because divalent cations have a higher charge density than monovalent cations, the divalents have a higher energy of hydration. Thus, in energetic terms, it takes more or stronger receptor binding sites to pull divalents away from their water of hydration than to pull away monovalents. This fact means that certain alterations of the basic structure of the molecule can make monovalent-over-divalent selectivity possible (Figure 8).

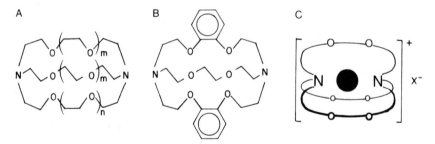

Figure 8. Structure of cation ligands of macrobicyclic type. These molecules contain an internal cavity into which metal cations may be taken up, forming cation inclusion complexes termed "cryptates." A. Generalized structure of which known cases are: *Ligand 1:* m = 0, n = 1; *2:* m = 1, n = 0; *3:* m = n = 1; *4:* n = 1, 2nd bridge: m = 0, 3rd bridge: $-(CH_2)_5-$; *5:* m = 1, 3rd bridge: $-(CH_2)_5-$; *6:* m = 1, 3rd bridge: $-(CH_2)_8-$. B. *Ligand 7,* related to *ligand 3.* C. A schematic representation of a cryptate-type inclusion complex in the case of *ligand 3* (X^- is the anion accompanying the complexed cation and located outside the complex). [Lehn]

One can achieve this type of selectivity (Lehn, 1973; Dietrich et al., 1973a) by (1) making the ligand very thick so that a thick layer or "skin" of organic groups envelops the cation and pushes away the polar molecules of the surrounding water medium; this results in a decrease of interaction between the cation and the water outside the ligand shell ("Born effect"), i.e., the stability of the complexes decreases as the "skin" gets thicker; the decrease is four times larger for doubly charged cations than for singly charged ones and thus destabilizes alkaline earth much more than alkali cation complexes; (2) removing receptor binding sites while keeping the cation entirely wrapped in the organic ligand; this also should decrease the stability of the bivalent much more than that of the monovalent complexes; (3) avoiding anionic binding sites (see also above).

This is illustrated by the fact that whereas ligand 3 (Figure 8) has K^+/Ba^{2+} selectivity of about 0.01, ligand 7 has $K^+/Ba^{2+} \sim 1$ (effect a), and ligand 6 has $K^+/Ba^{2+} > 200$ (effect b) (Dietrich et al., 1973a; Lehn, 1973; Lehn and Sauvage, 1976).

In the case of Li^+ itself these effects (a) and (b) can be used, too. However, it is sufficient to avoid charged binding sites and use only neutral ones as mentioned above. Thus, ligand $1,$ which contains an intramolecular cavity of appropriate size (about 0.8 A), is not only a highly stable Li^+ receptor (stability constant of about 10^5 in water and 5.10^7 in methanol), but it also has high Li^+/Mg^{2+} selectivity (about 1000) (Lehn and Sauvage, 1976).

Characteristics of a Lithium Carrier

In order to construct a molecule with good carrier properties for monovalents or Li^+, a different set of constraints must be met. Although the molecule must show a selective affinity for monovalents (in order to bind them at one aqueous interface), the molecule-monovalent complex must be sufficiently unstable to permit fast release at the aqueous interface on the other side of the hydrophobic barrier.

Knowing the size and charge of Li^+, one can derive an estimate of the stability of the Li-molecule complex necessary to make the molecule a good carrier for Li^+. Although ligand 1 is a good receptor for Li^+, the complex is too stable, and the exchange rate of Li^+ is too slow to make it a good Li^+ carrier.

Ligand $2,$ which has a cavity too large for Li^+, forms a less stable Li^+ complex than 1 and has fast Li^+ exchange rates (Lehn and Sauvage, 1975). Ligand 2 does indeed carry Li^+ efficiently through a bulk liquid membrane (a chloroform layer binding two water layers). It is, however, "poisoned" by both Na^+ and Ca^{2+}, which form very stable complexes with 2 (Kirch and Lehn, 1975).

The transformation of the Li^+, Na^+, K^+ receptors, *1*, *2*, and *3* respectively, into selective carriers of the same cations, can be achieved by a simple structural change: replacing one or two oxygen binding sites by CH_2 groups, i.e., *1* → *4*, *2* → *5*, *3* → *6* (Kirch and Lehn, 1975). Ligands *4*, *5*, *6* still complex Li^+, Na^+, K^+, respectively, but much less strongly than *1*, *2*, and *3*, and the cation exchange rates are much faster. Furthermore, whereas *2* and *3* are poisoned by alkaline-earth cations, the three ligands *4*, *5*, *6* complex these cations less than their preferred alkali cation. In other words, *4*, *5*, and *6* are efficient carriers of alkali cations and are little affected by the presence of Mg^{2+}, Ca^{2+}, Sr^{2+}, Ba^{2+}. In a typical experimental setup, the relative transport rates through a liquid ($CHCl_3$) membrane are given in Table 5 (Kirch and Lehn, 1975). It is seen that compound *4* is an efficient Li^+ carrier. It also transports Na^+ well. If a high Li^+/Na^+ selectivity is desired, further structural modification of *4* is required.

TABLE 5

Relative Transport Rates Through a $CHCl_3$
Membrane [Kirch and Lehn, 1975]

Carrier	Li^+	Na^+	K^+
4	1	1.8	--
5	0.03	3.5	--
6	--	1.6	3.6

Conclusion

Because the molecular mechanism of the neurobiological effects of the lithium cation is far from clear, the design of specific lithium receptors and carriers should be of help in its elucidation. The antipsychotic effects of Li^+ could be due to its action on an altered CNS receptor or carrier, which would normally function with a "biological" cation (Na^+, K^+, Mg^{2+}, Ca^{2+}) and react to Li^+ in the pathological state (see below "Possible Mechanisms of Action of Lithium from the Perspective of 'Receptor'-Li^+ Interaction"). Then, synthetic molecules that interact with Li^+ may have a double interest: (1) Li^+ receptors, strongly complexing Li^+ and removing it, may allow controlling Li^+ levels (and eventually producing Li^+ deprivation, if this is of any use). Their design (especially when of peptidic nature) might also give insight into the type of structure the altered CNS receptor might have. (2) Li^+ carriers, facilitating the flow of Li^+ through membranes, might be of pharmacological use in efficiently transferring the cations to an altered CNS receptor or in supplementing and amplifying the function of an altered CNS carrier.

In view of the complexity of the action mechanism as well as of the problems of testing and discerning the effects produced (not to mention the possible toxicity of the synthetic substance), there certainly is still a long way from the chemistry of Li^+ receptors and carriers to their neurobiology. Although chemical investigations approach the problem in a way very different from that of clinical observations, they may, nevertheless, help us to understand the molecular events involved in the neurobiological effects of lithium.

Ion Complexing with Natural and Synthetic Peptides: E.R. Blout

It has been possible to construct some specific cyclic peptides showing cation-binding properties. These compounds may be relevant to the study of biological systems, since living cells presumably use proteins as ionophores and ion carriers and receptors, and since these ionophores have been constructed with naturally occurring amino acids. The use of these peptides allows the study of conformational changes following the binding of certain cations, because the circular dichroism and NMR properties of the peptides and the peptide:ion complexes can be examined in solution.

The class of cyclic peptides being discussed possesses the general formula cyclo-(Pro-Gly)$_n$, using L-proline and glycine, where n = 2 through 5. Incorporation of proline residues serves to restrict the number of possible conformational states.

The peptide n = 2 is a rigid, asymmetric structure with no central cavity and hence no ion-complexing properties. Peptides n = 3, 4, and 5 do have central cavities and will complex a variety of cations. For the peptide n = 3, freedom of rotation is somewhat restricted but will vary depending on the nature of the solvent. Although the molecule is asymmetrical in water, it becomes symmetrical as it binds alkali monovalent ions. A diagram of (Pro-Gly)$_3$ is shown in Figure 9. Some binding constants for alkali and alkaline earth ions to this cyclic

TABLE 6

Cation Binding Constants for
cyclo-(Pro-Gly)$_3$ [Blout]

Ion*	K (M^{-1})
Li$^+$	1.8 × 10^2
Na$^+$	1.1 × 10^2
K$^+$	2.9 × 10^1
Ca^{2+}	1.4 × 10^3
Ba^{2+}	4.2 × 10^2

Solvent: 80% MeOH/20% water.
*Anion was perchlorate.
[*cyclo*-(Pro-Gly)$_3$] = 4.50 × 10^{-5} M.

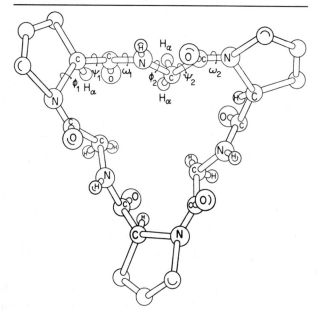

Figure 9. Diagrammatic representation of *cyclo*(Pro-Gly)$_3$. Pro (ϕ_1, ψ_1, ω_1) and Gly (ϕ_2, ψ_2, ω_2) residue rotation angles are indicated. [Deber et al., 1972]

peptide in aqueous and organic solvents are shown in Tables 6 and 7. As a receptor for Li$^+$, this compound has two drawbacks: Its selectivity for Li$^+$ over other monovalents is not great, and divalent cations are the preferred ligands.

TABLE 7

Binding Constants of Cations to cyclo-(Pro-Gly)$_3$ [Blout]

Cation*	Solvent	K (M^{-1})
Na$^+$	Water	2.2 ± 0.4
Ca^{2+}	Water	1.3 ± 0.1 × 10^2
Ca^{2+}	Acetonitrile	1.1 ± 0.4 × 10^5
Mg^{2+}	Acetonitrile	1.0 ± 0.6 × 10^5 (K$_1$)
		6.4 ± 1.8 × 10^2 (K$_2$)

*The anion was perchlorate.

The peptides n = 4 and n = 5 have larger central cavities (4 A and 6 A, respectively). They show even lower specificity toward Li$^+$, however.

Generally, these cyclic polypeptides can bind ions as a 1:1 complex of ion with polypeptide, as a "peptide sandwich" (2:1 complex), or as an "ion sandwich" (a 1:2 complex). The class of compounds has a wide range of binding constants for different cations but usually shows stability constants of the same order of magnitude for Li$^+$ and Na$^+$. Binding affinity for cations is increased in apolar solvents, suggesting that the compounds might serve as membrane-intercalated ionophores or receptors.

It is also of interest that the amino groups of amino acids or biogenic amines can be complexed by these cyclic polypeptides (the ammonium group fits into the central cavity). Some molecules can, for example, differentiate between D- and L-amino acid salts.

Kinetics of "Receptor"-Li$^+$ Interaction: R. Winkler

It seems reasonable to postulate that there exists a biological compound that can act as a receptor for Li$^+$. Given the nature of the Li$^+$ ion, we can make certain deductions about the mechanism and kinetics of the receptor-Li$^+$ interaction from model studies using antibiotics, which specifically interact with metal ions.

It is certainly true that the Li$^+$ ion is much less frequently involved in biochemical processes than its competitors, Na$^+$ and K$^+$. Chemically Li$^+$ belongs to the first main group of the periodic table, the alkali metals. The ions possess a noble-gas-like electron shell, which means that alkali cations behave quite indifferently towards ligands. In regard to ionic radii, the largest relative change clearly occurs between Li^+ and Na^+.

Li^+, the smallest among the alkali ions, has the highest electric field density at its surface, which corresponds to the largest energy of interaction with any ligand, as expressed in the free energy of hydration. It takes 122 kcal/mole to strip off all 6 H_2O molecules in the inner coordination sphere of the Li^+ cation. Nevertheless, the rate for the substitution of one single H_2O molecule by a ligand is very high, the rate constant of substitution being in the order of magnitude of 10^9 per sec. The fast exchange indicates a small activation energy for the substitution of the last H_2O molecule in an almost completed shell. This is due to the negative charges of the H_2O dipoles, which compensate for the metal ion charge very effectively, so that the last H_2O molecule can get off as easily for Li^+ as for Na^+, K^+, Rb^+, and Cs^+ (and also for Ca^{2+}, but not for Mg^{2+}). This fact will turn out to be of great importance in explaining the very fast substitution of the total coordination shell in chelate-forming complexes.

Since there is no specific chemistry distinguishing Li^+ from the more common alkali metal ions, one may draw the following conclusions:

1. There must exist a specific acceptor, which preferentially binds Li^+ and distinguishes it clearly from Na^+ and K^+.

2. The acceptor must exhibit a very favorable interaction with the Li^+ ion in order to compete with the binding of solvent molecules.

3. The acceptor must be of a chelate type, which means it must replace several of the solvent molecules from the inner coordination shell of the Li^+ ion. Only in this way can it gain sufficient specificity and distinguish Li^+ from Na^+ and the other alkali cations.

4. In order to bind Li^+ the chelate acceptor must be able to form a cavity, the dimensions of which are optimally adapted to the size of the unsolvated Li^+ ion.

Although the strength of binding between the acceptor and Li^+ is determined solely by the difference of the ligand and solvent binding energy, size is finally the only source for selective behavior.

Most of the dynamic studies have been carried out with antibiotics forming complexes with Na^+ and K^+. But conclusions with respect to discrimination of ions hold for Na^+ versus Li^+ as well. The model studies tell us about the magnitude of the rate and equilibrium

TABLE 8A

Stability and Rate Constants for Alkali Metal Ions
Forming Complexes with Murexide [Winkler]

Ion	k_{form} [$M^{-1} \times sec^{-1}$]	k_{diss} [sec^{-1}]	K_{stab} [M^{-1}]
Li^+	5.5×10^9	7.7×10^6	7.1×10^2
Na^+	1.5×10^{10}	5.9×10^6	2.6×10^3
K^+	$\sim 2.0 \times 10^{10}$ *	$\geq 10^7$	1.1×10^3

Solvent: methanol at 25°C.
*diffusion controlled..

TABLE 8B

Typical Example of Specificity of Alkali Ion Binding
Expressed in Rate and Stability Constants [Winkler]

	K_{stab} [M^{-1}]	k_{form} [$M^{-1} sec^{-1}$]	k_{diss} [sec^{-1}]
Na^+ with valinomycin	4.7	1.2×10^7	2.0×10^6
K^+ with valinomycin	3.0×10^4	3.5×10^7	1.3×10^3

Solvent: methanol at 25°C.

values generally to be expected for Li^+. Some characteristic data are summarized in Tables 8A and 8B.

The relatively high rate of complex formation immediately raises the question of what type of mechanism can account for the fact that all solvent molecules in the inner coordination shell of the metal ion are substituted by a multidentate ligand with such a high rate. Due to the relatively high energy of solvation, the removal of all solvent molecules prior to the entry of the ion into the cavity of the receptor would represent a quite slow process.

A more favorable energetic situation would apply if solvent molecules were gradually (i.e., in steps) replaced by receptor ligands. As this substitution occurs, the receptor would change conformation, shrinking down to a more compact structure as the ligands were drawn forward toward the metal ion in the central cavity. A nonflexible receptor, which could not "breathe" (expand and contract) as metal ions were drawn into and pushed out of the cavity, would show much lower rates of complex formation.

While we can understand how specificity could come about, we must also ask what phenomena could be triggered by the specific binding of Li$^+$. Equilibrium binding studies that refer to the final state of complexation will not tell us anything about the mechanism, but dynamic investigations do.

Let us assume that the specific binding site for Li$^+$ is some receptor sitting at a membrane. It will have to trigger some signal upon combination with Li$^+$. From what is known about receptors in other systems, it will most probably be a conformational change, which in turn affects the membrane structure and thus provides a signal to any suitable membrane-bound chemical process.

Possible Mechanisms of Action of Lithium from the Perspective of "Receptor"-Li$^+$ Interaction: M. Eigen

As noted previously, one can reasonably postulate that Li$^+$ must interact with specific "receptors" to produce its antipsychotic effects. Such a construct requires that (1) specific receptors exist, (2) the receptors specifically bind Li$^+$ in the presence of other cations known to exist in biological tissue in appreciable concentrations, and (3) binding of Li$^+$ to the receptor affects certain cells such that the psychotic process is suppressed.

Since the postulated cellular receptor must operate in an aqueous environment, it must form a complex of the chelate type with Li$^+$, in which the chelating groups in the receptor displace the water molecules in the ion's coordination shell. This places some constraints on the receptor, because its ligands must compete effectively with the water molecules. The *stability* of the receptor-ion complex is determined by the relative magnitudes of free energy of the complex as compared to the free energy of hydration of Li$^+$. The balance between these two free energies determines whether the receptor-ion complex will form or not.

In addition, the hypothetical Li$^+$ receptor must show *specificity*, a property determined by the size of the ion-containing cavity. The cavity in a Li$^+$ receptor would have a lower size limit of 0.8 A (corresponding to the radius of the metal ion). It should not have, on the other hand, a much larger size, because then ligands at the binding site could not favorably compete with the water molecules; and if water molecules are not substituted the interaction will not be sufficiently specific (as is shown in Winkler's work on antibiotics, see "Kinetics of 'Receptor'-Li^+ Interaction" above). The balance between the solvation and bonding energies noted above would thus determine the size of the cavity within quite narrow limits.

Given such a receptor system, differences in the stability constants for various metal cations may involve factors as large as 10^3 to 10^5, corresponding to something like 4 to 7 kcal/mole difference in bonding energies. Thus, such a receptor could indeed distinguish between Li^+ and such prevalent cations as extracellular Na^+ (100 mM) or intracellular K^+ (100 mM), provided that the concentration difference for Li^+ is only 10^2 (as in the therapeutic treatment). A priori, since large differences in concentration exist between Li^+ and other cations, any receptor sensitive to Li^+ must be capable of differentiating between cations at similar orders of magnitude, regardless of whether the receptor is defective or not.

Given such a receptor, Li^+ as used clinically could work its effects in a variety of ways:

1. Li^+ could be the effector ion in an unperturbed (normal) receptor system. This is unlikely, because Li^+ levels in normal people are at least 10^6 lower than those of Na^+ (extracellular) or K^+ (intracellular). Such a receptor would have a degree of specificity and stability for Li^+ probably higher than is possible in terms of free energy (see above). In this model, manic-depressive illness would lower the binding constant for Li^+, so that adding Li^+ would restore the system to normal. The 10^3-fold increase in serum Li^+, for example, might compensate for a 10^3-fold decrease in receptor specificity or stability.

2. Li^+ could be the effector in an unperturbed (normal) transport system. This model is also unlikely because of the constraints noted above.

3. Li^+ is not an effector in normal systems, but repairs a defect unique to manic-depressive illness.

a. The defect in the illness could be a substrate lack (ions of a certain *size* needed). It is true that ions such as Mg^{2+}, having the same ionic radius as Li^+, are not markedly deficient in manic patients; however, what might be significant is local concentration rather than the total concentration of ions.

b. The defect in the illness could be some alteration of a CNS receptor or carrier (due to a genetic defect). In this model, the active site of a protein could be altered so that its affinity for Ca^{2+}, Mg^{2+}, Na^+, or some amine was changed. Such an alteration would probably result in a changed cavity size, making it unsuited for carrying its normal ion substrate. The natural competitor would fit in the cavity, however, and hence if supplied could "fill" the defect. Such a model is reasonable.*

In regard to the therapeutic effects of lithium, it has been demonstrated that the disease symptoms are suppressed when there is still a 30-fold to 100-fold excess of intracellular concentrations of sodium over lithium. Since biological "receptors" can possess sufficient specificity to discriminate between the two ions at these orders of magnitude, it seems reasonable to assume that the lithium could be correcting some preexisting deficit. We can assume that Li^+ does compete effectively with Na^+ for any particular site (or set of sites), because the former and not the latter corrects whatever defect exists. The Li^+ could either (1) replace "some" ion which is not available where needed to permit normal functioning or (2) bind to a "receptor" (which has been changed by the illness to allow this binding) and permit it to function normally. If manic-depressives possess a defective, Li-correctable "receptor," the receptor-lithium interaction would need to be studied in manic-depressive subjects. Studies in normal situations could show only how the sequelae of receptor alteration can be minimized.

If manic-depressives lack "some" ion that is replaced by Li^+, one must ask which is the ion most likely to be replaced. Good candidates include Mg^{2+} (equal size to Li^+), Na^+ (equal charge to Li^+), or Ca^{2+} (size and charge larger than for Li^+, but interaction energy for ion-dipole interaction very similar to Li^+). Some sort of calcium-lithium interaction or competition seems quite likely, based both on much of the data presented here and on classical physicochemical considerations (energetics of dipole-ion interactions). Another promising possibility is that Li^+ may interact in some fashion with a receptor or carrier that normally binds or transports a biogenic amine but exists in an altered state in manic-depressive illness. This seems likely because both Ca^{2+} and Li^+ (as well as other ions, of course) have the potential for influencing the configuration of amine-carrying "holes" in carriers and receptors. Future research could profitably be directed toward investigating more critically the possibilities for just these types of interaction.

*A similar model has been proposed by Bunney et al., 1972a.

Ion Complexing with Proteins and Other Macromolecules:
R.J.P. Williams

No specific Li-binding protein is known, and therefore this section of the report on the effects of lithium on cellular proteins must be speculative. Again, there is little or no information on Na^+-, K^+-, or Mg^{2+}-binding proteins, and so we shall first focus on the calcium-binding proteins, about which much is known. This may well be very relevant to the action of lithium and may further afford us some appreciation of the selectivity of the binding between proteins and metal cations of the A-subgroup elements of the periodic table.

Calcium-Binding Proteins

Table 9 gives some details of the nature of the binding sites of calcium proteins. The binding ligands are all oxygen atoms appearing in carboxylate or carbonyl centers. Though not quantitatively related, the strength of binding is clearly somewhat dependent upon the number of carboxylate centers. The most stable complexes are found at protein sites presenting a cluster of four carboxylate residues. Even at such a site, the binding strength can be regulated by the actual structure (length and angle of the bonds formed with the metal cation). These bond lengths and angles are controlled by the balance between best conditions for the ligand-cation bonds and best internal energies of the protein in the presence of calcium. An optimum energy situation results. The relative positions of, say, the four carboxylate groups can

TABLE 9

Ca^{2+} Protein Binding [Williams]

Protein	Coordination number	log K*	No. of $-CO_2^-$	Reference
Parvalbumin	(a) 6 ? $+H_2O$	>7	4	Moews and Kretsinger,
	(b) 8	$\geqslant$7	4	1975
Thermolysin	6 - 8	~3	2 - 3	Edelman et al., 1972
Nuclease	6 ? $+H_2O$)	~4	3	Cotton et al., 1971
Concanavalin-A	6 ?	2 - 3	2	Matthews et al., 1974
Lysozyme	(?)	<2	1 - 2	Campbell et al., 1975

*K = binding constant for calcium.

be seen to affect the stability of a given element, here calcium, in a site cavity; but these positions are much more important in the adjustment of the relative binding power of that site for different cations. We approach the problem of the binding to proteins by looking first at the differences between the various metal cations. The extent to which cations are bound at a specific biochemical site depends, of course, not only on their charge and structural properties but also on their free concentrations in the compartment of a cell under discussion.

Structures

In each A-subgroup of the periodic table, cation size increases with atomic number. On a simple electrostatic view, all properties would be a simple function of size. This is true only to a limited extent. For example, the number of water molecules around a cation certainly increases down a group, e.g., from Be(4), to Mg(6), and Ca(8). Furthermore, structural studies show that in nearly all its compounds beryllium maintains a strict tetrahedron, magnesium maintains a strict octahedron, and that in both these cases respective bond lengths are always constant within close limits. However, there is no clear statement that can be made about calcium geometry. In fact, it appears that calcium accommodates to the demands of its surround much more readily than does either beryllium or magnesium. Protein sites must compete for metal cations with water, a monodentate ligand that adjusts readily to the demands of the central binding cation. A protein will not do this. The size and adjustability of Ca^{2+} permit it to shed its water and bind to irregularly placed protein anions, but magnesium does so only to a much smaller extent. Models illustrate this feature. Ethylene diaminetetraacetate (EDTA) binds calcium and magnesium equally well to its four carboxylate residues. In the ligand bis-ethylene-glycol diaminetetraacetate (EGTA), the four carboxylate groups are placed much further apart. From EDTA to EGTA, the stability of the magnesium complex drops by 10^4, while that of calcium is not affected. In the stability of model complexes, steric consideration are overwhelmingly important and must be dominant in selective protein-to-metal-ion binding.

Free Ion Concentration

Of course, binding depends upon free ion concentration. Some steady-state concentrations of cations in biological compartments are shown in Table 10. The importance of these observations

TABLE 10

Cation Concentrations Inside and Outside
Human Cells [Williams]

Ion	Concentration inside cell	Concentration outside cell
Li^+	1 - 5 mM	(highest drug dose) 1 - 5 mM
Na^+	5 - 10 mM	100 mM
Mg^{2+}	5 - 10 mM	3 mM
K^+	100 mM	10 mM
Ca^{2+}	less than 10^{-7} M	5 mM

emerges as we now examine the binding of multicarboxylate centers to calcium.

The first example of such groupings in intracellular calcium-binding proteins is that of the carp intracellular albumin. This has a binding constant for Ca^{2+} of $\sim 10^7$, which high affinity is necessary for the protein to bind Ca^{2+} effectively when the intracellular Ca^{2+} concentration is only 10^{-7} M. To achieve its specificity for Ca^{2+} despite the presence of intracellular Mg^{2+} levels $\sim 10^5$ times higher (5 to 10 mM), this protein utilizes a four-carboxylate-group chelating system of the correct size to "wrap around" the large Ca^{2+} ion but not to fit around the Mg^{2+} ion (see Table 9). Troponin, an intracellular calcium-binding protein, also contains such chelating carboxylate groups. Although this protein will not bind Ca^{2+} intracellularly when free Ca^{2+} ion levels approach 10^{-7} M, it will bind Ca^{2+} if intracellular free Ca^{2+} is raised to 10^{-6} M. Thus when muscle is "triggered" by the influx or release of Ca^{2+}, troponin can act to bind the added Ca^{2+}. The binding-site strengths and selectivities are nicely adjusted to a biological requirement for control over ion concentrations.

Lithium Binding

Although lithium has approximately the same size as magnesium, a surface potential somewhat similar to calcium, and the same charge as sodium, structurally it does not behave quite like any of these cations. Unlike magnesium but like calcium, lithium has a rather poorly defined coordination number and site geometry; but unlike calcium, the site geometry of lithium is based on a coordination number *lower* than the 6 of magnesium, but not so high as the 6 to 9 of calcium. Sodium ions are 6 coordinate or more. The principles outlined by Lehn, Eisenman, and Williams in this report imply that lithium can bind relatively selectively to a given center and, given a subtle choice of geometry at the site of binding, could bind more strongly than any of the other three cations. Again, an ionic model without polarization energies ("covalence" if you will) is insufficient to explain the difference of calcium from lithium and magnesium, for these two cations bind to nitrogen donors more strongly than calcium even when oxygen ligands like water are present in excess. In addition to binding-site size and stereochemistry discrimination, there can thus be ligand-type discrimination in favor of lithium. Again the ability of lithium to form tetrahedral coordination spheres gives its hydrate a size very like that of tetramethyl ammonium. Thus lithium could go into a binding site that normally bound, say, the choline head-group. In the context of the concentrations of Table 10, let us now look at lithium competition at the calcium-binding sites because these are the sites about which we know most.

In general, of all the monovalent cations only Li^+ could effectively compete for divalent (Ca^{2+}-binding) sites in a system using carboxyl groups as chelators. This holds true despite the rather great charge-density and ionic-radius differences that arise from the stereo-chemical differences between the two cations. Postulate, for example, a cellular protein system with binding constants for Mg^{2+} and Ca^{2+} of 10^2 and 10^6 respectively. Since Mg^{2+} is 10^4 to 10^5 times more concentrated inside the cell than Ca^{2+}, the two divalent cations under normal circumstances compete equally for such binding sites on the hypothetical protein, but the binding will be only very slight (see Table 10). If, however, free intracellular Ca^{2+} is increased by a factor of 10^2 (as in "triggering," for example), Ca^{2+} will bind preferentially to all the protein's ion-sensitive sites and displace any bound Mg^{2+}. Assume the hypothetical protein also has a binding constant for Li^+ of 10^3 (not an unreasonable figure). If, following Li^+ treatment, intra-cellular Li^+ is raised to 10^{-3} M, the Li^+ could compete effectively with Ca^{2+} at the ion-sensitive site. Since Li^+ can adjust its bond lengths more easily than Mg^{2+} (which usually forms 6 coordination bonds, each with a 2.1 A length), it would be capable of displacing even bound Mg^{2+}.

Lithium may compete with calcium in membranes as well as in proteins. High intracellular levels of free Ca^{2+} may stimulate secretion or release of neurotransmitters by serving as "intracellular cement," cross-linking vesicle membranes to the plasma membrane. Because Ca^{2+} can bond to several ligands without regard to symmetry and will accept bond lengths ranging from 2.4 A to 3.0 A, the calcium ion forms no true "coordination sphere" and is an excellent cross-linking agent. Because of the competition at these binding sites, Li^+ could interfere with this cross-linking function, prevent exocytosis, and, in effect, stabilize the vesicular membrane.

Structure and Action

There is also another biologically feasible mechanism by which Li^+ may act through proteins. Proteins exhibit striking conformational changes when they bind cations. Lysozyme, for example, changes its conformation (as indicated by shifts in the NMR spectrum of its tryptophan residues) when La^{3+} is added to its solutions. Other NMR studies indicate that as metals of varying radii are added to lysozyme or even to a simple small molecule (e.g., indole-β-acetic acid), the metal ion in the metal-ligand complex can change position with respect to the indole (tryptophan) ring, as in, for example, Figure 10. In a cellular protein forming a membrane pore, such a positional change could alter the geometry of the pore or channel through the cell membrane. If one position represents a closed and the other an open gate, a metal ion could thus influence the movement of itself and other ions through the membrane.

Action in chemistry or biology depends not just on binding but also demands the correct structures. We have looked first at the control

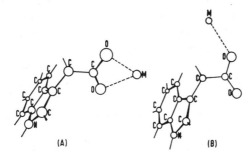

(A)   (B)

Figure 10. The change in the conformation of a complex from (A) to (B), really a movement of the metal ion with respect to the coordinating ligand, can be thought of as a change from a bidentate binding of a carboxylate to a monodentate binding at an ionic radius of ca 0.85 A. In the series Ge^{II}, Sn^{II}, Pb^{II} acetate complexes, the same change from bidentate to monodentate carboxylate coordination occurs at Sn^{II}, radius 1.15 ± 0.05 A. Whatever the cause of this change in structure with change in radius, it could be profoundly important in the case of biological ligands, not so much in terms of the thermodynamics of binding but in its kinetic consequences, see text. [Levine et al., 1974]

of action through binding strengths because binding is a "necessary" condition, but it is not a sufficient condition for action. We may write

$$\text{action} \propto \text{binding x rate constant}$$

where, as above, binding depends upon free-cation concentration and an equilibrium constant. The rate constant is, however, directly dependent upon the exact structure of the bound unit and perhaps on the ability of this structure to undergo precisely required transformations. We have stressed that lithium has pecularities of its own in these structural respects. Thus, while bound like other cations to a center, lithium could generate much more or much less of a specific activity critical to normal or abnormal function. In particular, we might think of the controlling roles of cations in membrane processes. As a possible further example, consider that calcium controls the action of tubulins, and their action assists such processes as exocytosis. The presence of lithium at 100 times the calcium concentration (see Table 10) could lead to some competitive binding, with steric differences producing quite noticeably different overall effects. Lithium/calcium competition for a protein could then be reflected in a host of cellular responses.

    Even the lipids in membranes may generate different or parallel selective actions of lithium and other cations. In general, the "leakiness" of membranes to cations is specific because of the differential energy required to pull off or replace water of hydration around these ions. In addition there exists a variety of biologically feasible schemes that permit *highly selective* (or nonselective) ion permeation. Membranes that are relatively permeable to ions (as in liver cells) may be composed of specific proteins that can act as dipoles and substitute their side-chains for the water of hydration. Some cells also have permeable membranes by virtue of the shorter-chain lipids used as membrane building blocks. (It is known that even lecithin liposomes can be made ion permeable by adding short-chain, less rigid lipids.) It is also possible that unsaturated double bonds (abundant in many brain lipids), or the pi-electron clouds of aromatic rings, can serve as polarizable ligands for certain cations and so facilitate their transport across membranes. Thus we may ask: Are the different membranes of different cells and organelles very differently sensitive specifically to lithium? Change of permeability could have a gross effect on membrane potentials.

The problem in biology is complicated by the fact that *multiple* interactions between cations are probably involved in cellular function; the relative steady-state "balance" between Na, K, Mg, and Ca (and however Li may affect these) probably governs how a system will behave at any one time. Thus, the only real hope for the inorganic chemist to contribute further lies in finding a biological system that retains Li^+ better than other cations. Rather than studying artificial molecules, then, one would search for natural Li-binding substances, perhaps by looking in bacteria or plants living in lithium-rich soil for a lithium-binding protein. There are two species of plants, *Ranunculae* and *Solanaceae,* that are known to have a high lithium content (Hewitt and Smith, 1974, p. 102). The physical chemist can help by examining what sort of known biological configurations might be capable of interacting with lithium, and how they do so.

Monovalent Cation Activation of Enzymes:
C.H. Suelter

In order to explore the effect of Li^+ on enzymes as a possible *modus operandi* for determining the therapeutic function of this cation in vivo, let us first examine the general effects of monovalent cations on enzymes and then examine possible mechanisms by which Li^+ might exert its physiological role.

Many enzymes require monovalent cations such as K^+, Na^+, NH_4^+, and Li^+ to express their maximum catalytic activity (Suelter, 1970; Evans and Sorger, 1966). Since all the cations usually activate, but to varying degrees, we will consider the cations as a group and concentrate on the reactions involved and the role of cations in the catalytic process.

Enzymes Activated By Monovalent Cations

Enzymes activated by monovalent cations may be divided into two broad classes: Class K-P and Class K-E (Suelter, 1970). The first class includes enzymes catalyzing phosphoryl transfer to the following functional groups:

$$O \qquad\qquad NH \qquad\qquad CH_2$$
$$\parallel \qquad\qquad \parallel \qquad\qquad\quad \parallel$$
$$-C-O^-, \quad -C-O^-, \text{ and } -C-O^-.$$

Thus, enzymic-catalyzed phosphorylation of carboxyl groups, enamines, and the enol-tautomer of compounds such as pyruvate normally requires monovalent cations to express maximum rate. The second group, Class K-E, includes a broad group of enzymes catalyzing elimination reactions. Included in this group are Class II aldolases, B_{12} enzymes catalyzing C-N or C-O bond cleavage, B_6 enzymes catalyzing α-β elimination reactions, and others too numerous to mention.

Activation of Specific Enzymes

Several purified enzymes requiring monovalent cations to express their maximum catalytic activity have been examined with regard to the mechanism by which monovalent cations activate. Three enzymes exemplifying different elements of activation will be examined.

Pyruvate kinase is essentially inactive in the absence of monovalent cations. The order of effectiveness of the cations with Mg^{2+} as the divalent cation is K^+ (1.00), NH_4^+ (0.81), Rb^+ (0.65), Na^+ (0.08), and Li^+ (0.02) (Kayne, 1971). Activation results from interaction of the cation with the enzyme and not the substrate, as indicated by identical K_a's of activation determined from kinetic data and data from enzyme difference spectra following interaction of cation with the protein (Suelter et al., 1966). The cation is bound within 5 to 8 A of the required divalent cation at the catalytic site (Reuben and Kayne, 1971). This close proximity accounts for the observation that the catalytic activity observed with each monovalent cation is influenced by the nature of the divalent cation (Kayne and Freedman, 1975).

Glycerol dehydrogenase is partially active in the absence of monovalent cations, showing 30% of its maximum observed activity in the presence of the preferred monovalent cation (McGregor et al., 1974). The cation increases the V_{max} and decreases the K_m for glycerol but has little or no effect on the K_m for nicotinamide adenine dinucleotide (NAD). The relative activating efficiency as measured by the maximum velocity is $NH_4^+ > K^+ > Rb^+$. Na^+ and Li^+ have no effect.

In the absence of monovalent cation activator but at saturating substrate concentration, 5'-AMP-aminohydrolase expresses its maximum catalytic activity (Smiley and Suelter, 1967). The effect of monovalent cation is noted only when subsaturating levels of substrate are used in the assay. The activation is affected by a change in the K_m

for 5′-AMP. The activity at subsaturating AMP does depend on the monovalent cation as well as on the source of the enzyme. Further, this is one of the few enzymes maximally activated by Li^+. For example, for rabbit muscle, $K^+ = Na^+ > Li^+ > Rb^+ = NH_4^+$ (Smiley et al., 1967); for rat liver, $Li^+ > Na^+ > K^+$ (Smith and Kizer, 1969); for bovine brain, $Li^+ > Na^+ > K^+ > NH_4^+ = Rb^+ > Cs^+$ (Rhoads, 1970); for human erythrocytes, $K^+ = Li^+ > Na^+$.* The dissociation constants for the cations are not available; 100 mM appears to be saturating in all cases.

In summary, one observes for systems in the absence of cations essentially no activity, partial activity, or complete activity. In general, all cations activate, with K^+, Rb^+, and NH_4^+ being the preferred activator; Li^+ and Na^+ are preferred in certain cases, but there is a limited number of such enzymes. The dissociation constants for these cations as activators (not listed above) range from 1 to 50 mM, depending on the cation and the enzyme. Activation usually involves an increase in V_{max} and a decrease in the K_m for one or more substrates. Sufficient evidence is not available to determine whether the cation binds at the active site and participates in the reaction per se, whether the effects are brought about by binding at sites distant from the catalytic site, or whether both mechanisms operate.

Possible Mechanism for Li⁺ Effect

Consideration of the most basic effect brought about by Li^+ leads one to suggest that the steady administration of this cation as a therapeutic agent would lead to altered steady-state levels of one or more metabolites critical for what we believe to be normal behavior. The question now is "How would Li^+ bring about altered levels of these metabolites?"

The most obvious effect to suggest is that Li^+ competes with other monovalent cations such as Na^+, K^+, or NH_4^+ for sites on an enzyme to alter the rate at which that enzyme processes its substrate. If Li^+ is a poorer activator than the other ions, inhibition will be observed; if Li^+ is a better activator, then additional activation will be observed. These altered rates of metabolism, assuming everything else is equal, should lead to altered steady-state levels of the affected metabolites in the cell. On the other hand, since monovalent cations are involved in (Na, K) ATPase and as a cosubstrate in the transport of

*S.L. Yun and C.H. Suelter, unpublished observations.

certain amino acids (Christensen, 1969), the cation may affect the steady-state levels of a metabolite in a cell by affecting its rate of entry or excretion.

The information available to date indicates that for most enzymes, Li^+ is a poorer activator than Na^+, K^+, or NH_4^+; very few enzymes are preferentially activated by Li^+. The one enzyme known to be preferentially activated by Li^+ is AMP aminohydrolase in brain (Rhoads, 1970) and liver (Smith and Kizer, 1969), although the implications of this observation are unknown. The observation of Dousa and Hechter (1970b) that Li^+ inhibited fluoride-stimulated brain adenyl cyclase has aroused considerable interest. However, as reviewed by Forn (1975), attempts to relate changes in cyclic AMP to mania are controversial.

If the amount of enzyme is rate limiting, then any effect of Li^+ that alters the rate of synthesis or degradation of one or more enzymes will alter the steady-state level of metabolites in a cell. Berg (1968) suggests that Li^+ affects protein synthesis at the transcription level, there being a decrease in DNA-dependent RNA. Other studies of protein synthesis in vitro have generally indicated a decreased protein synthesis when Li^+ is the activator instead of K^+ or NH_4^+ (see S. Johnson's review (1975) for a more detailed discussion of the effects of Li^+ on basic cellular processes).

It should be emphasized that any one single factor may not explain the effects of Li^+, but rather the sum total of all effects may work to alter levels of metabolites. In Suelter's opinion, more information on the effect of Li^+ on specific enzymes and an assessment of altered levels of metabolites and enzymes are needed to explore the therapeutic role of Li^+ more intelligently.

The Molecular Basis for Ion Selectivity and its Possible Bearing on the Neurobiology of Lithium: G. Eisenman

Since we do not understand the molecular basis of the affective disorders, it is hardly surprising that we cannot intuit why Li^+ should have its observed salutary effects. Nevertheless, the striking effects of Li^+ may provide us with a clue to the molecular biology of the disorder itself if we can answer the question: "What is special about Li^+ at the molecular level?" This is a question really of ion selectivity, and the lines along which it appears to be answerable are becoming apparent from selectivity studies on simple ion-complexing molecules such as the peptidelike ion carriers (Eisenman et al., 1973a), which contain the same functional carbonyl groups in their backbone that are likely to constitute the cation permeation pathways of cell membrane proteins and the ion-binding sites of cation-activated enzymes.

Two distinct aspects of Li^+ chemistry immediately stand out in these simple model systems. First, and more obvious, is its possible competitive ability to replace (or antagonize) such monovalent cations as Na^+, K^+, acetylcholine, the neurogenic amines, and, possibly, even H^+. For example, Li^+ is a well-known substitute for Na^+ in the sodium channel of nerve, as well as in the activation of nerve ATPase.

Second, and less obvious, is the possibility that Li^+ might compete for the "receptors" with such divalent cations as Ca^{2+} and Mg^{2+}. Theoretical considerations on model systems suggest that Li^+ should be the most effective monovalent competitor. Li^+ might in this way have a unique capability to interact with monovalent- and divalent-cation-dependent processes at the concentrations at which it is clinically effective. This general possibility has been noted by Schildkraut (1973) who pointed out the well-known chemical resemblance of Li^+ to Mg^{2+} and Ca^{2+} and suggested that some of its effects might strategically be considered as due to an action on various Ca^{2+}- and Mg^{2+}-dependent processes. Direct evidence that such a dual effect of Li^+ can actually occur in biological phenomena is given in the studies of Gardner and Frantz (1974) on ouabain binding to the glycoside binding sites of red blood cells. Not only were the expected specific effects of Li^+ found for the monovalent cation binding site, but Li^+ was observed to be able, uniquely among the group Ia cations, to compete for the divalent binding sites as well. Thus, although it seems that the sites subserving the divalent cation and monovalent cation functions of cells are likely to be distinct (and chemically different) structures, the above experimental data and the theoretical arguments presented below suggest that a possible element of uniqueness in the action of Li^+ might be its ability to interact at physiological concentrations with both monovalent- and divalent-dependent systems. A few concrete examples follow.

The competitive effects of Li^+ in relation to other monovalent cations are illustrated by considering the model (Figure 11) for monovalent cation selectivity (Eisenman, 1961) for singly negatively charged ion exchange sites, which has been generalized to neutral ligands (Eisenman et al., 1973b), including the model carbonyl group

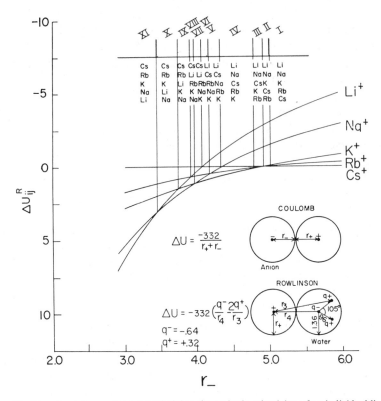

Figure 11. The atomistic asymmetry underlying the cationic selectivity of an individual ligand as illustrated by the hypothetical cation exchange between monopolar anion and a single multipolar water molecule. The radius of the oxygen is 1.4 A, and the values of the partial charges, the bond lengths, and the bond angle of the model water molecule are those proposed by Rowlinson (1951), with the value of partial charge at the oxygen atom, q_n, being -0.64 electron units and that at each of the two hydrogen atoms, $q_p/2$, being $+0.32$ electron units, with the O–H distance being 0.96 A and with the H–O–H angle being 105 degrees. Units in kcal/mole and A in all figures. Above the graph are tabulated the cationic sequences (increasing specificity downwards), corresponding to the eleven rank order designations, which in their particular progression as a function of decreasing radius, r_-, the model anion (increasing anionic field strength) comprises Eisenman's selectivity pattern. [Eisenman, 1961]

(Eisenman and Krasne, 1975) diagrammed in Figure 12. Figure 11 illustrates how, as a function of the anionic radius (more generally, of the "field strength") of a ligand group of the binding site, Li$^+$ can mimic any one of the other group Ia alkali metal cations. Thus the Li$^+$ isotherm can be seen successively to cross the Na, K, Rb, and Cs isotherms, from left to right, simply as a function of changing the radius of a model anionic ligand, which is a crude way of representing what happens when, more realistically, the electron density of such a

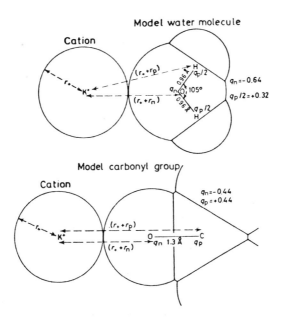

Figure 12. The charge distributions in a model water molecule and in a model carbonyl group. *Top:* a cation in contact with a single water molecule. *Bottom:* in contact with a single carbonyl. Outlines drawn to scale from CPK models (van der Waal's radius of oxygen is 1.4 A). The values of the partial charges, the bond lengths, and the bond angle of the model water molecule are the same as in Figure 11. The C=O bond length of the model carbonyl group, 1.3 A, is that proposed by Pauling (1960); and the value of partial charge at the oxygen atom, q_n, is −0.44 electron units and q_p is +0.44 electron units on the carbon. This value of partial charge was chosen so that the bond length multiplied by the partial charge would produce a dipole moment (2.75 debye) consistent with those observed for typical carbonyl-containing molecules. [Eisenman and Krasne, 1975]

ligand is changed. At the crossover point, where Li^+ intersects Na^+, Li^+ is indistinguishable from Na^+ (at least as far as its binding is concerned, although its effects, such as its mobility or its induction of electronic or molecular conformational changes on the binding molecule itself, might well be different). Presumably, for a site having this "field strength," Li^+ would be capable of mimicking a number of the properties of Na^+. At a somewhat lower "field strength" of the site, corresponding to a larger radius, r_-, the Li^+ isotherm can be seen to cross the K^+ isotherm, and we have here the situation in which Li^+ now can mimic (or compete with) K^+. From Figure 11 it should, therefore, be obvious that the particular effect to be expected of Li^+ is going to be a function of the chemical nature (i.e., "field strength," electron density, or acidity) of the site with which it is interacting, because for a high field strength

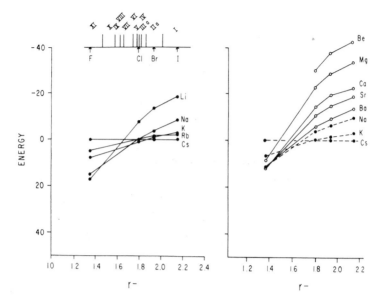

Figure 13. *Left:* Equilibrium selectivities for monovalent cations calculated in terms of free energies by the "thermochemical" method for a completely anhydrous model system having highly coordinated sites and counterions (the alkali halide crystals), but using internal energies as approximations to free energies. *Right:* Equilibrium selectivities for divalent cations for comparison similarly calculated by the "thermochemical" method for a completely anhydrous model system having highly coordinated sites and counterions (the alkali halide and alkaline earth halide crystals). The abscissa represents the anionic radius, r_-, in Ångström units. The ordinate is enthalpy in Kg-cal/g equiv. [Eisenman, 1965]

site it can mimic Na^+ whereas for a lower field strength site it can mimic K^+.

Similar considerations apply among the divalent cations, and between monovalent and divalent cations, as illustrated in Figures 13 and 14. Figure 13 presents the selectivity patterns computed from a "thermochemical" model (Eisenman, 1965) for group Ia cations (on the left) and group IIa cations (on the right). The details of these calculations will be found in the original reference; what is relevant here is that the divalent cations also show changes in their selectivity sequences as a function of the "field strength" of the detecting site and that the selectivities between divalent cations and monovalent cations are also a function of the "field strength" of the site. In addition, there are differences expected depending upon whether or not the competition involves an equivalent exchange of two monovalent cations for one divalent cation (Figure 14, left) or a molar, one-for-one exchange in

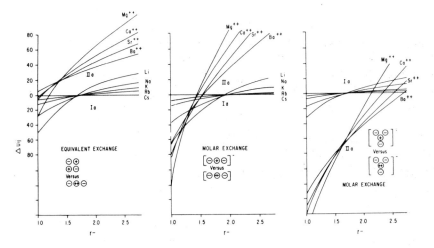

Figure 14. Comparison of an equivalent exchange (*left*) with the molar exchange of a model bidentate chelator (*middle*) and the molar exchange of a model tridentate chelator (*right*). The energies of the indicated configurations were calculated by Coulomb's law, and experimental values for the hydration energies of the cations were used throughout. [Eisenman, 1965]

which electroneutrality is not conserved microscopically, as illustrated in Figure 14 (middle). Monovalent cations are preferred over divalent cations for likely values of field strength in a model system undergoing an equivalent exchange (where one divalent cation exchanges for two monovalent cations, illustrated at the left). However, when the exchange takes place on a molar basis (one monovalent cation for one divalent cation, as illustrated in the center), the preference of monovalent over divalent cations is less pronounced, with divalent cations actually preferred at sites of higher field strength.* The effect of increasing the number of charged ligand groups from two to three is illustrated in Figure 14, at the right. In the case of three negatively charged ligand groups, divalent cations are preferentially selected over almost the entire range of reasonable site field strengths.

Note that in all these model situations, Li^+ is the monovalent cation that most effectively competes with those divalent binding sites that would selectively bind the smaller divalent cations, Mg^{2+} and Ca^{2+}, which is the manifestation in ligand exchange phenomena of the generalization that Li^+ can mimic Ca^{2+} and Mg^{2+} in a number of their classical chemical effects.

*Note that the competition between divalent and monovalent cations is complicated by a concentration dependence of the binding constant when the exchange takes place on an equivalent-for-equivalent rather than a mole-for-mole basis.

A further word about the possible effects of Li^+ on catechol-amine, indolamine, and acetylcholine receptors, releasers, and synthesis is in order. The ion-binding properties of valinomycin and its homologues provide clues to the types of molecular structures that might be involved. Thus, the observations (Eisenman et al., 1976a) on valinomycin- and hexadecavalinomycin-mediated membrane permeabi-lities of Li^+ and a number of substituted ammonium ions given in Figure 15 show that the backbone carbonyl ligands of these molecules, which Eisenman and his associates believe to be representative of polypeptide backbone ligands generally, have appropriate field strengths to interact quite well with a variety of substituted ammonium ions, including primary amines, as well as with the more familiar K^+ and Na^+ ions. Since the ligand groups are identical chemically in valinomycin and hexadecavalinomycin, Figure 15 illustrates the effect on selectivity of a pure variation in the size of the ion binding cavity. Particularly worth noting in regard to Li^+ is the parallelism between its selectivity (and that for Na^+) with the selectivities observed for the hydrazinium and hydroxylammonium cations. Hille (1971) has shown

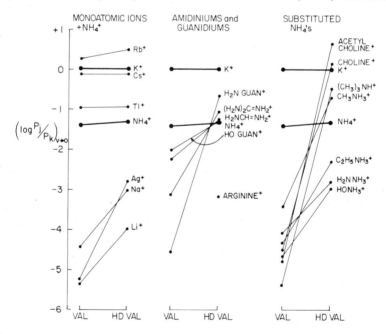

Figure 15. Permeability ratios of valinomycin and hexadecavalinomycin for a variety of monovalent cations in glyceryl dioleate/decane bilayers. [Eisenman et al., 1976a]

these to be the primary amines most similar to Na^+ and Li^+ for the sodium channel of nerve. Figure 15 also illustrates that understanding the selectivity among these various cations requires considerations of "field strength" as well as "fit," but a more detailed discussion would go beyond the scope of this contribution.

It should be pointed out that this discussion has only examined the *equilibrium* aspects of ion selectivity, which is only part of the story (compare Eisenman et al., 1976b) because such phenomena as ion permeation and enzyme activation also involve kinetic ion selectivity (through the rates of loading, unloading, and translocation as well as the velocity of the catalyzed enzyme reaction). This review has therefore been restricted to the affinity aspects of ion permeation and enzyme activation and has not considered the important kinetic effects manifested in "mobilities" of transport or "maximal velocities" of a reaction. Hille (1975a), however, has recently suggested how equilibrium selectivity considerations of the present type could be extended to apply to such kinetic selectivity phenomena by carrying out corresponding calculations for Eyring's "transition state" (Eyring et al., 1949) and has initiated a characterization of the transition state for the sodium channel of the squid axon (Hille, 1975b).

Channels and Ion Transport in Axons and Synapses: B. Hille

In addition to possessing areas that may be nonspecifically permeable to ions, mammalian cells have a variety of devices for effecting and controlling the entry and exit of specific cations (Figure 16). One type of specific permeability device, sometimes linked to the enzymatic hydrolysis of ATP, may be a mobile ionophoric carrier that can move through (or across) the cell membrane carrying one or more cations. Three examples of such devices are the sodium-potassium exchange pump, the calcium pump, and the sodium-calcium exchange device (Baker, 1972; Baker et al., 1969, 1971). A second type of device found primarily in excitable cells, the "channel," has been characterized as a pore extending through the cell membrane (Hille, 1970). The movement of cations through such channels is regulated by a "gating" phenomenon not well understood at present. Cells appear to have channels that are quite ion specific (e.g., the sodium channel, the potassium channel, and the calcium channel).

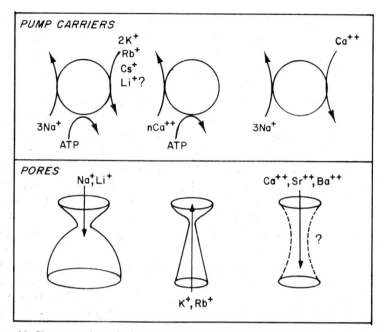

Figure 16. Plasma membrane ionic transport devices that could be affected by low levels of Li^+ ions. *Top:* Pump or carrier mechanisms that move ions against their electrochemical activity gradients. From left to right, the Na-K pumps of all animal cell membranes, the Ca pump, well studied in red blood cells, and the Na-Ca exchange carrier, well studied in excitable cells. *Bottom:* Electrically excitable pores of nerve and muscle membranes. From left to right, the Na channel, the K channel, and the Ca channel. [Hille]

Further, the movement of ions through the channels proceeds at a rate too rapid for a carrier mechanism (10^6 to 10^8 ions/sec, which approaches the theoretical limit of 10^9 ions/sec for a diffusion-mediated process).

Some general points about the nature of the sodium and potassium channels may be useful here, because they provide insight into the way in which cells "design" this type of ion carrier. The sodium channel is a pore with a channel size larger than the radius of a Na^+ ion. It will pass some larger ions like guanidinium (Hille, 1972). The potassium channel appears to be much more selective, and its pore may be smaller (Bezanilla and Armstrong, 1972; Hille, 1973). The selectivity may also be accounted for by lower pK_a's for the negative charges lining the channel, according to the theory of Eisenman (1961). This would produce a weaker negative field strength in the potassium channel than is present in the sodium channel.

It seems doubtful that either channel permits the movement of ions surrounded by their complete "clouds" of hydrating water. Nevertheless, their high turnover numbers indicate that the pore must provide an "aqueous environment" for the naked ions to sit in. Otherwise, the energy required to strip off each ion's water of hydration would be too large to permit such rapid transport. There is at present no direct chemical evidence that oxygen moieties line either channel, but such groups would make useful dipolar or negatively charged sites for "buffering" the positively charged ions as they move through the channels.

Several considerations suggest that ions inside the channels are not completely stripped of all their hydrating water molecules. The potassium channel, for example, appears to have a wide and not very selective opening on the inner side of the cell membrane (Figure 16). It is also quite long (approximately 3/4 the width of the membrane), with a relatively narrow "pore" facing the extracellular medium. Because the channel will accept tetraethylammonium and other ions from inside the cell, it must have a diameter of at least 8 A, large enough to permit a K^+ ion with a full hydration shell to enter. Once inside the channel, however, the K^+ ion probably loses some of its hydrating molecules, and in order to "exit" through the rather narrow pore at the extracellular surface of the membrane, it may be completely stripped (to become fully hydrated once again as soon as it passes through the pore). By stripping off hydrating molecules by degrees, the cell apparently takes advantage of the relatively small energy barriers to each step, as described previously in model systems (Eigen and Winkler, 1970).

How does Li^+ ion affect pores and carriers? The calcium pump and the sodium-calcium exchange device are not known to be strongly influenced by Li^+ ions. At the Na-K pump Li^+ has some K-like actions, suggesting that it may be partially pumped into cells. This suggestion, derived mostly from isolated membrane systems, seems directly at variance with the observations that in patients maintained on Li therapy the intracellular Li concentration in brain does not rise above that in serum, and the disagreement is all the more striking since the negative intracellular potential should concentrate cations even passively (see section above, "Clinical Prophylactic Effects and Clinical Pharmacology of Lithium"). Thus there remains a problem for physiologists.

Lithium ions can substitute for external Na^+ ions at the Na channel and are nearly equally permeant. Intracellular Li^+ does block K channels (Bezanilla and Armstrong, 1972). The Li^+ ion is apparently sucked down the channel by the voltage difference across the membrane. Pushed against the "pore," through which it cannot pass, the Li^+ ion does not have sufficient thermal energy to move itself back up the channel. Although K^+ ions can still enter the channel, they are prevented from approaching the pore by electrostatic repulsion with the Li^+ ion. The Ca^{2+} channel is not known to be affected by Li^+.

It seems clear that Li^+ may affect cell function by interacting with enzymes or ionophoric carriers and receptors of the type described previously (e.g., the ATPase-linked Na^+/K^+ exchange device). It should be borne in mind, however, that the interaction of Li^+ with cell channels may also be of great importance in determining the effects of Li^+ on cells—as illustrated here by the fact that Li^+ can cause blockage of the cell potassium channel.

IV. EFFECTS OF LITHIUM ON CELLULAR FUNCTIONS

Lithium has been demonstrated to interact with many biological systems and to affect cellular functions through alterations in enzyme activities, cell membrane transport, and receptor processes, including cyclic AMP-related events. Although lithium effects on many different cell systems have been studied (for reviews, see Schou, 1957, 1969, 1972, 1975a; Gershon and Shopsin, 1973; Johnson, 1975), only two broad areas are considered here: (1) the interactions of lithium with neurotransmitters at the cellular level, and (2) its involvement with the functions of the thyroid and the kidney.

A variety of evidence suggests that brain catecholamine and indolamine neurotransmitters may be involved in the affective disorders (Bunney and Davis, 1965; Schildkraut and Kety, 1967). Possible contributions of central acetylcholine-related functions to these disorders have also been suggested recently (Janowsky et al., 1972; Vizi et al., 1972). As the therapeutic effects of some antidepressant and neuroleptic drugs seem at least partly explicable on the basis of their interactions with brain neurotransmitter systems, studies of the effects of lithium on neurotransmitter release, re-uptake, metabolism, and receptor effects have been conducted.

While the effects of lithium on tissues other than brain may be less directly relevant to its behavioral and clinical effects, because of the complexity of the brain it is helpful to study simpler systems. The thyroid and the kidney are the organs studied in greatest detail in relation to lithium in animals and man, in part because lithium treatment may be associated with such side effects as goiter/myxedema and polyuria/polydipsia. The interference of lithium with cellular processes in these tissues, whose functions are well known, may provide some hints about its effects on cellular events in the central nervous system.

Effects of Lithium on Catecholamines and Other
Brain Neurotransmitters: D.L. Murphy

Lithium affects brain norepinephrine and dopamine metabolism at a number of sites. It also affects other brain neurotransmitters including serotonin, acetylcholine, and γ-aminobutyric acid (GABA), but there have been only a few studies of the non-amine neurotransmitters. While there is much circumstantial information relating the affective disorders and the effects of drugs used in their treatment to changes in central neurotransmitter function, it is by no means clear how lithium's multiple effects on these systems mediate the behavioral changes.

Catecholamine Neurotransmitter Release and Re-Uptake

Lithium reduces the release of norepinephrine induced by electrical stimulation from both brain tissue and peripheral adrenergic neurons (Katz et al., 1968, 1969; Bindler et al., 1971). Increased calcium concentrations in the perfusing medium reverse these lithium effects on brain slice preparations (Katz et al., 1969). Lithium given chronically also increases the transport of norepinephrine into brain synaptosomal preparations (Colburn et al., 1967; Baldessarini and Yorke, 1970; Kuriyama and Speken, 1970), a saturable, possibly carrier-dependent process that has been shown to require sodium and potassium gradients like other cell membrane transport processes for amino acids and glucose (Murphy and Kopin, 1972). Catecholamine metabolism in brain is shifted by lithium treatment towards the production of relatively more deaminated than O-methylated metabolites, a change compatible with increased intracellular degradation of the amines (Schildkraut et al., 1966, 1969) as would be expected if more neurotransmitter were accumulated and less were released.

Catecholamine Synthesis and Turnover

Studies of catecholamine levels and catecholamine synthesis rates yield a more complex picture than those of release and uptake, with several studies demonstrating reduced brain norepinephrine levels and an increase in the turnover of norepinephrine after both acute or chronic lithium administration (Corrodi et al., 1967; Stern et al., 1969; Greenspan et al., 1970), while other studies of chronic lithium treatment indicate no change in norepinephrine levels or turnover (Ho et al., 1970; Bliss and Ailion, 1970; Schildkraut, 1973). Dopamine levels and turnover do not seem to be affected by acute or chronic lithium administration (Corrodi et al., 1967; Stern et al., 1969; Ho et al., 1970; Bliss and Ailion, 1970; Schildkraut et al., 1969), although dopamine synthesis from ^{3}H-tyrosine was reported to be diminished after chronic (Friedman and Gershon, 1973) but not acute (Persson,

1970) lithium treatment in rats. Several issues may contribute to the variability in these turnover reports, including the small efficacy/toxicity ratio of lithium, probable treatment-time-dependent response differences (as discussed by Mandell below, "Effects of Lithium on Serotonin Synthesis"), and questions of whether the biochemical changes are primary or reflect differences in the neuronal activity in catecholamine pathways—for example, those secondary to behavioral changes induced by lithium through other mechanisms.

Catecholamine Receptor Responses

In addition to the effects of lithium on catecholamine uptake, release, and metabolism, there are some suggestions that lithium might modify adrenergic receptor responses. Reduced pressor responses to infused norepinephrine were observed in patients receiving lithium (Fann et al., 1972) and in anesthetized but not in conscious dogs treated with lithium (Sanghvi et al., 1973). Reductions in norepinephrine-induced phosphorylase a activity and in contractile force responses in the perfused guinea pig heart occurred with acute lithium administration (Frazer et al., 1972); however, in other studies with lithium, no changes in cat nictitating membrane responses to norepinephrine were observed (Sanghvi et al., 1970). Lithium produced an increase in the threshold for intracranial self-stimulation in the rat (Pick and Mills, 1971), a response that is apparently norepinephrine-dependent.

While some of these apparent "receptor" responses may, in fact, be mediated by lithium's effects on catecholamine uptake, release, or metabolism, a specific receptor response to norepinephrine that involves cyclic AMP production has been demonstrated to be affected by lithium. The stimulation of human platelet adenylate cyclase and cyclic AMP production by prostaglandin E_1 is markedly inhibited by norepinephrine. Lithium antagonizes both the norepinephrine and the prostaglandin E_1 responses, with higher concentrations of lithium required in acute, in vitro experiments than in chronic treatment studies (Murphy et al., 1973; Wang et al., 1974). Wang and his co-workers (1974) have shown that the effects of lithium on the cyclic AMP response to prostaglandin E_1 can be reversed by increasing the magnesium concentration in the medium. In brain, elevated cyclic AMP levels have generally been reported to occur in response to beta-receptor and possibly alpha-receptor catecholamine stimuli (Siggins et al., 1969; Chasin et al., 1971; Huang and Daly, 1972). Norepinephrine-prostaglandin E_1 antagonism is also observed, although this relationship is reversed in neuronal tissues, with prostaglandin E_1 inhibiting amine-induced alteration in cyclic AMP (Siggins et al., 1969; Chasin et al., 1971).

A lithium effect on one potential animal model for mania is of some interest because the behavioral changes in this model are thought to be mediated by catecholamines. D-Amphetamine in combination with chlordiazepoxide produces hyperactivity and other behavioral changes in rats. This hyperactivity is blocked by lithium treatment (Davies et al., 1974). Recently, it has been observed that chronic lithium treatment markedly attenuates the activation and euphoriant effects of amphetamine in depressed patients (van Kammen and Murphy, 1975). The close similarity of some of amphetamine's acute behavioral effects to hypomania and the effect of lithium on both spontaneous and amphetamine-induced activity and mood suggest that the lithium-amphetamine interaction may provide an interesting model for further study of lithium's mode of action. Similarly, some observations suggesting that rubidium and cesium may have effects on behavior and neurotransmitter function opposite or antagonistic to lithium (Stolk et al., 1970; Carroll and Sharp, 1971) may aid in the delineation of the mechanisms by which lithium and these other Group I cations act.

Acetylcholine, Glutamate, GABA, and Other Possible Neurotransmitters Affected by Lithium

In some acute in vitro experiments, lithium reduced brain tissue concentrations of GABA, glutamate, glutamine, and aspartic acid (De Feudis and Delgado, 1970; Berl and Clarke, 1972). Chronic lithium treatment, however, was associated with a small increase in glutamate in the amygdala and GABA in the hypothalamus (Gottesfeld et al., 1971).

No apparent effects of chronic lithium treatment were observed on choline or acetylcholine levels in the mouse brain (Krell and Goldberg, 1973). The release of acetylcholine from brain slices of rats chronically treated with lithium was no different from sodium-treated controls (Bowers and Rozitis, 1970). However, under conditions of higher lithium concentrations, especially in vitro, lithium may increase the release of acetylcholine and possibly inhibit its synthesis (Paton et al., 1971; Vizi et al., 1972). The acetylcholine-releasing effect of lithium was prevented by the omission of calcium from the medium, suggesting that calcium influx may mediate the lithium effects (Vizi et al., 1972). Decreased amplitude of cholinergic inhibitory post-synaptic potentials have also been observed with lithium (Waziri, 1968).

Many of these studies of acetylcholine and the amino acid neurotransmitter candidates have been carried out under in vitro or acute treatment situations using high concentrations of lithium, and their relevance to lithium in the clinic or to the cellular effects of lithium observed with lower drug concentrations are not readily interpretable. One exception is a study of a vagus nerve preparation revealing that lithium in concentrations of 1 to 5 mM decreased the conduction velocity of the action potential, possibly by inhibition of the Na-K membrane pump. A greater effect was observed at higher rates of electrical stimulation—an interesting model compatible with lithium's minimal effects on normal activity but modulating effects on hyperactivity (Ploeger, 1974).

Effects of Lithium on Serotonin Synthesis:
A.J. Mandell

In developing an animal model with which to explore the neurochemical mechanisms of action of lithium in relation to its clinical effects, several experimental constraints must be invoked. These include using dosages of lithium that produce blood levels of the drug comparable to those found clinically useful and studying the effect of the drug over time, because its antimanic effects occur within a few days but its prophylactic antidepressant effects require days or months. For the model to be discussed here, which involves a single neurotransmitter system, the serotonergic, there is an additional constraint: whatever the purported interaction between lithium and the neurotransmitter, it must account for both the antimanic and the antidepressant effects of the drug. In view of lithium's symmetrical effects, a unidirectional explanation will not suffice.

To assess the multiple interactions of the serotonin-synthesizing systems in the rat brain, Mandell's group measured four mechanisms simultaneously (Figure 17), and found that the serotonin-synthesizing capacity of the brain was affected by lithium in several sequential steps. As indicated in Figure 18, lithium administration to rats for one to 21 days at doses of 5 to 10 meq/kg/day led to augmentation of

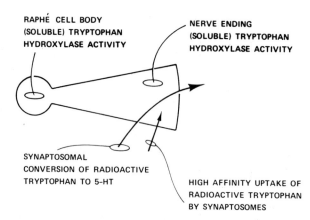

Figure 17. Four measures used in studies of lithium effects on the neuronal 5-HT biosynthetic system. [Mandell and Knapp, 1975b]

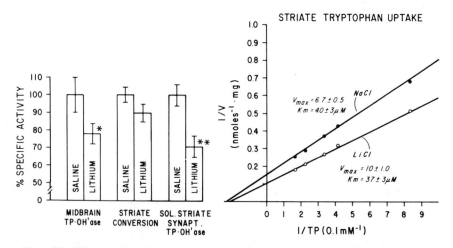

Figure 18. Effects of 21 daily lithium chloride injections on 4 parameters relevant to serotonin synthesis, measured simultaneously. The 3 bar graphs on the left show midbrain tryptophan hydroxylase activity, striate synaptosomal conversion of tryptophan to serotonin, and solubilized synaptosomal enzyme as percentages of their control specific activities, respectively: 574 ± 20, 200 ± 10, and 160 ± 5 pmol/mg/45 min. On the right, high affinity uptake of tryptophan is shown in a double reciprocal Linweaver Burk plot as nanomoles of labeled tryptophan retained/mg protein/4 min. The maximum velocity of the reaction (V_{max}) and Michaelis-Menten constant of the substrate (K_m) $\pm$ S.E.M. were estimated according to the method of Wilkinson (1961). * $p < 0.05$; ** $p < 0.001$. [Knapp and Mandell, 1975]

tryptophan uptake in striate synaptosomes (Knapp and Mandell, 1973, 1975). There are two synaptosomal uptake transport systems for tryptophan (Knapp and Mandell, 1973); lithium's effect was specific only for the high-affinity transport system. Facilitation of substrate uptake was also seen after preincubation of striate synaptosomes with lithium chloride in vitro. Apparently in direct response to the increased tryptophan uptake, an increase in the rate at which radioactive tryptophan is converted to serotonin also occurred during the first several days of lithium treatment.

Increments in tryptophan uptake and in conversion of tryptophan to serotonin were followed during subsequent days of lithium administration by a decrease in soluble tryptophan hydroxylase activity in the midbrain raphe system, the site of the serotonergic cell bodies. This change in enzyme activity was associated with a delayed return of synaptosomal tryptophan-to-serotonin conversion to the control rate. However, both the increase in synaptosomal tryptophan uptake and the reduction in midbrain tryptophan hydroxylase activity were maintained throughout the three-week study period (Figure 18). In contrast to the effects of lithium on tryptophan uptake in vitro, lithium additions had no direct effect on tryptophan hydroxylase activity in vitro. Studies with two artificial cofactors (2-amino-4-hydroxy-6,7-dimethyl-5,6,7,8-tetrahydropteridine (DMPH$_4$) and 2-amino-4-hydroxy-6-methyl-5,6,7,8-tetrahydropteridine (6-MPH$_4$)) yielded equivalent conclusions. In regard to some of the suggestions that lithium might alter biological processes by interacting with calcium, it is interesting to note that calcium stimulates tryptophan hydroxylase activity (Knapp et al., 1975).

The sequential changes reported here suggest that continued administration of lithium is associated with a feedback-related reduction in cell body tryptophan hydroxylase activity in response to a direct enhancing effect on tryptophan uptake and serotonin synthesis. If these changes contribute to the therapeutic effects of lithium, the establishment of a new steady state after continued lithium administration would be consistent with the 5- to 10-day delay in the clinical efficacy of lithium in patients with affective disorders. These sequential changes also are consonant with the observations of Goodwin and his colleagues (1975) that lithium treatment in patients with affective disorders is associated with two time-related changes in 5-hydroxyindolacetic acid (5-HIAA) accumulation in cerebrospinal fluid, measured with the probenecid technique. After short-term treatment (5 days), 5-HIAA in cerebrospinal fluid was increased; treatment continued for 21 days led to a reduction of this serotonin metabolite.

The relationships among serotonin synthesis, levels, turnover, and metabolism and behavioral states in animals and man are extremely complex, and it is possible that serotonin serves a regulatory role rather

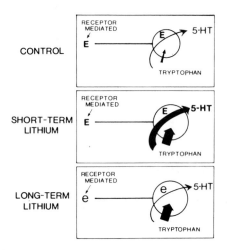

Figure 19. Hypothetical presynaptic mechanisms in the action of lithium. In the control neuron, tryptophan hydroxylase (E) is optimal both in the cell body and in the nerve ending. Tryptophan is taken up through the neuronal membrane and converted to serotonin (5-HT), which is released from the nerve ending. After short-term lithium treatment, substrate uptake is augmented and consequently synthesis and release of serotonin are increased, since intra-neuronal tryptophan hydroxylase is not saturated with regard to substrate. After long-term lithium treatment, the "amount" of enzyme has been reduced to compensate for the initial augmentation of serotonin released to the receptor. Tryptophan uptake remains augmented, but transmitter synthesis and release at the nerve ending have returned to control levels because of the enzyme deficit. [Mandell and Knapp, 1975b]

than a direct role with regard to behavior. Although no tidy hypothesis relating increases or decreases in serotonin synthesis to one or another pole of the affective continuum is possible at present, the serotonergic responses do suggest another possibility, which is diagrammed in Figure 19. The control levels of synaptosomal serotonin-synthesizing capacity after chronic lithium treatment represent the net effect of two maintained changes that were induced by the drug, i.e., the increase in the high-affinity uptake of tryptophan and the decrease in intra-synaptosomal rate-limiting enzyme activity. It is as though the uptake were elevated and stabilized at a ceiling, the intraneuronal enzyme activity were reduced and stabilized at the floor, and the bidirectional adaptive capacity were thus "used up," having returned the overall measure of nerve-ending biosynthetic capacity, the conversion rate, to baseline. Perhaps lithium's efficacy in preventing or dampening both manic and depressive episodes without changing many control level or normal behaviors in the intersymptomatic intervals is related to this way in which it influences the serotonergic system (Mandell and Knapp, 1975a,b).

An implication of this model for the action of lithium in treatment is the possibility that daily or regular tryptophan loads might be prophylactic in bipolar affective disorder. Recently it has been reported that tryptophan produces both antidepressant and antimanic effects in patients with bipolar affective disorders (Murphy et al., 1974) and that daily tryptophan loads can be used against affective disease in patients who show marked intolerance to lithium.*

Two pharmacological tests of this "buffering" theory of the action of lithium have been conducted recently in Mandell's laboratories. This group had reported (Knapp et al., 1974) that acute administration of amphetamine produced an adaptive decrease in tryptophan hydroxylase activity from the lateral raphe nuclei. Recent reports based upon earlier hypotheses (Bunney et al., 1972a) suggest that lithium prevents the euphoric "high" caused by acutely administered amphetamine and cocaine in man (van Kammen and Murphy, 1975).† In the case of amphetamine, Mandell's model would predict that the adaptive decrease in tryptophan hydroxylase activity already induced by lithium would prevent further decrease in the enzyme as well as inhibit further behavioral effects. Such findings have been forthcoming (Mandell and Knapp, 1975b; Segal et al., 1975). Cocaine blocks uptake of tryptophan into synaptosomes, reduces conversion of tryptophan to serotonin, and leads to an adaptive increase in raphe tryptophan hydroxylase (Knapp and Mandell, 1972‡). Lithium, as might have been expected from this model, antagonizes all three changes in this cocaine-induced sequence (Mandell and Knapp, 1975b‡).

Much more work must be done at basic and clinical levels before it will be clear whether the clinical actions of lithium can, in fact, be explained by this kind of "buffering" and/or "cross-tolerance" for abnormally high or low amounts of functioning neurotransmitter.

Effects of Lithium on Brain Cell Electrical
Responses to Neurotransmitters: F.E. Bloom

Electrodes can be used to study modifications produced by drugs like lithium on the electrical responses of specific brain cells to neurotransmitters. Two well-studied cell groups are the cerebellar

---

*N. Kline, personal communication.
†Also, W.E. Bunney, Jr., personal communication.
‡Also S. Knapp and A.J. Mandell, manuscript in preparation.

Purkinje cells and the hippocampal pyramidal cells, both of which receive norepinephrine-specific terminals from the locus coeruleus. Norepinephrine applied by iontophoresis reduces the firing rate of these cells via a beta-adrenergic receptor. Cyclic AMP administration mimics the effects of norepinephrine, while norepinephrine's effects can be blocked by prostaglandin E_1 (Bloom et al., 1975).

Lithium chloride applied by iontophoresis blocks the inhibitory effect of norepinephrine on hippocampal pyramidal cells (Figure 20).

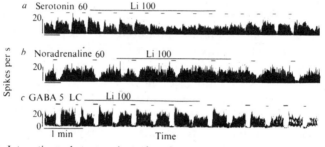

Figure 20. Interactions between iontophoretic application of Li^+, several putative neurotransmitters, and locus coeruleus (LC) stimulation. Hippocampal cellular activity in the pyramidal layer was integrated over 1-sec intervals and recorded on an ink recorder. *a*. The effects of Li^+ on the responses to serotonin applied with an injection current of 60 nA at fixed regular intervals (bars). The concurrent application of Li^+ (with current of 100 nA), for 2-3 min caused a slowing of the spontaneous firing, but also blocked the response to serotonin. This response was reinstated 1-2 min after termination of Li^+ current. *b*. Same as in (*a*), with a different cell, Li^+ antagonized the response to norepinephrine with no noticeable effect on spontaneous activity. *c*. Li^+ effects tested against the iontophoretic application of GABA and stimulation of LC. Stimulation parameters: pulses of 0.1 msec, 0.4 nA, applied through a concentric stimulating electrode at a rate of 10 per sec for 5 sec. Li^+ had no effect on the response to GABA but there was an antagonism of the response to LC stimulation. Note the difference in time scale between (*a*), (*b*), and (*c*). [Segal, 1974]

The inhibitory effect on the firing rate of the pyramidal cells produced by stimulation of the nucleus locus coeruleus (which contains the cells of origin of the noradrenergic projection to the cerebellum) is also blocked by lithium. The norepinephrine-like inhibitory response to cyclic AMP was not modified by lithium, suggesting that lithium acts at some step prior to cyclic AMP, perhaps via the calcium-dependent step in cyclic AMP synthesis.

In regard to other transmitters capable of affecting these cells, neither the excitatory effects of acetylcholine nor the inhibitory effects of GABA on pyramidal cells was affected by lithium. Some blunting of the inhibitory response to serotonin was observed, however.

Similar experiments of neurotransmitter-induced changes in firing rates of brain cells have not yet been accomplished in animals treated chronically with lithium. Also, it is not known whether magnesium or calcium changes would modify the effects of lithium. This system might profitably be explored in temporal conjunction with some biochemical studies of neurotransmitter metabolism such as those described above in the section, "Effects of Lithium on Serotonin Synthesis."

Lithium Effects on Water Metabolism: I. Singer

Lithium has many complicated actions on water and electrolyte metabolism, some of which are clinically important. For example, one prominent side effect of lithium's clinical use is increased urine output. However, when various clinical and laboratory observations are examined in detail, it is clear that lithium-induced polyuria may result from actions at several different sites, within both the kidney and the central nervous system (Cox and Singer, 1975). Analysis of these mechanisms of lithium action on water metabolism provides some insights into how lithium might affect other lithium-sensitive physiological systems that are less accessible to experimental investigation (Singer and Rotenberg, 1973).

In the majority of cases, lithium-related polyuria and the associated reduction in urine osmolality are resistant to the effects of exogenous antidiuretic hormone (ADH; vasopressin). In these cases, the polyuria must be of nephrogenic (related to the renal response to ADH), rather than of central (related to the production or release of ADH) origin. In order to concentrate the urine, the kidney must generate and maintain an osmotic gradient in the medullary region, principally by the transport of electrolyte (and urea) into the interstitium; then the kidney must utilize the gradient appropriately by responding to ADH, which allows the reabsorption of water from the collecting ducts. Therefore, a lithium-induced failure to respond to ADH may be due to the failure to create, to maintain, or to utilize the osmotic gradient.

Although lithium is concentrated in the kidney, with a corticomedullary gradient of approximately 1 to 2.5 formed for lithium, there is no evidence that lithium alters the corticopapillary gradient for sodium chloride (Solomon, 1967; Forrest et al., 1974). Lithium can also reduce sodium reabsorption or transport in man and in animals, with the production of an early natriuresis (Thomsen and Schou, 1968; Thomsen et al., 1974), but the glomerular filtration rate and electrolyte-free water clearance remain normal during chronic lithium administration (Singer et al., 1972). Thus, the ability to deliver electrolyte to the concentrating mechanism, the ability to separate electrolyte and water, and the ability to create and maintain an osmotic gradient thereby seem unimpaired.

The remaining possibility, that lithium impairs ADH-responsiveness by affecting gradient utilization, seems more likely. ADH is thought to induce osmotic water flow by stimulating the enzyme adenylate cyclase to generate cyclic AMP (cAMP, Figure 21)

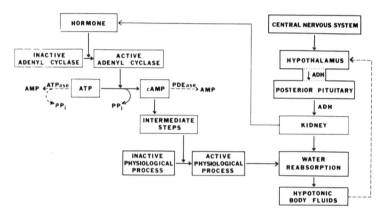

Figure 21. Mechanisms of action of ADH. ADH = antidiuretic hormone; ATP = adenosine triphosphate; AMP = adenosine monophosphate; cAMP = cyclic adenosine 3′,5′-monophosphate; PPi = pyrophosphate; ATPase = adenosine triphosphatase; PDEase = cAMP phosphodiesterase. [Cox and Singer, 1975]

from adenosine triphosphate (ATP) (Handler and Orloff, 1973). Cyclic AMP reproduces virtually all of the actions of ADH in vitro, and ADH increases cAMP levels in ADH-responsive renal tissues. The level of cAMP is also controlled by two other enzymes: phosphodiesterase (PDEase), which converts cAMP to AMP, and adenosine triphosphatase (ATPase), which converts ATP to AMP. PDEase inhibitors, such as theophylline, increase cAMP levels and physiological responses to ADH. Lithium could interfere with any of the steps required to generate cAMP, could accelerate the destruction of cAMP, or could interfere with the action of cAMP.

Lithium has more than one action on these intrarenal mechanisms. Lithium clearly lowers ADH-induced increases in renal medullary cAMP levels (Dousa and Hechter, 1970a; Geisler et al., 1972). Although lithium can increase (Na-K)-dependent ATPase activity (Willis and

Fang, 1970; Gutman et al., 1973), this action alone cannot explain the lower cAMP levels because lithium's actions are not affected when an ATP-regenerating system is added to the assay (Wraae et al., 1972). There is also no evidence that lithium can lower basal cAMP levels or stimulate PDEase activity in human renal medulla (Dousa, 1973). These biochemical data confirm physiological observations suggesting that lithium acts by inhibiting ADH-induced increases in cAMP levels. For example, lithium reversibly inhibits ADH-induced, but not dibutyryl-cAMP-induced, osmotic water flow in toad urinary bladder (Singer et al., 1972; Singer and Franko, 1973). These biochemical and physiological effects were observed at urinary lithium levels that are achieved in lithium-treated patients. Furthermore, there is evidence that lithium has more than one physiological site of action. For example, Forrest and his co-workers (1974) have found that lithium-induced polyuria in rats is completely unresponsive to ADH and partially unresponsive to cAMP, suggesting impairments both before and after cAMP generation.

In a few cases, lithium-related polyuria does respond (at least partially) to the exogenous administration of ADH (Singer et al., 1972; Forrest et al., 1974). In addition, lithium is concentrated in the pituitary of some animals (Wittrig et al., 1970) and can deplete neurosecretory material from the pituitary and the supraoptic nuclei (Ellman and Gan, 1973; Hochman and Gutman, 1974). These clinical and laboratory observations suggest that lithium can cause central as well as nephrogenic diabetes insipidus. Moreover, there is some evidence that lithium can induce primary polydipsia in animals, with a secondary polyuria (Smith et al., 1970; Smith and Balagura, 1972). However, primary polydipsia has not yet been documented in lithium-treated patients.

In summary, it is clear that lithium can cause both nephrogenic and central diabetes insipidus in man and also primary polydipsia in animals. The most common clinical condition, nephrogenic diabetes insipidus, does not correlate well with serum lithium levels, but urinary levels may be more important. Both the central and the renal effects of lithium may be due to lowered hormone-induced increases in cAMP levels, with lithium actions both before and after cAMP generation. Other effects of lithium, including its partial substitution for other extracellular and intracellular cations, may underlie its effects on the adenylate cyclase system and on both water and electrolyte metabolism.

Effects of Lithium on Thyroid Gland Function: J. Wolff

Clinically, lithium treatment can produce goiter and hypo-thyroidism. This side effect of lithium's use in psychiatry has recently been employed in the treatment of thyrotoxicosis (Temple et al., 1972). Lithium decreases the release of thyroidal ^{131}I and leads to slightly decreased plasma levels of thyroxine (T_4). In some individuals, a compensatory increase in thyroid-stimulating hormone (TSH) occurs, at least transiently.

The possible sites of lithium's actions on thyroid physiology have been explored in some detail. There is no evidence at present to implicate the brain mechanisms involved at the hypothalamic level (thyrotropin-releasing hormone) or the pituitary (TSH), although lithium is accumulated in the pituitary (and also in the thyroid gland itself) to concentrations 3 to 5 times higher than those in plasma (Berens et al., 1970b). Most of the evidence points to an inhibition of the release of T_4 from the thyroid gland as the single most important effect of lithium (Sedvall et al., 1968, 1969; Berens et al., 1970a; Berens and Wolff, 1975).

It was originally hypothesized that the specific mode of action of lithium on T_4 secretion resulted from an inhibition of thyroid adenylate cyclase, which was shown to occur at lithium concentrations of 4 mM in bovine thyroid membrane fractions (Wolff et al., 1970) (Figure 22). TSH activates this enzyme to produce cyclic AMP, which

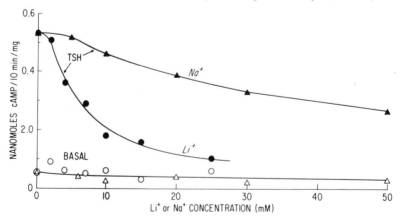

Figure 22. The inhibitory effect of Li⁺ and Na⁺ ions on beef thyroid adenyl cyclase. The Mg^{2+} concentration is 2.5 mM. o—o and ●—●: Li⁺ experiments; △—△ and ▲—▲: Na⁺ experiments; o—o and △—△: basal activity; ●—● and ▲—▲: cyclase activity stimulated with 200 mu/ml of bovine TSH. [Wolff et al., 1970]

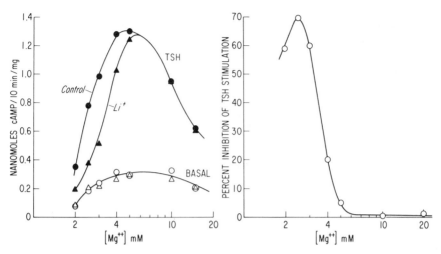

Figure 23. The effect of Mg^{2+} concentration on the Li^+-inhibition of TSH-stimulated adenyl cyclase activity. Li^+ concentration is 10 mM, TSH concentration 200 mu/ml. *Left panel,* o−o and ●−●: controls; △−△ and ▲−▲: Li^+ experiments. o−o and △−△: basal activity; ●−● and ▲−▲: TSH-stimulated adenyl cyclase. *Right panel,* Percent inhibition is expressed as

$$1 - \frac{\text{TSH} - \text{basal activity (with } Li^+)}{\text{TSH} - \text{basal activity (without } Li^+)} \quad .$$

[Wolff et al., 1970]

then mediates the release of T_4. The reduction in adenylate cyclase activity produced by lithium was sensitive to small changes in the magnesium concentration of the medium; lowered Mg markedly enhanced the enzyme's sensitivity to lithium and increased Mg abolished lithium's inhibitory effects (Figure 23). Of interest is the fact that membrane Na-K ATPase was not affected by lithium in these studies (Wolff et al., 1970). Although lithium's action on thyroid adenylate cyclase may be an important clue to understanding its effects on other cell systems, more recent data has indicated that this alteration may not explain its antithyroid effects, since lithium inhibits secretion stimulated by cyclic AMP, i.e., lithium can act at a step beyond adenylate cyclase (J.A. Williams et al., 1971).

It may be that lithium directly affects the thyroid cell membrane process of T_4 secretion. This may or may not be a good analogy for lithium's effects on neural membrane mechanisms, because T_4 secretion does not occur by exocytosis but rather by the endocytotic release of a 670,000 molecular weight protein, thyroglobulin. Endocytosis at the apex of a follicle cell involves the formation and protrusion of pseudopods, with the pinching off of colloid droplets. Lithium can completely abolish the accumulation of colloid droplets and endocytosis (J.A. Williams et al., 1971). While other drugs besides lithium can also affect endocytosis, little is known about their mechanism, although there are some suggestions that the process is calcium dependent. As noted previously, a calcium-lithium interaction is a distinct possibility.

V. LITHIUM AND THE BIOLOGY OF MANIC-DEPRESSIVE ILLNESS: S.S. Kety

The Biology of Mania

There is convincing evidence today from psychopharmacology that the putative catecholamine neurotransmitters, norepinephrine and dopamine, are in some way involved in the manic process. Drugs that would be expected to elevate synaptic concentrations of brain norepinephrine and dopamine include monoamine oxidase inhibitors, some tricyclic antidepressants, and L-dopa. All of these drugs have been associated with the triggering of manic episodes. On the other hand, certain substances that should act to decrease functional activity of catecholamines have been associated with decreased manic symptomatology. These include α-methyl-p-tyrosine (AMPT), which competitively inhibits the rate-limiting enzyme in the formation of dopamine and norepinephrine; some phenothiazines and butyrophenones, which block catecholamine receptors; and lithium carbonate, which in some animal studies was shown to decrease release of norepinephrine at the presynaptic nerve endings and to facilitate its reuptake into the presynaptic nerve.

Lithium Carbonate in Mania

Substantial evidence suggests that there are one or more genetic defects underlying manic-depressive illness. Lithium may act in some way to correct these defects. A common theme of several studies of the action of lithium involves norepinephrine or cyclic AMP, and the observations are such as to explain this ion's action in mania by some diminution of catecholamine synaptic action. However, the various studies are not entirely consistent with that hypothesis. More important, if lithium acts in that way to reduce the symptoms of mania, a different and, in fact, opposite action on catecholamines must be invoked to explain the antidepressant and prophylactic actions of lithium. There is a way out of this dilemma, however, in a hypothesis (Kety, 1971) that takes into account the mounting evidence that serotonin is also invoked in manic-depressive illness.

Studies on the brain (post-mortem) and on cerebrospinal fluid indicate a diminished activity of serotonin in depression and in both phases of manic-depressive illness. Tryptophan administration has been found by some to enhance the antidepressant effects of monoamine oxidase inhibitors. Behavioral effects in animals associated with serotonin potentiation are more compatible with stabilization than with activation. It is possible that serotonin plays a homeostatic role at synapses, damping the effects of other transmitters such as the catecholamines. Manic-depressive illness could be viewed primarily as a deficiency in the serotonin-governed stabilization of mood in which the normal fluctuations mediated by norepinephrine or other transmitters go out-of-bounds. Although mania or depression would respond to drugs that antagonized or enhanced respectively the effects of norepinephrine, both states might be prevented or treated by a single agent that potentiated the action of serotonin. The studies reported by Mandell suggest that lithium may be such an agent. He and his co-workers observed an increase in the uptake of tryptophan by synaptosomes prepared from lithium-treated animals, and an augmented synthesis of serotonin (Knapp and Mandell, 1973, 1975). It is true that in these animals continued lithium treatment caused a feedback-induced diminution in tryptophan hydroxylase activity and a consequent reduction of serotonin synthesis to its unstimulated rate, but these were normal rats. It is possible that, in manic-depressive patients whose illness may be the result of some initial inadequacy in serotonin synthesis or in its synaptic activity, the continued administration of lithium would stabilize serotonin activity at a higher level.

Our knowledge of the role of these and many other neurotransmitters in the various components of behavior is still very fragmentary, and the application of inadequate knowledge to the clinical problems of affective disorder can only be speculative and is undoubtedly simplistic. To the extent that those speculations are heuristic, however, they may be warranted.

VI. MODE OF ACTION OF Li IN TREATING AFFECTIVE DISORDERS–NEUROBIOLOGICAL CONSIDERATIONS:
D.L. Murphy, J.L. Costa, and W.E. Bunney, Jr.

A neurobiological understanding of the affective disorders, mania and depression, has not yet been achieved. Mania and depression are most simply conceptualized as recurrent extremes of mood and motor activity. Cognitive, physiological, and complex psychological changes that may be of psychotic magnitude also occur as part of the syndromes. Among the various affective disorder subtypes, cyclic bipolar (manic-depressive) and recurrent unipolar depressive disorders are those most clearly responsive to lithium treatment.

While possible mechanisms by which lithium might act in achieving its remarkable therapeutic and prophylactic effects necessarily remain speculative in the absence of etiological knowledge, increased understanding of how a simple cation like lithium might affect human behavior has been sought at many levels. Stabilizing or dampening effects on some brain system involved in the regulation of mood, motor activity, and biorhythms have been looked for as lithium's most likely mode of action. This line of thought is supported by apparent dampening effects of lithium on physiological processes that contribute to two other human disorders, both characterized by failure of hormonal regulatory mechanisms—thyrotoxicosis and CNS-related polyuria.

Lithium has many effects on brain neurotransmitter systems and hormonal functions that are capable of affecting mood, cognition, motor activity, and biorhythms. Some of these differing effects may result from common actions of lithium on cellular processes, such as membrane transport and release phenomena or the cyclic AMP second messenger and intracellular signal amplification mechanisms. Ultimately, of course, lithium must interact at the molecular level with biological tissue sites, broadly conceptualized as lithium "receptors," which may, in fact, be sites ordinarily occupied by other physiological cations such as Mg^{2+}, Ca^{2+}, Na^+, or K^+. The concept that lithium's behavioral effects may be explicable in terms of its physical and chemical properties is supported by the occurrence of definite effects on motor activity, aggression, and other interactional behavior in animals produced by the two other Group I alkali metals, rubidium and cesium. Indeed, possible beneficial psychoactive effects of rubidium are now under study in man.

Lithium's Physical-Chemical Properties in Simple Systems

Model systems utilizing synthetic macropolycyclic polyethers, synthetic peptides, antibiotic ionophores, and artificial membranes are proving to be useful in more closely specifying how lithium's unique physical properties, including size, charge, energy of hydration, and solvent characteristics, might predict its other chemical interactions.

Model systems, wherein details of molecular structure can be closely defined and, in some instances, molecular structure systematically varied, provide a most valuable approach to understanding the characteristics of lithium "receptors," the sites at which lithium interacts at the molecular level in biological tissues. A proposed "lithium receptor" should have certain characteristics: (1) It must have sufficient specificity for lithium to permit binding in the presence of the other cations that are usually present in higher concentrations in biological tissues than lithium. (2) The receptor must form a cavity compatible with the size of the lithium ion; specifically, it must have a lower size limit of 0.8 A, which is the radius of the nonhydrated lithium ion. There have been comparatively few studies yet of lithium's interactions in simple biological systems such as DNA solutions, bilayer artificial membranes, or purified enzyme preparations.

Cellular Effects of Lithium

Lithium's effects on more complex cellular systems have been widely investigated because of the promise of unraveling its whole-organism effects through actions on fairly well understood cell functions. Lithium has been demonstrated to be capable of affecting nerve and erythrocyte cell membrane events, mitochondrial and other cellular energy metabolism, as well as a number of enzymes in vivo. However, many of these effects occur only at lithium concentrations far higher than those used therapeutically. Hence there has been greater interest in several cellular processes that a growing number of studies have demonstrated to be affected by lithium in concentrations of 1 to 5 mM. Most prominent among these effects are: (1) on adenylate cyclase activity and cyclic AMP, as well as on some intracellular effects of cyclic AMP; (2) on secretion and release processes, which are calcium-dependent and modulated by magnesium concentrations in many cases; and (3) on the cellular membrane transport of amino acids, glucose, biogenic amines, and cations.

The many hormone effects that are dampened by lithium's action on adenyl cyclase or other components of the cyclic AMP system are particularly noteworthy. There are data implicating cAMP changes in the behavioral switch process into mania, and the role of cAMP as a cellular signal amplification mechanism makes such hypotheses attractive. As hormones have long-term cyclic effects on behavior, the neuroendocrine effects of lithium certainly require further exploration. Moreover, the growing understanding of similar cAMP functions in pre- and post-synaptic neurotransmitter receptor functions, some of which are altered by lithium, makes this system an especially likely prospect for being involved in lithium's behavioral effects.

Lithium's Interactions with Other Cations

Lithium may affect adenylate cyclase through magnesium-dependent processes, just as a number of other cellular transport and release mechanisms appear to be affected by lithium via its effects on the divalent cations, magnesium and calcium. A particularly critical synaptic function, the release of neurotransmitters from synaptic vesicles, appears to depend upon an increase of free intracellular calcium; and lithium's antagonistic effects on this system could readily be expected to lead to a reduction in behavioral functions modulated by neurotransmitters contained in synaptic vesicles, at least acutely. There have been very few studies of the effects of lithium on the intracellular concentrations and metabolism of calcium and magnesium in man, although some appropriate techniques to approach this question are available. Additionally, other model systems for magnesium-calcium interactions should be studied for lithium effects.

Lithium's ability to alter cellular membrane ATPase, Na/K transport, and possibly intracellular sodium concentrations provide another potential locus of action for lithium's behavioral effects. There are, in fact, a few reports of increased "residual" (intracellular plus bone) sodium in manic and depressive patients, and it has been suggested that intracellular lithium-sodium interactions might affect transport gradients for biogenic amines or other neurotransmitters capable of affecting behavior. They might also affect the conformational state of cellular receptors for neurotransmitters and other cell signal molecules, many of which have been demonstrated to be sensitive to sodium or lithium concentration changes. The interesting example of a modulatory effect on a vagus nerve preparation whose Na/K membrane pump and nerve conduction velocity is reduced by lithium, particularly at higher rates of electrical stimulation, ought to lead to a search for similar regulatory effects of lithium in other model systems.

Lithium's Effects on Brain Neurotransmitters and Behavior

Consideration of the way lithium affects behavior has naturally focused on the brain neurotransmitter systems most clearly implicated in the regulation of psychomotor activity, emotional and aggressive behavior, sleep, and other functions altered in mania and depression. These include the dopamine, norepinephrine, serotonin, and possibly the GABA and acetylcholine neurotransmitter systems. Some of the cellular effects of lithium on brain amine neurotransmitter function (decreased release and increased amine reuptake) are congruent with its antimanic actions, although it is much less clear how lithium's antidepressant activity and its prophylactic effects on recurrent manic and depressive cycles might be mediated. The suggestion that the serotonergic neurotransmitter systems might provide such a regulatory role is of great interest and, in fact, has been partially validated by studies in man of cerebrospinal fluid levels of serotonin metabolites. The availability of this serotonergic model system and of a catecholaminergic model for mania based upon amphetamine-induced hyperactivity reversible by lithium, which has also been validated in man, may aid in the further delineation of genuinely analogous models. Lithium's effects can be studied further at behavioral, cellular, and molecular levels by the use of such models.

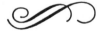

ABBREVIATIONS

ADH	antidiuretic hormone
AMP	adenosine monophosphate
AMPT	α-methyl-p-tyrosine
ATP	adenosine triphosphate
ATPase	adenosine triphosphatase
cAMP	cyclic adenosine $3',5'$-monophosphate
CNS	central nervous system
$DMPH_4$	2-amino-4-hydroxy-6,7-dimethyl-5,6,7,8-tetrahydropteridine
DNA	deoxyribonucleic acid
Dopa	dihydroxyphenylalanine
EDTA	ethylene diaminetetraacetate
EGTA	bis-ethyleneglycol diaminetetraacetate
GABA	γ-aminobutyric acid
Gly	glycine
5-HIAA	5-hydroxyindoleacetic acid
5-HT	5-hydroxytryptamine (serotonin)
$6\text{-}MPH_4$	2-amino-4-hydroxy-6-methyl-5,6,7,8-tetrahydropteridine
NAD	nicotinamide adenine nucleotide
NMR	nuclear magnetic resonance
PDEase	phosphodiesterase
PPi	pyrophosphate
Pro	proline
RNA	ribonucleic acid
T_4	thyroxine
TSH	thyroid-stimulating hormone

BIBLIOGRAPHY

This bibliography contains two types of entries: (1) citations given or work alluded to in the report, and (2) additional references to pertinent literature by conference participants and others. Citations in group (1) may be found in the text on the pages listed in the right-hand column.   Page

Adelmann, H.B. (1936): The problem of cyclopia. *Q. Rev. Biol.* 11:161-182.

Angrist, B.M., Gershon, S., Levitan, S.J., and Blumberg, A.G. (1970): Lithium-induced diabetes insipidus-like syndrome. *Compr. Psychiatry* 11:141-146.

Baastrup, P.C., Poulsen, J.C., Schou, M., Thomsen, K., and Amdiesen, A. (1970):   188
Prophylactic lithium: Double-blind discontinuation in manic-depressive and recurrent-depressive disorders. *Lancet* 2:326-330.

Baastrup, P.C. and Schou, M. (1967): Lithium as a prophylactic agent. Its effect against recurrent depressions and manic-depressive psychosis. *Arch. Gen. Psychiatry* 16:162-172.

Baer, L., Durell, J., Bunney, W.E., Jr., Levy, B.S., Murphy, D.L., Greenspan, K., and Cardon, P.V. (1970): Sodium balance and distribution in lithium carbonate therapy. *Arch. Gen. Psychiatry* 22:40-44.

Baker, P.F. (1972): Transport and metabolism of calcium ions in nerve. *Prog.*   161
Biophys. Mol. Biol. 24:179-223.

Baker, P.F., Blaustein, M.P., Hodgkin, A.L., and Steinhardt, R.A. (1969): The   161
influence of calcium on sodium efflux in squid axons. *J. Physiol.* 200:431-458.

Baker, P.F., Hodgkin, A.L., and Ridgway, E.B. (1971): Depolarization and calcium   161
entry in squid giant axons. *J. Physiol.* 218:709-755.

Baldessarini, R.J. and Yorke, C. (1970): Effects of lithium and of pH on   123,166
synaptosomal metabolism of noradrenaline. *Nature* 228:1301-1303.

Behr, J.-P. and Lehn, J.-M. (1973): Transport of amino acids through organic liquid membranes. *J. Am. Chem. Soc.* 95:6108-6110.

Benjamin, W.B., Fish, S.T., and Singer, I. (1974): Insulin-induced adenosine 3':5'-cyclic monophosphate-independent phosphorylation of a fat-cell protein: Effect of starving and re-feeding. *Trans. Biochem. Soc.* 2:920-922.

Bentley, P.J. and Wasserman, A. (1972): The effects of lithium on the permeability of an epithelial membrane, the toad urinary bladder. *Biochim. Biophys. Acta* 266:285-292.

Berens, S.C., Bernstein, R.S., Robbins, J., and Wolff, J. (1970a): Antithyroid   178
effects of lithium. *J. Clin. Invest.* 49:1357-1367.

Berens, S.C., Williams, J.A., and Wolff, J. (1971): Dissociation of thyrotropin-stimulated hormone secretion and glucose oxidation in thyroid glands by lithium and colchicine. *Biochim. Biophys. Acta* 252:314-323.

Neurosciences Res. Prog. Bull., Vol. 14, No. 2   189

Page

Berens, S.C. and Wolff, J. (1975): The endocrine effects of lithium. *In: Lithium Research and Therapy*. Johnson, F.N., ed. New York: Academic Press, pp. 443-472.   123,178

Berens, S.C., Wolff, J., and Murphy, D.L. (1970b): Lithium concentration by the thyroid. *Endocrinology* 87:1085-1087.   178

Berg, W.E. (1968): Effect of lithium on the rate of protein synthesis in the sea urchin embryo. *Exp. Cell Res.* 50:133-139.   154

Berl, S. and Clarke, D.D. (1972): Effects of Li^+ on the metabolism in brain of glutamate, glutamine, aspartate and GABA from $[1\text{-}^{14}C]$ acetate *in vitro. Brain Res.* 36:203-213.   168

Berneis, K.H., Pletscher, A., and Da Prada, M. (1969): Metal-dependent aggregation of biogenic amines: A hypothesis for their storage and release. *Nature* 224:281-282.

Bezanilla, F. and Armstrong, C.M. (1972): Negative conductance caused by entry of sodium and cesium ions into the potassium channels of squid axons. *J. Gen. Physiol.* 60:588-608.   162,164

Bindler, E.H., Wallach, M.B., and Gershon, S. (1971): Effect of lithium on the release of ^{14}C-norepinephrine by nerve stimulation from the perfused cat spleen. *Arch. Int. Pharmacodyn. Ther.* 190:150-154.   166

Bliss, E.L. and Ailion, J. (1970): The effect of lithium upon brain neuroamines. *Brain Res.* 24:305-310.   166

Bloom, F.E. (1972): Amino acids and polypeptides in neuronal function. *Neurosciences Res. Prog. Bull.* 10:122-251. Also *In: Neurosciences Research Symposium Summaries, Vol. 7.* Schmitt, F.O. et al., eds. Cambridge, Mass.: M.I.T. Press, 1974, pp. 122-251.

Bloom, F.E. (1974): To spritz or not to spritz: The doubtful value of aimless iontophoresis. *Life Sci.* 14:1819-1834.

Bloom, F.E., Siggins, G.R., Hoffer, B.J., Segal, M., and Oliver, A.P. (1975): Cyclic nucleotides in the central synaptic actions of catecholamines. *In: Advances in Cyclic Nucleotide Research, Vol. 5.* (Second International Conference on Cyclic AMP, Vancouver, July 8-11, 1974.) Drummond, G.I., Greengard, P., and Robison, G.A., eds. New York: Raven Press, pp. 603-618.   174

Blout, E.R., Deber, C.M., and Pease, L.G. (1974): Cyclic peptides. *In: Peptides, Polypeptides, and Proteins*. Blout, E.R., Bovey, F.A., Goodman, M., and Lotan, N., eds. New York: John Wiley and Sons, Inc., pp. 266-281.

Bowers, M.B., Jr. and Rozitis, A. (1970): Acetylcholine release from cortical brain slices of rats injected with lithium. *J. Pharm. Pharmacol.* 22:647.   168

Brodie, H.K.H., Murphy, D.L., Goodwin, F.K., and Bunney, W.E., Jr. (1971): Catecholamines and mania: The effect of alpha-methyl-para-tyrosine on manic behavior and catecholamine metabolism. *Clin. Pharmacol. Ther.* 12:218-224.   130

Buchsbaum, M., Goodwin, F.K., Murphy, D., and Borge, G. (1971): AER in affective disorders. *Am. J. Psychiatry* 128:19-25.

Bunney, W.E., Jr. and Davis, J.M. (1965): Norepinephrine in depressive reactions. A review. *Arch. Gen. Psychiatry* 13:483-494.   165

Bunney, W.E., Jr., Gershon, E.S., and Winokur, G. (1976): X linkage in manic-depressive psychosis. *Neurosciences Res. Prog. Bull.* 14:46-53.   125

Bunney, W.E., Jr., Goodwin, F.K., Davis, J.M., and Fawcett, J.A. (1968): A behavioral-biochemical study of lithium treatment. *Am. J. Psychiatry* 125:499-512.   127,128

Bunney, W.E., Jr., Goodwin, F., and Murphy, D. (1972a): The 'switch process' in manic-depressive illness; III. Theoretical implications. *Arch. Gen. Psychiatry* 27:312-317.   125,144, 173

Bunney, W.E., Jr., Goodwin, F.K., Murphy, D.L., House, K.M., and Gordon, E.K. (1972b): The "switch process" in manic-depressive illness. II. Relationship to catecholamines, REM sleep, and drugs. *Arch. Gen. Psychiatry* 27:304-309.   125

Bunney, W.E., Jr. and Hartmann, E.L. (1965): Study of a patient with 48-hour manic-depressive cycles. *Arch. Gen. Psychiatry* 12:611-618.   126

Bunney, W.E., Jr. and Murphy, D.L. (1973): The behavioral switch process and psychopathology. *In: Biological Psychiatry.* Mendels, J., ed. New York: John Wiley and Sons, Inc., pp. 345-367.

Burgermeister, W., Wieland, T., and Winkler, R. (1974): Antamanide. Dynamics of metal-complex formation. *Eur. J. Biochem.* 44:305-310.

Burgermeister, W., Wieland, T., and Winkler, R. (1974): Antamanide. Relaxation study of conformational equilibria. *Eur. J. Biochem.* 44:311-316.

Cade, J.F.J. (1949): Lithium salts in the treatment of psychotic excitement. *Med. J. Aust.* 2:349-352.   117,124

Campbell, I.D., Dobson, C.M., and Williams, R.J.P. (1975): Nuclear magnetic resonance studies on the structure of lysozyme in solution. *Proc. Roy. Soc. A* 345:41-59.   145

Campbell, I.D., Dobson, C.M., Williams, R.J.P., and Xavier, A.V. (1973): The determination of the structure of proteins in solution: lysozyme. *Ann. N.Y. Acad. Sci.* 222:163-174.

Campbell, I.D., Dobson, C.M., Williams, R.J.P., and Xavier, A.V. (1974): New nmr techniques for the quantitative determination of the structure of proteins in solution applied to hen egg-white lysozyme (HEWL). *In: Lysozyme.* Osserman, E.F., Canfield, R.E., and Beychok, S., eds. New York: Academic Press, pp. 219-227.

Neurosciences Res. Prog. Bull., Vol. 14, No. 2   **191**

Page

Carlson, H.E., Robbins, J., and Murphy, D.L. (1974): The effect of lithium on thyroid iodine release in patients with primary affective disorder. *Psychopharmacologia* 35:249-256.

Carroll, B.J. and Sharp, P.T. (1971): Rubidium and lithium: opposite effects on amine-mediated excitement. *Science* 172:1355-1357.   168

Casteels, R., Droogmans, G., and Hendrickx, H. (1973): Effect of sodium and sodium-substitutes on the active ion transport and on the membrane potential of smooth muscle cells. *J. Physiol.* 228:733-748.

Chasin, M., Rivkin, I., Mamrak, F., Samaniegg, S.G., and Hess, S.M. (1971): α- and β-adrenergic receptors as mediators of accumulation of cyclic adenosine 3',5'-monophosphate in specific areas of guinea pig brain. *J. Biol. Chem.* 246:3037-3041.   167,168

Cheney, J. and Lehn, J.-M. (1972): Proton cryptates. *J. Chem. Soc. (Lond.) Chem. Commun.* 487-489.   133

Cheney, J., Lehn, J.M., Sauvage, J.P., and Stubbs, M.E. (1972): [3]-Cryptates: Metal cation inclusion complexes with a macrotricyclic ligand. *J. Chem. Soc. (Lond.) Chem. Commun.* 1100-1101.   133

Child, C.M. (1940): Lithium and echinoderm exogastrulation: With a review of the physiological-gradient concept. *Physiol. Zool.* 13:4-42.

Christensen, H.N. (1969): Some special kinetic problems of transport. *Adv. Enzymol.* 32:1-20.   154

Colburn, R.W., Goodwin, F.K., Bunney, W.E., Jr., and Davis, J.M. (1967): Effect of lithium on the uptake of noradrenaline by synaptosomes. *Nature* 215:1395-1397.   166

Colburn, R.W. and Maas, J.W. (1965): Adenosine triphosphate-metal-norepinephrine ternary complexes and catecholamine binding. *Nature* 208:37-41.

Coppen, A., Noguera, R., Bailey, J., Burns, B.H., Swani, M.S., Hare, E.H., Gardner, R., and Maggs, R. (1971): Prophylactic lithium in affective disorders. Controlled trial. *Lancet* 2:275-279.   120

Corrodi, H., Fuxe, K., Hökfelt, T., and Schou, M. (1967): The effect of lithium on cerebral monoamine neurons. *Psychopharmacologia* 11:345-353.   123,166

Corrodi, H., Fuxe, K., and Schou, M. (1969): The effect of prolonged lithium administration on cerebral monoamine neurons in the rat. *Life Sci.* 8(Part I):643-651.   123

Cotton, F.A., Bier, C.J., Day, V.W., Hazen, E.E., Jr., and Larsen, S. (1971): Some aspects of the structure of staphylococcal nuclease. *Cold Spring Harbor Symp. Quant. Biol.* 36:243-255.   145

Cox, M. and Singer, I. (1975): Lithium and water metabolism. *Am. J. Med.*   175,176
59:153-157.

Cundall, R.L., Brooks, P.W., and Murray, L.G. (1972): A controlled evaluation of   120
lithium prophylaxis in affective disorders. *Psychol. Med.* 2:308-311.

Davies, C., Sanger, D.J., Steinberg, H., Tomkiewicz, M., and U'Prichard, D.C.   168
(1974): Lithium and α-methyl-p-tyrosine prevent "manic" activity in rodents.
Psychopharmacologia 36:263-274.

Davis, J.M. and Fann, W.E. (1971): Lithium. *Annu. Rev. Pharmacol.* 11:285-302.

Deber, C.M., Blout, E.R., Torchia, D.A., Dorman, D.E., and Bovey, F.A. (1972):
Proton and ^{13}C NMR studies of conformations of *cyclo*(-Pro-Gly-)$_3$. *In:
Chemistry and Biology of Peptides.* Meienhofer, J., ed. Ann Arbor, Mich.: Ann
Arbor Science Publishers, pp. 39-43.

Deber, C.M., Torchia, D.A., Wong, S.C.K., and Blout, E.R. (1972): Conformational   138
interconversions of the cyclic hexapeptide *cyclo*(Pro-Gly)$_3$. *Proc. Nat. Acad. Sci.*
69:1825-1829.

DeFeudis, F.V. and Delgado, J.M.R. (1970): Effects of lithium on amino-acids in   168
mouse brain *in vivo. Nature* 225:749-750.

Diem, K. and Lentner, C., eds. (1970): *Documenta Geigy. Scientific Tables,* 7th Ed.
Ardsley, N.Y.: Geigy Pharmaceuticals, pp. 109-123.

Dietrich, B., Lehn, J.M., and Sauvage, J.P. (1973a): Cryptates: Control over   133,134,
bivalent/monovalent cation selectivity. *J. Chem. Soc. (Lond.) Chem. Commun.*   135
15-16.

Dietrich, B., Lehn, J.M., and Sauvage, J.P. (1973b): Cryptates—XI. Complexes   133
macrobicycliques, formation, structure, propriétés. *Tetrahedron* 29:1647-1658.

Dietrich, B., Lehn, J.M., Sauvage, J.P., and Blanzat, J. (1973c): Cryptates—X.
Synthèses et propriétés physiques de systèmes diaza-polyoxa-macrobicycliques.
Tetrahedron 29:1629-1645.

Dousa, T.P. (1973): Lithium: interaction with ADH dependent cyclic AMP system   177
of human renal medulla. *Clin. Res.* 21:282.

Dousa, T. and Hechter, O. (1970a): The effect of NaCl and LiCl on vasopressin-   176
sensitive adenyl cyclase. *Life Sci.* 9(Part I):765-770.

Dousa, T. and Hechter, O. (1970b): Lithium and brain adenyl cyclase. *Lancet*   154
1:834-835.

Edelman, G.M., Cunningham, B.A., Reeke, G.N., Jr., Becker, J.W., Waxdal, M.J.,   145
and Wang, J.L. (1972): The covalent and three-dimensional structure of
concanavalin A. *Proc. Nat. Acad. Sci.* 69:2580-2584.

Neurosciences Res. Prog. Bull., Vol. 14, No. 2   **193**

Page

Eigen, M. (1963): Fast elementary steps in chemical reaction mechanism. *Pure Appl. Chem.* 6:97-115.

Eigen, M. and De Maeyer, L. (1971): Carriers and specificity in membranes. *Neurosciences Res. Prog. Bull.* 9:299-437. Also *In: Neurosciences Research Symposium Summaries, Vol. 6.* Schmitt, F.O. et al., eds. Cambridge, Mass.: M.I.T. Press, 1972, pp. 299-437.

Eigen, M. and Wilkins, R.G. (1965): The kinetics and mechanism of formation of metal complexes. *In: Mechanisms of Inorganic Reactions. Advances in Chemistry Series No. 49.* Gould, R.F., ed. Washington, D.C.: American Chemical Society, pp. 55-80.

Eigen, M. and Winkler, R. (1970): Alkali-ion carriers: Dynamics and selectivity. *In: The Neurosciences: Second Study Program.* Schmitt, F.O., editor-in-chief. New York: Rockefeller University Press, pp. 685-696.   163

Eisenman, G. (1961): On the elementary atomic origin of equilibrium ionic specificity. *In: Membrane Transport and Metabolism* (Proceedings of a symposium held in Prague, August 22-27, 1960). Kleinzeller, A. and Kotyk, A. eds. New York: Academic Press, pp. 163-179.   155,156, 162

Eisenman, G. (1965): Some elementary factors involved in specific ion permeation. Proceedings of the XXIIIrd International Congress of Physiological Sciences, Tokyo, *87*: 489-506.   158,159

Eisenman, G., Ciani, S.M., and Szabo, G. (1968): Some theoretically expected and experimentally observed properties of lipid bilayer membranes containing neutral molecular carriers of ions. *Fed. Proc.* 27:1289-1304.

Eisenman, G. and Krasne, S. (1973): The selectivity of carrier antibiotics for substituted ammonium ions. *Biophys. Soc.* 244a. (abstr.)   156,157

Eisenman, G. and Krasne, S.J. (1975): The ion selectivity of carrier molecules, membranes and enzymes. *In: MTP International Review of Science, Biochemistry Series, Vol. 2. The Biochemistry of Cell Walls and Membranes.* Fox, C.F., ed. London: Butterworth, Inc., pp. 27-59.

Eisenman, G., Krasne, S., and Ciani, S. (1976a): Further studies on ion selectivity. *In: Proceedings of the International Workshop on Ion-Selective Electrodes and on Enzyme Electrodes in Biology and in Medicine.* Kessler, M., Clark, L., Lübbers, D., Silver, I., and Simon, W., eds. Munich, Berlin, Vienna: Urban and Schwarzenberg. (In press)   160

Eisenman, G., Krasne, S., and Ciani, S. (1976b): The kinetic and equilibrium components of selective ionic permeability mediated by nactin- and valinomycin-type carriers having systematically varied degrees of methylation. *In: International Conference on Carriers and Channels in Biological Systems. Ann. N.Y. Acad. Sci.* 264:34.   161

Eisenman, G., Szabo, G., Ciani, S., McLaughlin, S.G.A., and Krasne, S. (1973a): Ion binding and ion transport produced by lipid soluble molecules. *Prog. Surf. Memb. Sci.* 6:139-241.   155

Eisenman, G., Szabo, G., McLaughlin, S.G.A., and Ciani, S.M. (1973b): Molecular   155
basis for the action of macrocyclic carriers on passive ionic translocation across
lipid bilayer membranes. *J. Bioenerg.* 4:93-148.

Ellman, G.L. and Gan, G.L. (1973): Lithium ion and water balance in rats. *Toxicol.*   177
Appl. Pharmacol. 25:617-620.

Evans, H.J. and Sorger, G.J. (1966): Role of mineral elements with emphasis on the   151
univalent cations. *Annu. Rev. Plant Physiol.* 17:47-76.

Eyring, H., Lumry, R., and Woodbury, J.W. (1949): Some applications of modern   161
rate theory to physiological systems. *Recent Chem. Prog.* 10:100-114.

Fann, W.E., Davis, J.M., Janowsky, D.S., Cavanaugh, J.H., Kaufmann, J.S., Griffith,   167
J.D., and Oates, J.A. (1972): Effects of lithium on adrenergic function in man.
Clin. Pharmacol. Ther. 13:71-77.

Forn, J. (1975): Lithium and cyclic AMP. *In: Lithium Research and Therapy.*   154
Johnson, F.N., ed. New York: Academic Press, pp. 485-497.

Forn, J. and Valdecasas, F.G. (1971): Effects of lithium on brain adenyl cyclase
activity. *Biochem. Pharmacol.* 20:2773-2779.

Forrest, J.N., Jr., Cohen, A.D., Torretti, J., Himmelhoch, J.M., and Epstein, F.M.   175,177
(1974): On the mechanism of lithium-induced diabetes insipidus in man and the
rat. *J. Clin. Invest.* 53:1115-1123.

Frazer, A., Hancock, A., Mendels, J., and MacIntire, R. (1972): Effect of lithium   167
on catecholamine-induced responses in the isolated perfused guinea pig heart.
Biol. Psychiatry 5:79:87.

Friedman, E. and Gershon, S. (1973): Effect of lithium on brain dopamine. *Nature*   166
243:520-521.

Gardner, J.D. and Frantz, C. (1974): Effects of cations on ouabain binding by   155
intact human erythrocytes. *J. Membr. Biol.* 16:43-64.

Geisler, A., Wraae, O., and Olesen, O.V. (1972): Adenyl cyclase activity in kidneys   123,176
of rats with lithium-induced polyuria. *Acta Pharmacol. Toxicol.* 31:203-208.

Genefke, I.K. (1972): The concentration of 5-hydroxytryptamine (5-HT) in   123
hypothalamus, grey and white brain substance in the rat after prolonged oral
lithium administration. *Acta Psychiatr. Scand.* 48:400-404.

Gershon, E.S., Bunney, W., Jr., Leckman, J., Van Eerdewegh, M., and DeBauche, B.   125
(1976): The inheritance of affective disorders: a review of the data and
hypothesis. *Behav. Genet.* (In press)

Gershon, E.S., Dunner, D.L., and Goodwin, F. (1971): Toward a biology of   125
affective disorders: Genetic contributions. *Arch. Gen. Psychiatry* 25:1-15.

Gershon, S. and Shopsin, B., eds. (1973): *Lithium: Its Role in Psychiatric Research*   165
and Treatment. New York: Plenum Press.

Neurosciences Res. Prog. Bull., Vol. 14, No. 2

195

Page

Gilman, H. and Eisch, J.J. (1963): Lithium. *Sci. Am.* 208(1):89-102.

Goodwin, F.K. and Ebert, M.H. (1973): Lithium in mania: Clinical trials and controlled studies. *In: Lithium: Its Role in Psychiatric Research and Treatment.* Gershon, S. and Shopsin, B., eds. New York: Plenum Press, pp. 237-252.

Goodwin, F.K., Murphy, D.L., and Bunney, W.E., Jr. (1969): Lithium-carbonate treatment in depression and mania. *Arch. Gen. Psychiatry* 21:486-496.

Goodwin, F.K., Murphy, D.L., Dunner, D.L., and Bunney, W.E., Jr. (1972): Lithium response in unipolar versus bipolar depression. *Am. J. Psychiatry* 129:44-47.　　　129

Goodwin, F.K., Sack, R.L., and Post, R.M. (1975): Clinical evidence for neurotransmitter adaptation in response to antidepressant therapy. *In: Neurobiological Mechanisms of Adaptation and Behavior.* Mandell, A.J., ed. New York: Raven Press, pp. 33-45.　　　171

Gordon, M.W. and van der Velde, C.D. (1974): Metabolic adaptation in the manic-depressive. *Nature* 247:160-162.

Gottesfeld, Z., Ebstein, B.S., and Samuel, D. (1971): Effect of lithium on concentrations of glutamate and GABA levels in amygdala and hypothalamus of rat. *Nature New Biol.* 234:124-125.　　　168

Greenspan, K., Aronoff, M.S., and Bogdanski, D.F. (1970): Effects of lithium carbonate on turnover and metabolism of norepinephrine in rat brain—correlation to gross behavioral effects. *Pharmacology* 3:129-136.　　　166

Greenspan, K., Goodwin, F.K., Bunney, W.E., and Durell, J. (1968): Lithium ion retention and distribution. Patterns during acute mania and normothymia. *Arch. Gen. Psychiatry* 19:664-673.

Gustafson, T. (1950): Survey of the morphogenetic action of the lithium ion and the chemical basis of its action. *Rev. Suisse Zool.* 57(Suppl.):77-91.

Gustafson, T. and Lenicque, P. (1952): Studies on mitochondria in the developing sea urchin egg. *Exp. Cell Res.* 3:251-274.

Gutman, Y., Hochman, S., and Wald, H. (1973): The differential effect of lithium on microsomal ATPase in cortex, medulla and papilla of the rat kidney. *Biochim. Biophys. Acta* 298:284-290.　　　177

Handler, J.S. and Orloff, J. (1973): The mechanism of action of antidiuretic hormone. *In: Handbook of Physiology. Sec. 8. Renal Physiology.* Orloff, J. and Berliner, R.W., eds. Baltimore, Md.: Williams and Wilkins, pp. 791-814.　　　176

Hansen, H.H. and Zerahn, K. (1964): Concentration of lithium, sodium and potassium in epithelial cells of the isolated frog skin during active transport of lithium. *Acta Physiol. Scand.* 60:189-196.

Harris, C.A. and Jenner, F.A. (1972): Some aspects of the inhibition of the action of antidiuretic hormone by lithium ions in the rat kidney and bladder of the toad, *Bufo marinus. Br. J. Pharmacol.* 44:223-232.　　　123

Hemphill, R.M., Zielke, C.L., and Suelter, C.H. (1971): 5,'-adenosine monophosphate aminohydrolase. Evidence for anomalous substrate saturation kinetics at low enzyme concentrations. *J. Biol. Chem.* 246:7237-7240.

Henderson, R., Ritchie, J.M., and Strichartz, G.R. (1973): The binding of labelled saxitoxin to the sodium channels in nerve membranes. *J. Physiol.* 235:783-804.

Henderson, R., Ritchie, J.M., and Strichartz, G.R. (1974): Evidence that tetrodotoxin and saxitoxin act at a metal cation binding site. *Proc. Nat. Acad. Sci.* 71:3936-3940.

Herrera, F.C. (1972): Inhibition of lithium transport across toad bladder by amiloride. *Am. J. Physiol.* 222:499-502.

Hewitt, E.J. and Smith, T.A. (1974): *Plant Mineral Nutrition.* New York: Halsted   151
Press.

Hille, B. (1970): Ionic channels in nerve membranes. *Prog. Biophys. Mol. Biol.*   161
21:1-32.

Hille, B. (1971): The permeability of the sodium channel to organic cations in   160
myelinated nerve. *J. Gen. Physiol.* 58:599-619.

Hille, B. (1972): The permeability of the sodium channel to metal cations in   162
myelinated nerve. *J. Gen. Physiol.* 59:637-658.

Hille, B. (1973): Potassium channels in myelinated nerve. Selective permeability to   162
small cations. *J. Gen. Physiol.* 61:669-686.

Hille, B. (1975a): A four barrier model of the sodium channel. *Biophys. J.* 15:164a. 161
(Abstr.)

Hille, B. (1975b): Ionic selectivity of Na and K channels of nerve membranes. *In:*   161
Membranes. Vol. 3. Lipid Bilayers and Biological Membranes: Dynamic Processes. Eisenman, G., ed. New York: Marcel Dekker, pp. 255-323.

Ho, A.K.S., Loh, H.H., Craves, F., Hitzemann, R.J., and Gershon, S. (1970): The   166
effect of prolonged lithium treatment on the synthesis rate and turnover of monoamines in brain regions of rats. *Eur. J. Pharmacol.* 10:72-78.

Ho, A.K.S. and Tsai, C.S. (1975): Lithium and ethanol preference. *J. Pharm.*   131
Pharmacol. 27:58-59.

Hochman, S. and Gutman, Y. (1974): Lithium: ADH-antagonism and ADH   177
independent action in rats with diabetes insipidus. *Eur. J. Pharmacol.*
28:100-107.

Hörstadius, S. and Gustafson, T. (1948): On the developmental physiology of the
sea urchin. *Symp. Soc. Exp. Biol.* 2:50-56.

Huang, M. and Daly, J.W. (1972): The accumulation of cyclic adenosine   167
monophosphate in incubated slices of brain tissue: I. Structure-activity relationships of agonists and antagonists of biogenic amines and of tricyclic tranquilizers and antidepressants. *J. Med. Chem.* 15:458-463.

Hullin, R.P., McDonald, R., and Allsopp, M.N.E. (1972): Prophylactic lithium in recurrent affective disorders. *Lancet* 1:1044-1046.   120

Janowsky, D.S., Davis, J.M., El-Yousef, M.K., and Sekerke, H.J. (1972): A cholinergic-adrenergic hypothesis of mania and depression. *Lancet* 2:632-635.   165

Johnson, F.N., ed. (1975): *Lithium Research and Therapy*. New York: Academic Press.   165

Johnson, S. (1975): The effects of lithium on basic cellular processes. *In: Lithium Research and Therapy*. Johnson, F.N., ed. New York: Academic Press, pp. 533-556.   154

Katz, R.I., Chase, T.N., and Kopin, I.J. (1968): Evoked release of norepinephrine and serotonin from brain slices: Inhibition by lithium. *Science* 162:466-467.   166

Katz, R.I. and Kopin, I.J. (1969): Release of norepinephrine-^{3}H and serotonin-^{3}H evoked from brain slices by electrical-field stimulation—calcium dependency and the effects of lithium, ouabain and tetrodotoxin. *Biochem. Pharmacol.* 18:1935-1939.   166

Kayne, F.J. (1971): Thallium (I) activation of pyruvate kinase. *Arch. Biochem. Biophys.* 143:232-239.   152

Kayne, F.J. and Freedman, R. (1975): Monovalent-divalent cation interactions in pyruvate kinase. *Fed. Proc.* 34:566. (Abstr.)   152

Kety, S.S. (1971): Brain amines and affective disorders. *In: Brain Chemistry and Mental Disease. Advances in Behavioral Biology, Vol. 1*. Ho, B.T. and McIsaac, W.M., eds. New York: Plenum Press, pp. 237-244.   181

Kirch, M. and Lehn, J.M. (1975): Selective transport of alkali metal cations through a liquid membrane by macrobicyclic carriers. *Angew. Chem.* 14:555-556.   135,136

Kline, N.S., Wren, J.C., Cooper, T.B., Varga, E., and Canal, O. (1974): Evaluation of lithium therapy in chronic and periodic alcoholism. *Am. J. Med. Sci.* 268:15-22.   131

Knapp, S. and Mandell, A.J. (1972): Narcotic drugs: Effects on the serotonin biosynthetic systems of the brain. *Science* 177:1209-1211.   173

Knapp, S. and Mandell, A.J. (1973): Short- and long-term lithium administration: Effects on the brain's serotonergic biosynthetic systems. *Science* 180:645-647.   170,182

Knapp, S. and Mandell, A.J. (1974): Serotonin biosynthetic capacity of mouse C-1300 neuroblastoma cells in culture. *Brain Res.* 66:547-551.

Knapp, S. and Mandell, A.J. (1975): Effects of lithium chloride on parameters of biosynthetic capacity for 5-hydroxytryptamine in rat brain. *J. Pharm. Exp. Ther.* 193:812-823.   170,171, 182

Knapp, S., Mandell, A.J., and Bullard, W.P. (1975): Calcium activation of brain tryptophan hydroxylase. *Life Sci.* 16:1583-1594.

Knapp, S., Mandell, A.J., and Geyer, M.A. (1974): Effects of amphetamines on   173
regional tryptophan hydroxylase activity and synaptosomal conversion of
tryptophan to 5-hydroxytryptamine in rat brain. *J. Pharmacol. Exp. Ther.*
189:676-689.

Krell, R.D. and Goldberg, A.M. (1973): Effect of acute and chronic administration   168
of lithium on steady-state levels of mouse brain choline and acetylcholine.
Biochem. Pharmacol. 22:3289-3291.

Kuechler, E. and Rich, A. (1969): Sequential synthesis of messenger RNA and
antibodies in rabbit lymph nodes. *Nature* 222:544-547.

Kuechler, E. and Rich, A. (1969): Two rapidly labeled RNA species in the
polysomes of antibody-producing lymphoid tissue. *Proc. Nat. Acad. Sci.*
63:520-527.

Kuriyama, K. and Speken, R. (1970): Effect of lithium on content and uptake of   166
norepinephrine and 5-hydroxytryptamine in mouse brain synaptosomes and
mitochondria. *Life Sci.* 9:1213-1220.

Leblanc, G. (1972): The mechanism of lithium accumulation in the isolated frog
skin epithelium. *Pfluegers Arch.* 337:1-18.

Lee, G., Lingsch, C., Lyle, P.T., and Martin, K. (1974): Lithium treatment strongly   123
inhibits choline transport in human erythrocytes. *Br. J. Clin. Pharmacol.*
1:365-370.

Lehn, J.-M. (1973): Design of organic complexing agents. Strategies towards   133,134,
properties. *In: Structure and Bonding, Vol. 16.* Dunitz, J.D. et al., eds. Berlin: 135
Springer-Verlag, pp. 2-69.

Lehn, J.-M. and Sauvage, J.P. (1976): Stability and selectivity of alkali and   135
alkaline-earth (2)-cryptate complexes. *J. Am. Chem. Soc.* (In press)

Lehn, J.-M., Sauvage, J.P., and Dietrich, B. (1970): Cryptates: Cation exchange   133
rates. *J. Am. Chem. Soc.* 92:2916-2918.

Lehn, J.-M., Simon, J., and Wagner, J. (1973a): Mesomolecules. Polyaza-polyoxa   133
macropolycyclic systems. *Angew. Chem.* 12:578-579.

Lehn, J.-M., Simon, J., and Wagner, J. (1973b): Molecular and cation complexes of   133
macrotricyclic and macrotetracyclic ligands. *Angew. Chem.* 12:579-580.

Levine, B.A., Thornton, J.M., and Williams, R.J.P. (1974): Conformational studies   149
of lanthanide complexes with carboxylate ligands. *J. Chem. Soc. (Lond.) Chem.*
Commun. pp. 669-670.

Lindvall, O. and Björklund, A. (1974): The organization of the ascending
catecholamine neuron systems in the rat brain as revealed by the glyoxylic acid
fluorescence method. *Acta Physiol. Scand.* Suppl. 412.

Neurosciences Res. Prog. Bull., Vol. 14, No. 2   **199**

Page

McGregor, W.G., Phillips, J., and Suelter, C.H. (1974): Purification and kinetic   152
characterization of a monovalent cation-activated glycerol dehydrogenase from
Aerobacter aerogenes. J. Biol. Chem. 249:3132-3139.

McMahon, D. (1974): Chemical messengers in development: A hypothesis. *Science*
185:1012-1021.

Madison, V., Attreyi, M., Deber, C.M., and Blout, E.R. (1974): Cyclic peptides. IX.
Conformations of a synthetic ion-binding cyclic peptide, *cyclo*-(Pro-Gly)$_3$, from
circular dichroism and ^{1}H and ^{13}C nuclear magnetic resonance. *J. Am. Chem.
Soc.* 96:6725-6734.

Mandell, A.J. (1973a): Neurobiological barriers to euphoria. *Am. Sci.* 61:565-573.

Mandell, A.J. (1973b): Redundant macromolecular mechanisms in central synaptic
regulation. *In: New Concepts in Neurotransmitter Regulation.* Mandell, A.J., ed.
New York: Plenum Press, pp. 259-277.

Mandell, A.J. and Knapp, S. (1974): Regulation of function of tryptophan
hydroxylase. *In: Neuropsychopharmacology of Monoamines and Their Regulatory Enzymes.* Usdin, E., ed. New York: Raven Press, pp. 177-188.

Mandell, A.J. and Knapp, S. (1975a): A model for the neurobiological mechanisms   172
of action involved in lithium prophylaxis of bipolar affective disorder. *In:
Aminergic Hypotheses of Behavior: Reality or Cliche?* Bernard, B.K., ed.
Washington, D.C.: NIDA Res. Monograph Series 3, pp. 97-197.

Mandell, A.J. and Knapp, S. (1975b): Neurobiological mechanisms in lithium   170,172,
prophylaxis of manic-depressive disease: an hypothesis. *In: Chemical Tools in*   173
Catecholamine Research, Vol. 2. Almgren, O., Carlsson, A., and Engel, J., eds.
Amsterdam: North-Holland Publishing Co., pp. 9-16.

Mandell, A.J., Knapp, S., and Hsu, L.L. (1974): *Minireview.* Some factors in the
regulation of central serotonergic synapses. *Life Sci.* 14:1-17.

Mandell, A.J., Segal, D.S., Kuczenski, R.T., and Knapp, S. (1972): Some
macromolecular mechanisms in CNS neurotransmitter pharmacology and their
psychobiological organization. *In: The Chemistry of Mood, Motivation and
Memory. Advances in Behavioral Biology, Vol. 4.* McGaugh, J.L., ed. New York:
Plenum Press, pp. 105-148.

Marshall, M.H., Neumann, C.P., and Robinson, M. (1970): Lithium, creativity, and   121
manic-depressive illness: Review and prospectus. *Psychosomatics* 11:406-408.

Matthews, B.W., Weaver, L.H., and Kester, W.R. (1974): The conformation of   145
thermolysin. *J. Biol. Chem.* 249:8030-8044.

Mazia, D., Petzelt, C., Williams, R.O., and Meza, I. (1972): A Ca-activated ATPase
in the mitotic apparatus of the sea urchin egg (isolated by a new method). *Exp.
Cell Res.* 70:325-332.

Melia, P.I. (1970): Prophylactic lithium: A double-blind trial in recurrent affective   120
disorders. *Br. J. Psychiatry* 116:621-624.

Mendels, J. and Frazer, A. (1973): Intracellular lithium concentration and clinical
response: Towards a membrane theory of depression. *J. Psychiatr. Res.* 10:9-18.

Mendlewicz, J. and Fleiss, J.L. (1974): Linkage studies with X-chromosome   125
markers in bipolar (manic-depressive) and unipolar (depressive) illnesses. *Biol.
Psychiatry* 9:261-294.

Moews, P.C. and Kretsinger, R.H. (1975): Refinement of the structure of carp   145
muscle calcium-binding parvalbumin by model building and difference Fourier
analysis. *J. Mol. Biol.* 91:201-228.

Murphy, D.L., Baker, M., Goodwin, F.K., Miller, H., Kotin, J., and Bunney, W.E.,   173
Jr. (1974): L-Tryptophan in affective disorders: indoleamine changes and
differential clinical effects. *Psychopharmacologia* 34:11-20.

Murphy, D.L. and Bunney, W.E., Jr. (1971): Total body potassium changes during
lithium administration. *J. Nerv. Ment. Dis.* 152:381-389.

Murphy, D.L., Colburn, R.W., Davis, J.M., and Bunney, W.E., Jr. (1969a):
Stimulation by lithium of monoamine uptake in human platelets. *Life Sci.*
8:1187-1193.

Murphy, D.L., Colburn, R.W., Davis, J.M., and Bunney, W.E., Jr. (1970):
Imipramine and lithium effects on biogenic amine transport in depressed and
manic-depressed patients. *Am. J. Psychiatry* 127:339-345.

Murphy, D.L., Donnelly, C., and Moskowitz, J. (1973): Inhibition by lithium of   167
prostaglandin E_1 and norepinephrine effects on cyclic adenosine monophosphate production in human platelets. *Clin. Pharmacol. Ther.* 14:810-814.

Murphy, D.L., Goodwin, F.K., and Bunney, W.E., Jr. (1969b): Aldosterone and
sodium response to lithium administration in man. *Lancet* 2:458-461.

Murphy, D.L., Goodwin, F.K., and Bunney, W.E., Jr. (1971): Leukocytosis during
lithium treatment. *Am. J. Psychiatry* 127:1559-1561.

Murphy, D.L. and Kopin, I.J. (1972): The transport of biogenic amines. *In:*   166
Metabolic Transport. Metabolic Pathways, Vol. 6. 3rd Ed. Hokin, L.E., ed. New
York: Academic Press, pp. 503-542.

Natochin, Y.V. and Leont'ev, V.G. (1965): Pituitrin stimulation of active transport
of lithium by wall of frog urinary bladder. *Fed. Proc.* 24:T403-T407.

Olesen, O.V. and Thomsen, K. (1974): Effect of prolonged lithium ingestion on   123
glucagon and parathyroid hormone responses in rats. *Acta Pharmacol. Toxicol.*
34:225-231.

Paton, W.D.M., Vizi, E.S., and AbooZar, M. (1971): The mechanism of acetyl-   168
choline release from parasympathetic nerves. *J. Physiol.* 215:819-848.

Neurosciences Res. Prog. Bull., Vol. 14, No. 2   **201**

Page

Pauling, L. (1960): *The Nature of the Chemical Bond and the Structure of Molecules and Crystals: An Introduction to Modern Structural Chemistry.* 3rd Ed. Ithaca, N.Y.: Cornell University Press.   157

Pearson, I.B. and Jenner, F.A. (1971): Lithium in psychiatry. *Nature* 232:532-533.

Persson, T. (1970): Drug induced changes in ^{3}H-catecholamine accumulation after ^{3}H-tyrosine. *Acta Pharmacol. Toxicol.* 28:378-390.   166

Petersen, V., Hvidt, S., Thomsen, K., and Schou, M. (1974): Effect of prolonged thiazide treatment on renal lithium clearance. *Br. Med. J.* 13:143-145.   122

Pick, G. and Mills, W.A. (1971): The effects of lithium and amphetamine on threshold of intracranial reinforcement. Presented at the 42nd Annual Meeting of the Eastern Psychological Assoc.   167

Plenge, P., Mellerup, E.T., and Rafaelsen, O.J. (1970): Lithium action on glycogen synthesis in rat brain, liver, and diaphragm. *J. Psychiatr. Res.* 8:29-36.   123

Ploeger, E.J. (1973): The effects of lithium on excitable cell membranes. I. The effect on the ionic distribution and the resting potential of rat striated muscle fibres. *Eur. J. Pharmacol.* 21:21-23.

Ploeger, E.G. (1974): The effects of lithium on excitable cell membranes: On the mechanism of inhibition of the sodium pump of non-myelinated nerve fibres of the rat. *Eur. J. Pharmacol.* 25:316-321.   169

Ploeger, E.J. and Den Hertog, A. (1973): The effects of lithium on excitable cell membranes. II. The effect on the electrogenic sodium pump of non-myelinated nerve fibres of the rat. *Eur. J. Pharmacol.* 21:24-29.

Polatin, P. and Fieve, R.R. (1971): Patient rejection of lithium carbonate prophylaxis. *J. Am. Med. Assoc.* 218:864-866.   121

Prien, R.F., Caffey, E.M., Jr., and Klett, C.J. (1973a): Prophylactic efficacy of lithium carbonate in manic-depressive illness. *Arch. Gen. Psychiatry* 28:337-341.   120

Prien, R.F., Klett, C.J., and Caffey, E.M., Jr. (1973b): Lithium carbonate and imipramine in prevention of affective episodes. A comparison in recurrent affective illness. *Arch. Gen. Psychiatry* 29:420-425.   120

Ranzi, S. (1962): The proteins in embryonic and larval development. *Adv. Morphog.* 2:211-257.

Reuben, J. and Kayne, F.J. (1971): Thallium-205 nuclear magnetic resonance study of pyruvate kinase and its substrates. Evidence for a substrate-induced conformational change. *J. Biol. Chem.* 246:6227-6234.   152

Rhoads, D.G. (1970): Study on adenylate deaminase from calf brain. Doctoral dissertation, Brandeis University, Waltham, Mass.   153,154

Rogawski, M.A., Knapp, S., and Mandell, A.J. (1974): Effects of ethanol on
   tryptophan hydroxylase activity from striate synaptosomes. *Biochem. Pharmacol.* 23:1955-1962.

Rose, B. and Loewenstein, W.R. (1971): Junctional membrane permeability.
   Depression by substitution of Li for extracellular Na, and by long-term lack of
   Ca and Mg; restoration by cell repolarization. *J. Membr. Biol.* 5:20-50.

Ross, V. and Rich, A. (1969-1970): Nuclear magnetic resonance analysis of
   neurotransmitter and drug-nucleotide interactions. *In: N.M.R. Preliminary
   Studies of Lithium–Neurotransmitters–Nucleotide Interactions: M.I.T. Biology
   Dept. Summaries,* pp. 102-103.

Rowlinson, J.S. (1951): The lattice energy of ice and the second virial coefficient   156
   of water vapour. *Trans. Faraday Soc.* 47:120-129.

Runnström, J. and Immers, J. (1970): Heteromorphic budding in lithium-treated
   sea urchin embryos. *Exp. Cell Res.* 62:228-238.

Runnström, J. and Markman, B. (1966): Gene dependency of vegetalization in sea
   urchin embryos treated with lithium. *Biol. Bull.* 130:402-414.

Samuel, D. and Gottesfeld, Z. (1973): Lithium, manic-depression, and the
   chemistry of the brain. *Endeavour* 32:122-128.

Sanghvi, I., Geyer, H.M., and Gershon, S. (1973): The effect of lithium on   167
   adrenergic function in dog. *Life Sci.* 12:337-344.

Sanghvi, I., Urquiaga, X., and Gershon, S. (1970): The effect of acute and chronic   167
   lithium administration on the superior cervical ganglion of the cat. *Pharmacol.
   Res. Commun.* 2:361-368.

Schildkraut, J.J. (1965): The catecholamine hypothesis of affective disorders: A
   review of supporting evidence. *Am. J. Psychiatry* 122:509-522.

Schildkraut, J.J. (1973): Pharmacology–the effects of lithium on biogenic amines.   155,166
   In: Lithium: Its Role in Psychiatric Research and Treatment. Gershon, S. and
   Shopsin, B., eds. New York: Plenum Press, pp. 51-73.

Schildkraut, J.J. and Kety, S.S. (1967): Biogenic amines and emotion. *Science*   165
   156:21-30.

Schildkraut, J.J., Logue, M.A., and Dodge, G.A. (1969): Effects of lithium salts on   166
   turnover and metabolism of norepinephrine in rat brain. *Psychopharmacologia*
   14:135-141.

Schildkraut, J.J., Schanberg, S.M., and Kopin, I.J. (1966): The effects of lithium   166
   ion on H^3-norepinephrine metabolism in brain. *Life Sci.* 5:1479-1483.

Schou, M. (1956): Lithiumterapi ved mani. Praktiske retningslinier. *Nord. Med.*   117
   55:790-794.

Page

Schou, M. (1957): Biology and pharmacology of the lithium ion. *Pharmacol. Rev.*   165
9:17-58.

Schou, M. (1968): Lithium in psychiatric therapy and prophylaxis. *J. Psychiatr.*   121
Res. 6:67-95.

Schou, M. (1969): The biology and pharmacology of lithium: A bibliography.   165
Psychopharmacol. Bull. 5:33-62.

Schou, M. (1972): A bibliography on the biology and pharmacology of lithium—   165
Appendix I. *Psychopharmacol. Bull.* 8:36-62.

Schou, M. (1973a): Possible mechanisms of action of lithium salts: Approaches and
perspectives. *Biochem. Soc. Trans.* 1:81-87.

Schou, M. (1973b): Practical problems of lithium maintenance treatment.
Psychiatr. Neurol. Neurochir. (Amst.) 76:511-522.

Schou, M. (1973c): Preparations, dosage, and control. *In: Lithium: Its Role in*
Psychiatric Research and Treatment. Gershon, S. and Shopsin, B., eds. New
York: Plenum Press, pp. 189-199.

Schou, M. (1973d): Prophylactic lithium maintenance treatment in recurrent   117,119
endogenous affective disorders. *In: Lithium: Its Role in Psychiatric Research*
and Treatment. Gershon, S. and Shopsin, B., eds. New York: Plenum Press,
pp. 269-294.

Schou, M. (1976): A bibliography on the biology and pharmacology of lithium—   165
Appendix II. *Psychopharmacol. Bull.* 12:49-74.

Schou, M. (1976): Current status of lithium therapy in affective disorders and other
diseases. *In: Lithium in Psychiatry. A Synopsis.* Villeneuve, A., ed. Quebec: Les
Presses de l'Université Laval. (In press)

Schou, M. and Baastrup, P.C. (1973): Personal and social implications of lithium   121
maintenance treatment. *In: Psychopharmacology, Sexual Disorders and Drug*
Abuse. Ban, T.A. et al., eds. Amsterdam: North-Holland Publishing Co.,
pp. 65-68.

Schou, M. and Thomsen, K. (1975): Lithium prophylaxis of recurrent endogenous   117,120
affective disorders. *In: Lithium Research and Therapy.* Johnson, F.N., ed. New
York: Academic Press, pp. 63-84.

Sedvall, G., Jönsson, B., and Petterson, U. (1969): Evidence of an altered thyroid   178
function in man during treatment with lithium carbonate. *Acta Psychiatr. Scand.*
Suppl. 207:59-66.

Sedvall, G., Jönsson, B., Petterson, U., and Levin, K. (1968): Effects of lithium   178
salts on plasma protein bound iodine and uptake of I^{131} in thyroid gland of
man and rat. *Life Sci.* 7(Part I):1257-1264.

Page

Segal, D.S., Callaghan, M., and Mandell, A.J. (1975): Alterations in behaviour and   173
catecholamine biosynthesis induced by lithium. *Nature* 254:58-59.

Segal, M. (1974): Lithium and the monoamine neurotransmitters in the rat   174
hippocampus. *Nature* 250:71-73.

Siggins, G.R., Hoffer, B.J., and Bloom, F.E. (1969): Cyclic adenosine monophos-   167,168
phate: possible mediator for norepinephrine effects on cerebellar Purkinje cells.
Science 165:1018-1020.

Sinclair, J.D. (1974): Lithium-induced suppression of alcohol drinking by rats.   131
Med. Biol. 52:133-136.

Singer, I. and Franko, E.A. (1973): Lithium-induced ADH resistance in toad   177
urinary bladders. *Kidney Int.* 3:151-159.

Singer, I. and Goodman, S.J. (1966): Mammalian ependyma: Some physicochemical determinants of ciliary activity. *Exp. Cell Res.* 43:367-380.

Singer, I. and Rotenberg, D. (1973): Mechanisms of lithium action. *N. Engl. J. Med.*   175
289:254-260.

Singer, I., Rotenberg, D., and Puschett, J.B. (1972): Lithium-induced nephrogenic   176,177
diabetes insipidus: In vivo and in vitro studies. *J. Clin. Invest.* 51:1081-1091.

Small, J.G., Milstein, V., Perez, H.C., Small, I.F., and Moore, D.F. (1972): EEG and   121
neurophysiological studies of lithium in normal volunteers. *Biol. Psychiatry*
5:65-77.

Smiley, K.L., Jr., Berry, A.J., and Suelter, C.H. (1967): An improved purification,   153
crystallization, and some properties of rabbit muscle 5'-adenylic acid deaminase.
J. Biol. Chem. 242:2502-2506.

Smiley, K.L., Jr. and Suelter, C.H. (1967): Univalent cations as allosteric activators   152
of muscle adenosine 5'-phosphate deaminase. *J. Biol. Chem.* 242:1980-1981.

Smith, D.F. and Balagura, S. (1972): Sodium appetite in rats given lithium. *Life*   177
Sci. 11(Part I):1021-1029.

Smith, D.F., Balagura, S., and Lubran, M. (1970): "Antidotal thirst": A response to   177
intoxication. *Science* 167:297-298.

Smith, L.D. and Kizer, D.E. (1969): Purification and properties of rat liver AMP   153,154
deaminase. *Biochim. Biophys. Acta* 191:415-424.

Solomon, S. (1967): Action of alkali metals in papillary-cortical sodium gradient of   175
dog kidney. *Proc. Soc. Exp. Biol. Med.* 125:1183-1186.

Stallone, F., Shelley, E., Mendlewicz, J., and Fieve, R.R. (1973): The use of lithium   120
in affective disorders, III: A double-blind study of prophylaxis in bipolar illness.
Am. J. Psychiatry 130:1006-1010.

Neurosciences Res. Prog. Bull., Vol. 14, No. 2   205

Page

Stern, D.N., Fieve, R.R., Neff, N.H., and Costa, E. (1969): The effect of lithium   166
chloride administration on brain and heart norepinephrine turnover rates.
Psychopharmacologia 14:315-322.

Stolk, J.M., Nowack, W.J., and Barchas, J.D. (1970): Brain norepinephrine: 168
enhanced turnover after rubidium treatment. *Science* 168:501-503.

Suelter, C.H. (1970): Enzymes activated by monovalent cations. *Science*   151
168:789-795.

Suelter, C.H. (1974): Monovalent cations in enzyme-catalyzed reactions. *In: Metal
Ions in Biological Systems, Vol. 3. High Molecular Complexes.* Sigel, H., ed. New
York: Marcel Dekker, pp. 201-251.

Suelter, C.H., Kovacs, A.L., and Antonini, E. (1968): Time dependence of
activation of muscle AMP-aminohydrolase by substrate and potassium ion. *FEBS
Letters* 2:65-68.

Suelter, C.H., Singleton, R., Jr., Kayne, F.J., Arrington, S., Glass, J., and Mildvan,   152
A.S. (1966): Studies on the interaction of substrate and monovalent and
divalent cations with pyruvate kinase. *Biochemistry* 5:131-139.

Tasaki, I., Singer, I., and Takenaka, T. (1965): Effects of internal and external ionic
environment on excitability of squid giant axon. A macromolecular approach. *J.
Gen. Physiol.* 48:1095-1123.

Temple, R., Berman, M., Carlson, H.E., Robbins, J., and Wolff, J. (1972): The use   178
of lithium in Graves' disease. *Mayo Clin. Proc.* 47:872-878.

Temple, R., Berman, M., Robbins, J., and Wolff, J. (1972): The use of lithium in
the treatment of thyrotoxicosis. *J. Clin. Invest.* 51:2746-2756.

Teorell, T. (1954): Rhythmical potential and impedance variations in isolated frog
skin induced by lithium ions. *Acta Physiol. Scand.* 31:268-382.

Thomas, E.L., Shao, T.-C., and Christensen, H.N. (1971): Structural selectivity in
interaction of neutral amino acids and alkali metal ions with a cationic amino
acid transport system. *J. Biol. Chem.* 246:1677-1681.

Thomsen, K. (1970): Lithium-induced polyuria in rats. *Int. Pharmacopsychiatry*   123
5:233-241.

Thomsen, K., Jensen, J., and Olesen, O.V. (1974): Lithium-induced loss of body   122,175
sodium and the development of severe intoxication in rats. *Acta Pharmacol.
Toxicol.* 35:337-346.

Thomsen, K., Jensen, J., and Olesen, O.V. (1976a): Effect of prolonged lithium   122
ingestion on the response to mineralocorticoids in rats. *J. Pharmacol. Exp. Ther.*
(In press)

Thomsen, K., Olesen, O.V., Jensen, J., and Schou, M. (1976b): The mechanism of   122
gradually developing lithium intoxication in rats. *In: Current Developments in
Psychopharmacology.* Valzelli, L. and Essman, W.B., eds. New York: Spectrum
Publ. (In press)

Thomsen, K. and Schou, M. (1968): Renal lithium excretion in man. *Am. J.* 122,175
Physiol. 215:823-827.

Thomsen, K. and Schou, M. (1973): The effect of prolonged administration of 122
hydrochlorothiazide on the renal lithium clearance and the urine flow of
ordinary rats and rats with diabetes insipidus. *Pharmakopsychiatr. Neuropsycho-*
pharmakol. 6:264-269.

van Kammen, D.P. and Murphy, D.L. (1975): Attenuation of the euphoriant and 131,168,
activating effects of d- and l-amphetamine by lithium carbonate treatment. 173
Psychopharmacologia 44:215-224.

Vizi, E.S., Illés, P., Rónai, A., and Knoll, J. (1972): The effect of lithium on 165,168,
acetylcholine release and synthesis. *Neuropharmacology* 11:521-530. 169

Wacker, W.E.C. and Williams, R.J.P. (1968): Magnesium/calcium balances and
steady states of biological systems. *J. Theor. Biol.* 20:65-78.

Wang, Y.-C., Pandey, G.N., Mendels, J., and Frazer, A. (1974): Effect of lithium on 167
prostaglandin E_1-stimulated adenylate cyclase activity of human platelets.
Biochem. Pharmacol. 23:845-855.

Waziri, R. (1968): Presynaptic effects of lithium on cholinergic synaptic trans- 169
mission in *Aplysia* neurons. *Life Sci.* 7:865-873.

Wilkinson, G.N. (1961): Statistical estimations in enzyme kinetics. *Biochem. J.*
80:324-332.

Williams, J.A., Berens, S.C., and Wolff, J. (1971): Thyroid secretion *in vitro:* 179
Inhibition of TSH and dibutyryl cyclic-AMP stimulated ^{131}I release by Li^+.
Endocrinology 88:1385-1388.

Williams, R.J.P. (1970a): The biochemistry of sodium, potassium, magnesium, and
calcium. *Q. Rev. Lond. Chem. Soc.* 24:331-365.

Williams, R.J.P. (1970b): Cation distributions and the energy status of cells.
Bioenergetics 1:215-225.

Williams, R.J.P. (1972): A dynamic view of biological membranes. *Physiol. Chem.*
Phys. 4:427-439.

Williams, R.J.P. (1973): The chemistry and biochemistry of lithium. *In: Lithium:* 116
Its Role in Psychiatric Research and Treatment. Gershon, S. and Shopsin, B.,
eds. New York: Plenum Press, pp. 15-31.

Williams, R.J.P. (1974): Calcium ions: Their ligands and their functions. *Biochem.*
Soc. Symp. 39:133-138.

Williams, R.J.P. (1975): The binding of metal ions to membranes and its
consequences. *In: Biological Membranes.* Parsons, D.S., ed. Oxford: Oxford
University Press, pp. 106-121.

Neurosciences Res. Prog. Bull., Vol. 14, No. 2   207

Page

Willis, J.S. and Fang, L.S.S. (1970): Lithium stimulation of ouabain-sensitive   177
respiration and (Na$^+$-K$^+$)-ATPase of kidney cortex of ground squirrels. *Biochim. Biophys. Acta* 219:486-489.

Winkler, R. (1972): Kinetics and mechanism of alkali ion complex formation in solution. *In: Structure and Bonding, Vol. 10.* Dunitz, J.D. et al., eds. Berlin: Springer-Verlag, pp. 1-24.

Wittrig, J., Woods, A.E., and Anthony, E.J. (1970): Mechanisms of lithium action.   177
Dis. Nerv. System 31:767-771.

Wolff, J., Berens, S.C., and Jones, A.B. (1970): Inhibition of thyrotropin-   178,179
stimulated adenyl cyclase activity of beef thyroid membranes by low concentration of lithium ion. *Biochem. Biophys. Res. Commun.* 39:77-82.

Wraae, O., Geisler, A., and Olesen, O.V. (1972): The relation between vasopressin   123,177
stimulation of renal adenyl cyclase and lithium-induced polyuria in rats. *Acta Pharmacol. Toxicol.* 31:314-317.

Zerahn, K. (1955): Studies on the active transport of lithium in the isolated frog skin. *Acta Physiol. Scand.* 33:347-358.

NEURON-TARGET CELL INTERACTIONS

Based on an NRP Work Session
held June 22-24, 1975, and updated by participants

by

Barry H. Smith
Neurosciences Research Program
Boston, Massachusetts

and

Georg W. Kreutzberg
Max Planck Institute for Psychiatry
Munich, Federal Republic of Germany

Yvonne M. Homsy
NRP Writer-Editor

CONTENTS

PARTICIPANTS

Edson X. Albuquerque
Department of Pharmacology and
    Experimental Therapeutics
University of Maryland
    School of Medicine
660 West Redwood Street
Baltimore, Maryland 21201

Barry Arnason
Department of Neurology
Massachusetts General Hospital
Boston, Massachusetts 02114

Mark A. Bisby
Division of Medical Physiology
University of Calgary
2920 24th Avenue, NW
Calgary, Alberta T2N 1N4, Canada

Ira B. Black
Department of Neurology
The New York Hospital-Cornell
    Medical Center
525 East 68th Street
New York, New York 10021

Floyd E. Bloom
Arthur V. Davis Center for
    Behavioral Neurobiology
Salk Institute
P.O. Box 1809
San Diego, California 92112

Jack Diamond
Department of Neurosciences
McMaster University Medical Center
1200 Main Street West
Hamilton, Ontario L8S 4J9, Canada

Mac V. Edds, Jr.*
Neurosciences Research Program
165 Allandale Street
Jamaica Plain, Massachusetts 02130

Bernice Grafstein
Department of Physiology
Cornell University Medical College
1300 York Avenue
New York, New York 10021

Lloyd A. Greene
Department of Neuroscience
Children's Hospital Medical Center
300 Longwood Avenue
Boston, Massachusetts 02115

Lloyd Guth
Department of Anatomy
University of Maryland
    School of Medicine
29 S. Greene Street
Baltimore, Maryland 21201

Karl Herrup
Department of Neuroscience
Children's Hospital Medical Center
300 Longwood Avenue
Boston, Massachusetts 02115

Asao Hirano
Department of Pathology
Montefiore Hospital and Medical Center
111 East 210th Street
Bronx, New York 10467

Georg W. Kreutzberg
Max Planck Institute for Psychiatry
Kraepelinstrasse 2
8 Munich 23
Federal Republic of Germany

Lynn T. Landmesser
Department of Biology
Yale University
New Haven, Connecticut 06520

*Deceased November 29, 1975.

Jennifer LaVail
Department of Neuroscience
Children's Hospital Medical Center
300 Longwood Avenue
Boston, Massachusetts 02115

Thomas L. Lentz
Section of Cytology
Yale University School of Medicine
333 Cedar Street
New Haven, Connecticut 06510

Gary Lynch
Department of Psychobiology
University of California, Irvine
Irvine, California 92664

Michael A. Moskowitz
Department of Nutrition and
    Food Science
Massachusetts Institute of
    Technology, 56-245
Cambridge, Massachusetts 02139

Paul Patterson
Department of Neurobiology
Harvard Medical School
25 Shattuck Street
Boston, Massachusetts 02115

Geoffrey Raisman
Laboratory of Neurobiology
National Institute for Medical Research
The Ridgeway, Mill Hill
London NW7 1AA, England

Stephen A. Rudolph
Department of Pharmacology
Yale University School of Medicine
333 Cedar Street
New Haven, Connecticut 06510

Francis O. Schmitt
Neurosciences Research Program
165 Allandale Street
Jamaica Plain, Massachusetts 02130

Peter Schubert
Max Planck Institute for Psychiatry
Kraepelinstrasse 2
8 Munich 23
Federal Republic of Germany

Barry H. Smith
Neurosciences Research Program
165 Allandale Street
Jamaica Plain, Massachusetts 02130

Hans Thoenen
Department of Pharmacology
Biocenter of the University of Basel
Klingelbergstrasse 70
CH-4056 Basel, Switzerland

Frederic G. Worden
Neurosciences Research Program
165 Allandale Street
Jamaica Plain, Massachusetts 02130

Richard J. Wurtman
Department of Nutrition and
    Food Science
Massachusetts Institute of
    Technology, 56-245
Cambridge, Massachusetts 02139

Note: NRP Work Session reports are reviewed and revised by participants prior to publication.

I. INTRODUCTION

The neuron is most commonly thought of as a receiver, processor, and transmitter of electrical signals. Indeed, this view, which is found in textbooks, neglects an evolutionarily older neuronal attribute: "secretory function." This function was best demonstrated by Bargmann (1949a,b) when he elucidated the neurosecretory pathway from the hypothalamus to the pituitary in mammals. With the subsequent documentation of both antero- and retrograde axonal and dendritic transport, as well as of the transsynaptic movement of nontransmitter molecules, this secretory activity (as well as more general release phenomena) has become recognized as a fundamental neuronal property that is by no means restricted to a few specialized neurosecretory cells, or even to a single region of such a cell. Furthermore, evidence has been obtained that there is actually a bidirectional, transsynaptic, and transcellular interchange between neurons and their target cells (including other neurons, glia, and a variety of peripheral or end-organ cells). This molecular transfer is critical to the continued health and even the viability of the cells involved. The potential significance of such an interchange in neuronal circuitry, whether for transcellular nutrition, metabolic coupling within a given circuit, or even information processing, is great. After in-depth discussions of these ideas at NRP planning sessions, it became readily apparent that a Work Session was needed to explore further the full potential of molecular flux in neuronal circuitry.

Historical Perspectives

Not only is the concept of neurotrophic function an old one, but the term "trophism" has been used in different ways by various authors. For example, the trophic functions of neurons were discussed in the pathology literature of the nineteenth century. The first evidence for a theory of the trophic function of the nervous system was provided by Magendie (1824), the great experimental physiologist, while experimenting with irritation of the trigeminal nerve to produce corneal ulcerations. Confirming and expanding on Magendie's experiments, Samuel (1860) in his book, *Die trophischen Nerven,* concluded that there is a special "trophic nervous system" in the organism. After close examination of secretory nerves and much experimental work, Heidenhain (1878) demonstrated the trophic influences of the nervous system and postulated the existence of trophic fibers in the composition of sympathetic nerves. In 1874, the French neurologist Charcot was able to state:

> Rien de mieux établi en pathologie, que l'existence de ces troubles trophiques consécutifs aux lésions de centres nerveux ou de nerfs.*

The precise nature of neurotrophism, of course, was not made explicit in this early research. Much of the subsequent data came from the examination of war injuries (nerve trauma) resulting in neuromas, trophic ulcers, vasomotor disturbances, etc. The efforts of the French physiologist, Claude Bernard, were mainly directed at determining the influence of the nervous system on general metabolism. In 1922 Pavlov† published an article devoted to postoperative gastrointestinal tract pathology in dogs; he regarded these processes as a disorder of neurotrophism secondary to an operative injury of the nervous system. Loewi (1921), collecting wash fluid from a stimulated heart, found that the fluid had the same direct effect on a normal heart as nerve stimulation. This "vagusstoff" was, of course, the neurotransmitter acetylcholine. Although most recent definitions try to differentiate between transmitter and neurotrophic effects (see the NRP Work Session, *"Trophic" Effects of Vertebrate Neurons* (Guth, 1969)), transmitters were very much considered part of the earlier view of neurotrophism.‡

Interest in neurotrophic phenomena was widespread in the first decades of the twentieth century. Ramón y Cajal (1928), in his *Degeneration and Regeneration of the Nervous System,* referred to the neuronal soma as a trophic center and viewed Wallerian degeneration of the peripheral nerve stump as "trophic degeneration." That this phenomenon is actually transcellular, as well as intraneuronal, is evidenced by the changes in myelin. Ramón y Cajal (1928, p. 77) recognized this

---

*"Nothing in pathology is better established than the existence of these trophic disturbances resulting from lesions of the nerve centres or nerves" (as quoted by Speransky, 1943, p. 339).
†See Pavolv's *Works on Physiology of Digestion* printed in 1952.
‡Even today, the exact role played by transmitters in the range of neurotrophic phenomena is not entirely clear. Since these molecules may have nontransmitter functions, they may have to be included in our present definitions. This question is considered throughout this publication.

phenomenon long before it was known that the myelin sheath is part of a nonneuronal cell, as demonstrated by his statement:

> All that one may say is that the morphological alterations of the myelin precede those of the axon, and that its fragmentation and degeneration are influenced, like those of the axon, by the suspension of the trophic action of the mutilated neurone. This trophic action is perhaps exercised through some product of catabolism given out by the axon when the trophic current flows. This trophic current, as Heidenhain suggested . . . must not be confused with the ordinary nervous impulse.

Whereas the early foundations of neurotrophism rested on clinical data, the 1900's saw increasing emphasis on experimental paradigms. Not the least of these was that of the neuronal control of the development and maintenance of taste buds (see Guth, 1971a, 1974b; Zalewski, 1974). In 1920 Olmstead proposed that nerve is a causative factor in the formation of taste buds, and the subsequent experimental analysis of this phenomenon led Torrey (1934) to propose that the source of the neural influence on taste bud formation was a "neurosubstance" that originated in the nerve cell body and passed down the nerve fiber to the tongue to transform epithelial cells of the papillae into taste cells. His vision of axoplasmic transport has since been amply documented.

Other studies to determine which types of nerves can maintain taste buds have shown a specificity restricted to the chorda tympani, glossopharyngeal, and vagus nerves (i.e., nerves normally innervating taste buds). Other sensory, motor, and autonomic nerves were found to be ineffective (Lashkov, 1945; Guth, 1958; Oakley, 1970; Zalewski, 1969, 1970). Work is continuing on this problem, and the new simplifying techniques of organ culture (Farbman, 1974; see also Lentz in Chapter II) should provide insight into the mechanisms of this neuron-target cell interaction.

Another critical area of neurotrophic research has been the regulation of amphibian limb regeneration (see reviews by Singer, 1952; Thornton, 1968, 1970; Guth, 1974b). The amputated limb does not regenerate if the regional nerves are transected before or shortly after amputation.* It is the sensory nerves that are the most effective in regeneration, although motor nerves are also effective if they are

---

*There is a possibility that the neurotrophic influence is realized as an increase in vascularization and that the increased blood supply is the important factor supporting limb regeneration (Smith and Wolpert, 1975).

present in sufficient numbers in the blastema. Isolated sensory ganglia or fragments of CNS tissue implanted locally into a denervated stump will support normal regeneration. In contrast to the neural specificity of taste bud development, a nonspecific trophic factor seems critical here. Neither the taste bud nor amphibian nerve stump regeneration, however, appears dependent on a transmitter for the trophic effect (Singer, 1952, 1974).

The neuromuscular junction has been studied to elucidate the trophic influences of nerve or muscle and also as a model for the central synapse. The atrophy of muscle after motor nerve injury is a clinical fact; but, because the nerve impulse, transmitter, and putative neurotrophic influences travel in the same direction and are probably delivered at the same site, it has been difficult to sort out the various factors and establish a nontransmitter, nonactivity neurotrophic influence. Studies on (1) the regulation of the resting membrane potential in rats (Albuquerque et al., 1971a) and in normal and hibernating squirrels,* (2) acetylcholine sensitivity (Miledi, 1960; Albuquerque and McIsaac, 1970; Albuquerque et al., 1972; Lømo, 1974), and (3) cholinesterase activity (Guth, 1969; Lentz, 1974a) support the existence of distinct neurotrophic factors (see Chapter II).

The Evolution of Molecular Signals

From an evolutionary point of view, the secretory activity of nerve cells originated very early. Thus, we should not be surprised that neurons release materials other than transmitters. It has even been suggested that nerve cells arose from the secretory cells of the metazoan ectoderm; the development of long processes enabled these primitive cells to send their molecular message to distant target cells (Lentz, 1968). Moreover, with the appearance of such cells, the successful concept of cellular asymmetry was introduced.

Morphological studies of sponges by Pavans de Ceccaty (1974) revealed networks of elongated neuroid cells. These interconnected cells contact the neighboring epithelia by means of close appositions, i.e., "press-button-like" articulations and structures resembling gap junctions. Such contacts are equipped to carry out a directional movement of substances or signals along circuits from cell to cell. The cell bodies, themselves, show specialized features for secretion and contraction in

---

*E. X. Albuquerque, L. Guth, and S. S. Deshpande, unpublished observations.

the form of granules and filamentous structures. Although action potentials have not been recorded from these neuroid cells, electrotonic spread and coupling, as well as changes in resting potentials and membrane conductance, have been described. The latter characteristics are related to changes in ionic gradients, which are considered important auxiliary mechanisms for the release of neurohumoral substances. Thus, in neuroid cells of sponges, electrical phenomena may be the epiphenomena of a secretory mechanism.

Secretory material is probably released at the intercellular junctions as well as into the extracellular space. Lentz (1968) identified in neural-like cells in sponges substances such as Gomori-positive neurosecretory material, catecholamines, serotonin, acetylcholine, and acetylcholinesterase — all of which are known to exist in higher organisms. These findings stress the significance of secretory mechanisms not only for the chemical synapse but also for the activity of the nervous tissue as a trophic system. From his studies, Lentz (1968, p. 123) concluded that at least in some cases "the functions of the primitive nerve cell were largely hormonal and it [cell] most closely resembled a neurosecretory cell." It would seem that this secretory function, already present in the protonervous integrator system of sponges, precedes that of electrogenesis. The architectural and functional principles of neurosecretion were not forgotten during evolution and seem to be as basic as those of neural electrical function.

The New Perspective

Russian investigators have long had a strong interest in neurotrophism and, as noted above, have contributed greatly to the development of the subject: Razumovsky (1884) on atrophic processes in bones, Pavlov (1885) on heartbeat regulation, Molotkov (1925) on neural dystrophism in surgical pathology, and Shamov (see Speransky, 1943, p. 336) on trophic ulcers and the sympathetic nervous system. In his book, *A Basis for the Theory of Medicine,* Speransky (1943, p. 343) took a rather broad view when he wrote:

> ... *there are no non-trophic nerve elements in the organism, i.e., elements that have neither direct nor indirect connection with metabolism.* In actual work the question that has to be put is not that of the trophic nervous system as such, but of the *nervous component of processes* which are very diverse in external form.

. . . the nervous component remains from beginning to end the factor that determines their [the processes] *general state.* It, as it were, unites the separate elements into a whole, it forms the cement, any change in which inevitably alters the appearance of the process in all its other parts . . . . *Apart from memory, we do not know of a single nervous function which can be realised by itself, without change in the state of some other organ . . . .*

While there is much in the detailing of Speransky's view with which we would not agree, we readily concur with his emphasis on the pervasiveness and importance of such processes. We know now that neuron-target interactions are complex and are not polarized or unidirectional. The fact that changes in the target organ have profound effects on both developing and mature spinal motor neurons, including control of cell death, was first pointed out in 1909 by Shorey (see also Hamburger, 1934; Prestige, 1970; Price, 1974) and has since been extended by Thoenen, Raisman, and Landmesser (see Chapter IV). These data serve to emphasize that both the neuron and its target cell are interdependent, with molecular signals traveling between them in the maintenance of a dynamic balance.

Such considerations made it clear that the concept of neuro-trophism was too narrow and that a broader view was needed; this led to the Work Session being organized around the theme of "neuron-target cell interactions." What has become evident is that the system of molecular signals, as reflected in the mutual interdependency of neurons and their target cells, is as important as (and sometimes more than) the electrical signaling system. Nowhere is such a chemical communication system likely to be of more significance than in the dendrodendritic interactions of the local circuit neurons that Ramón y Cajal thought responsible for the higher integration functions of the brain, such as learning and memory (Rakic, 1975). Ultimately, such an exchange is coupled to actual information processing.

The number and variety of molecular signals already described are confusing. In this brief introduction, several substances were mentioned and the list grows with each ensuing chapter. As we ascend in phylogeny, the number of substances released by neurons increases steadily. In mammals the multitude of known and assumed molecular signals used in communication between neurons, and between neurons and other cells, is a taxonomic challenge.

Since intercellular molecular interactions can be organized with respect to time, Kreutzberg felt it might be helpful to order the various known molecular signals in a matrix of concentric circles with time

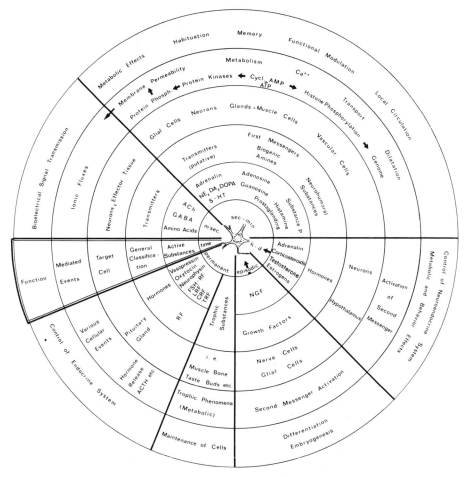

Figure 1. Some examples of the secretory activity of neurons, including the actions of various molecular signals. Categories of items in the different concentric circles are given in the double-lined segment. The inner circle shows the approximate time range in which the molecular interaction between neurons and target cells is operative. The second circle names some identified substances, which are usually grouped under certain headings, such as neurotransmitters, hormones, first messengers, etc., as shown in the third circle. The fourth circle indicates the target cell for the molecular signals either released by neurons or released by other cells for neurons. The fifth circle gives examples of the chemical events mediated by the molecular signals. Some are well known, e.g., ionic fluxes, membrane changes, activation of second messengers, polysome aggregation, and microtubule assembly. The functional meaning of such molecular processes for the appropriate system or the whole organism is shown in the outer circle. ACh = acetycholine; ACTH = adrenocorticotropic hormone; ATP = adenosine triphosphate; CRF = corticotropin-releasing factor; cyl. AMP = cyclic adenosine monophosphate; DA = dopamine; FSH-RF = follicle-stimulating hormone; GABA = γ-aminobutyric acid; 5-HT = 5-hydroxytryptophan; LRF = luteinizing hormone-releasing factor; NE = norepinephrine; NGF = nerve growth factor; RF = releasing factor; TRF = thyrotropin-releasing factor. [Kreutzberg]

providing the circumferential axis (Figure 1). This scheme is not complete since it fails to depict the complex interactions of one group of signals with another and, undoubtedly, leaves out some signals. To depict the interactions adequately would require a multidimensional matrix and, indeed, this will be necessary as we progress in our knowledge. For the moment, the simple two-dimensional representation is useful as a framework in which the available data and concepts can be arranged.

At the NRP Work Session, the data presented demonstrated the rapid growth of this field and, particularly, the plethora of signals identified, as well as their complex interactions. Organization of the wide variety of data reported into a meaningful whole is the task of this review. An attempt has been made to identify the major themes and areas of particular promise and/or problems. Chapter II deals with the proof of trophism, which is a problem decades old; yet it is the foundation of our discussion. The problem is replete with lessons for present and future experiments. Chapters III to VI take up the questions of synthesis, transport, delivery, and the functional and developmental significance of the molecular signals. Chapter VII deals with the pathology resulting from the failure of the molecular signal system and, in so doing, portrays a relatively untapped resource with great potentiality for both the basic and clinical scientist. Chapter VIII delves into what is known about the mechanisms by which the exchanged signals exert their effects; thus, it receives considerable attention in the *Bulletin*. Chapter IX deals with some lessons learned and proposes future research strategies in this exciting field of neuron-target cell interactions.

II. THE PROOF OF TROPHISM

For more than 50 years, the term "trophic" has been used to describe a variety of phenomena. In 1968 at an NRP Work Session on *Trophic Effects of Vertebrate Neurons* (Guth, 1969), it was agreed that, for scientific as well as historical reasons, this undeniably vague term should be retained. At that 1968 meeting, the following questions were asked: (1) "Is there a 'trophic' function of the neuron that is distinct from its role in impulse conduction and transmission?" (2) "Is the 'trophic' function a property of nervous tissue in general, or do nerves differ in their trophic capabilities?" (3) "Are there alternative explanations to the observed facts that do not require us to invoke an hypothesis of 'trophic' nerve function?" (4) "Should all influences of the nerve on the metabolism of the end-organ be considered 'trophic'?" For the most part, these questions have not been wholly resolved since that earlier NRP meeting.

In answer to the first question, Guth (1974b) has recently itemized the evidence that he considers most persuasive. Although there is no point in repeating his detailed discussion of this evidence, it is worth emphasizing his statement that the regulation of taste buds provides one of the best evidences of a trophic function that is distinct from transmission. In this case, taste buds degenerate when their sensory nerve supply is interrupted and they reappear when the nerve regenerates. Stimulation of the cut end of the nerve actually hastens the loss of the taste buds. A transmitter is not known to be involved here. However, the nerve does not function independently of other physiological regulations, and its ability to regulate the differentiation of the taste bud is, itself, dependent on, and modified by, the presence of extrinsic hormonal factors, such as testosterone and a specific gustatory epithelium.

Another demonstration of neurotrophism is provided by the regulation of amphibian limb regeneration. The nervous system is critical to this process, and, in fact, regeneration does not occur if the regional nerves are transected before or shortly after amputation.*

---

*The neural influence may, however, act through the process of vascularization (Smith and Wolpert, 1975).

According to Singer (1952; see also reviews by Thornton, 1968, 1970), both sensory and motor nerves are effective in this regard, although the former are much more potent. Neural activity per se is not important because CNS connections can be severed proximal to the sensory ganglia. When CNS fragments or isolated sensory ganglia are locally implanted, they are sufficient for regeneration to occur. The suggestion must be, then, that there is a nontransmitter neuroplasmic factor (or factors) that is the necessary and sufficient agent.

In the case of neuronal regulation of the physiological and metabolic properties of muscle, the picture is much less clear. The exact role of transmitters, particularly acetylcholine (ACh), has been the subject of many experiments and much debate. The issue is whether transmitters may have actions other than that of transmission, i.e., "trophic-like" actions on metabolism. Indeed, we should not be too quick to rule out transmitters in this role. Although the evidence is not complete, it does appear that cholinergic transmission plays a significant (but not exclusive) role in the metabolic relationships between motor nerves and skeletal muscle. Drachman (1974a,b) was able to conclude that cholinergic transmission is a *necessary* condition for the neural maintenance of muscle.

At the Work Session, Albuquerque discussed an experiment by Hawken and co-workers (1974) in which a rat left hemidiaphragm preparation was denervated. Within 24 hours in vitro, depolarization of the corresponding muscle occurred. If the denervated left hemidiaphragm was incubated with the right hemidiaphragm while the right phrenic nerve was being stimulated, the denervation-induced fall in resting membrane potential was inhibited. This action could not be attributed to muscle contraction because the same result was also obtained when the experiments were performed in the presence of sufficient d-tubocurarine (5 mg/1) to abolish muscle contractions. Hawken and collaborators suggest that stimulation of the phrenic nerve releases a soluble substance into the bathing solution that could be termed a trophic factor since it inhibited a fall in resting membrane potential. Furthermore, the resting potential can be maintained with norepinephrine or dibutyryl cyclic adenosine monophosphate. It is possible that one of the trophic factors is a transmitter agent. However, a transmitter, by itself, is not sufficient for the maintenance of all normal muscle properties.

Control of Pre- and Postsynaptic Membrane Properties: Studies with Batrachotoxin and 6-Aminonicotinamide: E. X. Albuquerque

Albuquerque, who has been very interested in sorting out the problems of use-disuse and the role of neurotransmitters as well as of other trophic substances, has articulated a number of arguments that there are trophic effects that are distinct from transmitter effects at the nerve-muscle junction. In published evidence he has included the following points: (1) Extrajunctional ACh sensitivity can occur even in the presence of spontaneous transmitter release (Albuquerque et al., 1974b). (2) Partial depolarization of the postsynaptic membrane, whose time of appearance is dependent on the length of the nerve stump and occurs while transmitter release is still active, cannot be an ACh effect (Albuquerque et al., 1971b). (3) The reinnervation of skeletal muscle following nerve crush is associated with an increase in the membrane potential before the ACh system returns to normal (McArdle and Albuquerque, 1973). (4) In a study of the effects of ouabain on chronically denervated and dystrophic muscles of the mouse, a loss of membrane sensitivity to ouabain, independent of ACh activity (d-tubocurarine block), was shown to occur (McArdle and Albuquerque, 1975). Albuquerque believes that the nerve releases a trophic factor that regulates the activity of the electrogenic sodium pump. (5) The extrajunctional receptors induced by chronic denervation of skeletal muscle show differences from the junctional receptors in their quantitative pharmacological interactions (such as various cholinolytic agents), suggesting neurotrophic and not simply ACh control (Albuquerque and McIsaac, 1969). (6) Experimental studies of dystrophic chicken muscle, which show a decreased rate of rise of the action potential and increased membrane resistance, membrane capacitance, and duration of miniature end-plate potentials (MEPP's), suggest altered membrane sodium permeability that is under neurotrophic control (Albuquerque and Warnick, 1971; Lebeda et al., 1974). Taken together, the data support the view that changes in electrical properties may be correlated with a lack of neurotrophic factor (or factors) regulating ionic membrane mechanisms.

Reasoning that trophic substances secreted by the neuron are likely to be transported from the soma to the periphery, Albuquerque and collaborators (1972, 1974b) applied colchicine and vinblastine to the sciatic nerve and measured neural junction and muscle properties at various times thereafter. There was no change in the ability of the nerve to maintain muscle activity, but chemical and electrical changes of the muscle included depolarization of the membrane, development of extrajunctional sensitivity to acetycholine, and the appearance of tetrodotoxin (TTX)-resistant action potentials — all changes of functional denervation. In fact, 7 days after application of vinblastine and colchicine, MEPP's were slightly more frequent. The induced membrane depolarization, after colchicine and vinblastine application, occurred in the absence of any major alteration or blocking of ionic conductances and before the appearance of extrajunctional ACh sensitivity and the increase in membrane resistance that follows denervation. Again, it may be that the electrogenic pump is defective.

Despite the evidence presented, there has been some criticism of the colchicine experiments. In confirmation of the above findings, Lømo (1974) demonstrated an increase in extrajunctional sensitivity and a fall in resting membrane potential after colchicine application to innervated skeletal muscles. In addition, he showed that similar changes developed in denervated soleus muscle that was kept active by direct stimulation. Since direct stimulation, in the absence of colchicine, has been shown to prevent such changes (Lømo and Rosenthal, 1972), it would seem that colchicine may have some effects on the muscle membrane that are not mediated by the nerve. However, when results from the cuff method were compared to those from the intraperitoneal injection of ^{3}H-colchicine, it was revealed that, in the latter experiment, there was a two-fold increase in the concentration of colchicine in muscle over that found in the cuff application, but no denervation changes were recorded (Kauffman et al., 1974).

Cangiano (1973; Cangiano and Fried, 1974,1976) has found that after injection of 1 to 5 μl of 0.2 M colchicine solution into the subepineural space of the sciatic nerve, the entire extensor digitorum longus (EDL) muscle membrane becomes sensitive to iontophoretically applied acetylcholine, and the muscle action potentials become resistant to tetrodotoxin despite normal innervation. Under these conditions, the same changes appear in the contralateral muscles, indicating a systemic action of colchicine. Although there was a partial block of the axonal transport of ^{3}H-labeled proteins in the treated sciatic nerve, which correlated with a partial paralysis of the ipsilateral leg, supersensitivity developed in the contralateral leg muscle where axoplasmic transport was found to be normal. When colchicine was applied with a silicone cuff, denervation-like changes were confined to the ipsilateral EDL muscle. However, impulse conduction block at the level of the cuff was usually observed. On the basis of these experiments, Cangiano concluded that (1) colchicine can produce denervation-like changes in normally active muscle by a direct action on the muscle membrane without blocking axoplasmic transport and that (2) the colchicine cuff experiments do not provide unambiguous evidence supporting the existence of neurotrophic influences on the muscle membrane.

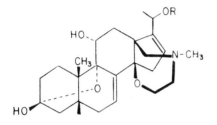

a. R = H

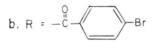

b. R = —C—⬡—Br

Figure 2. Structures of (a) batracho-toxinin A, (b) the 20α-p-bromobenzoate of batrachotoxinin A, (c) batrachotoxin, and (d) homobatrachotoxin. [Albuquerque et al., 1971a]

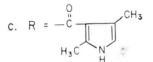

c. R =

d. R =

In an effort to shed some further light on this problem, Albuquerque has conducted other experiments, which he reported at the Work Session. Using hibernating animals, Albuquerque and collaborators found that inactivity did not cause any sign of denervation to occur.* In another study batrachotoxin (BTX), a steroidal alkaloid (Figure 2) derived from the skin of the Columbian poison arrow frog, *Phyllobates aurotaenia* (Albuquerque et al., 1973), was used to cause an

*E. X. Albuquerque, S. S. Deshpande, and J. Garcia, unpublished data.

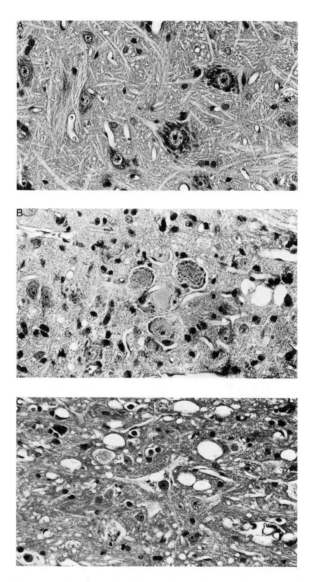

Figure 3. A. Saline-injected control after 3 days. Anterior horn of lumbar level shows normal cellularity and density of neuropil. Hemotoxylin and eosin stain. ×250. B. Six hours after subarachnoid injection of BTX. Anterior horn of lumbar level with marked spongiosis; most neurons show swollen, vacuolar profiles; others appear shrunken. Hemotoxylin and eosin stain ×250. C. Lumbar anterior horn 3 days after subarachnoid injection of BTX. There are increased numbers of hyperchromatic inflammatory cells; many neurons show central chromatolysis. Hemotoxylin and eosin stain. ×250. [Garcia, Pence, Deshpande, and Albuquerque]

irreversible depolarization of rat spinal cord motoneurons, as well as a blockade of both slow flow and fast axoplasmic transport (Ochs and Worth, 1975). BTX achieves its action by producing an increase in sodium conductance in muscles and axons (Albuquerque et al., 1971a,c; Hogan and Albuquerque, 1971; Narahashi et al., 1971; Warnick et al., 1971). It is particularly useful because a very small number of molecules (20 ng in 20 μl) can be used in these studies. A rather dramatic effect is obtained without any question of the substance affecting the muscle membrane directly. BTX administration results in a marked depolarization and a swelling of the motoneuron soma and axon, presumably because of the sodium influx (Albuquerque and Warnick, 1972). Other changes include displacement of the nucleus, disorganization of the organelles, splitting of myelin, and an apparent increase in neurofilaments (Figures 3 and 4; Garcia et al., 1975).

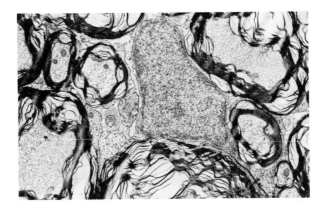

Figure 4. Subpial lateral tract 24 hours after subarachnoid injection of BTX. Myelin splitting, increased neurofilaments, and reduced numbers of microtubules are evident in large myelinated axons. ×8,000. [Garcia, Pence, Deshpande, and Albuquerque]

Under conditions of complete hindlimb paralysis and lack of axonal transport in the rat, differences in the changes in the properties exhibited by slow and fast muscles were observed by Albuquerque. Within 24 hours, the EDL muscle showed a drop in membrane potential of nearly 20 mV; this drop was similar to that seen when the nerve was cut to achieve denervation (Figure 5A). The soleus muscle, meanwhile, showed no change in membrane potential over 20 days. During this time, the MEPP's increased in amplitude for both the fast and slow

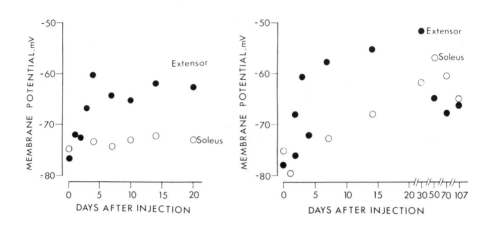

Figure 5. Mean resting membrane potentials of surface fibers of the extensor and soleus muscles at various days after injection of BTX (A) or 6-aminonicotinamide (B) into the subarachnoid space of the spinal cord. Membrane potentials were recorded from 10 to 20 fibers for each muscle. A. Each point is the mean for at least 3 rats except for Day 20 (2 rats). B. Each point is the mean for 3 to 4 rats for Days 4, 7, 14, and 70 and for 1 to 2 rats for the remaining periods. [Albuquerque et al., 1975]

muscles (see Figure 6 and Table 1). With acetylcholinesterase, there was a junctional decrease in both muscles at the same time. The quantal content at end-plate regions was normal. Both the muscle and the presynaptic regions showed no alteration; thus, if BTX did reach a nerve terminal, it did not destroy it (Jansson et al., 1974). Furthermore, there was increased extrajunctional acetylcholine sensitivity as in denervation, an effect that is observed in both muscles equally. On the basis of these findings, there seem to be two aspects to neurotrophism: (1) The neural control of acetylcholinesterase is common to both muscles, and (2), on the other hand, there is a differential neural control of the membrane potential in the fast and slow muscles, the slow muscle being much less affected by motoneuron depolarization and blockade of axoplasmic flow.

To clarify further the role of activity, Albuquerque and co-workers (1975) studied the effects of direct muscle or nerve stimulation in the presence of BTX. In the case of direct muscle stimulation, the resting membrane potential remained low, but there was decreased ACh extrajunctional sensitivity. With nerve stimulation, facilitation of recovery of the muscle membrane potential occurred (Table 2). According to Albuquerque, this stimulation also helped to

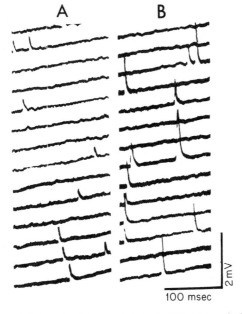

Figure 6. Miniature end-plate potentials recorded from extensor muscle fibers in control (A) and 7 days after injection of BTX (B). Vertical calibration: 2.0 mV; horizontal calibration: 100 msec. [Albuquerque et al., 1975]

TABLE 1

Amplitude, Half-Decay Time, and Frequency of Miniature End-Plate
Potentials after Injection of BTX into the Subarachnoid
Space of the Spinal Cord
[Albuquerque et al., 1975]

Muscle	Days after injection	Amplitude, mV	Half-decay time, msec	Frequency, sec^{-1}
Extensor	Control (3)*	0.56 ± 0.01†	1.50 ± 0.03	2.70 ± 0.28
	1 (3)	0.57 ± 0.02	1.66 ± 0.06	2.96 ± 0.42
	7 (5)	0.57 ± 0.02	1.81 ± 0.14	2.68 ± 0.35
	12-15 (3)	0.74 ± 0.03	2.37 ± 0.15	1.33 ± 0.36
	21 (2)	0.74 ± 0.02	2.46 ± 0.05	4.30 ± 0.80
Soleus	Control (3)	0.45 ± 0.01	1.71 ± 0.04	1.16 ± 0.15
	1 (3)	0.41 ± 0.02	1.66 ± 0.04	1.55 ± 0.13
	7 (5)	0.65 ± 0.04	2.60 ± 0.11	0.70 ± 0.07
	12-15 (3)	0.82 ± 0.03	2.61 ± 0.08	1.30 ± 0.25
	21 (2)	0.92 ± 0.04	2.48 ± 0.64	1.10 ± 0.17

*The numbers in parentheses represent the number of rats.

† All values represent means ± S.E.M. The recordings were made from at least 3 fibers (50-100 MEPP's/fiber) from each muscle.

TABLE 2

Effects of Direct and Indirect Stimulation on the Membrane Potential of Rats
Injected with BTX into the Subarachnoid Space of the Spinal Cord
[Albuquerque et al., 1975]

Muscle	Days after injection	Directly stimulated	Nonstimulated	Muscle	Days after injection	Indirectly stimulated	Nonstimulated
Extensor	8	-59 ± 0.8*	-65 ± 0.9	Extensor	8	-74 ± 0.7	-57 ± 0.8
Soleus	12	-69 ± 1.3	-67 ± 0.8	Soleus	8	-75 ± 0.6	-68 ± 0.4

*The values are the means ± S.E.M.

remove the toxin and promote the regeneration of the motoneuron in the spinal cord. If the nerve is transected and stimulated distally, restoration of the muscle membrane potential is much less, suggesting that the spinal cord needs afferent input for its own recovery and that the motoneuron itself, and not activity alone, is necessary.*

Albuquerque and his collaborators have also looked at the effects of 6-aminonicotinamide. This agent has long been known to cause pronounced neurotoxic effects, and, in fact, Sternberg and Philips (1958) showed that 6-aminonicotinamide injected intraperitoneally produces marked destruction of anterior horn cells. In the spinal cord, these effects were seen as early as 24 hours after injection and were maximal by 4 days. A single injection of 6-aminonicotinamide into the lumbar spinal cord of rats produced a rigid paralysis of both hindlimbs with a latency of 24 to 36 hours and a duration of at least 5 months. In contrast to the effects obtained with BTX, flaccidity and rigidity are characteristic of the paralysis obtained with 6-aminonicotinamide.

Again, a decrease in membrane potential was the first event to occur in these rats. Within 48 hours the membrane potential in the extensor muscles was reduced by approximately 9 mV. Soleus muscles were unaffected until 14 days later, when the membrane potential in the extensor and soleus muscles was -57 and -68 mV, respectively (see Figure 5B). After 40 days, the membrane potential in extensor muscles recovered partially, while soleus muscles continued to undergo marked membrane depolarization. These findings confirm that the extensor (fast) muscle is more susceptible to neural regulation of its membrane potential than is the soleus muscle. 6-Aminonicotinamide likewise caused a marked increase in MEPP amplitude and time course, indirectly reflecting a decrease in junctional cholinesterase and membrane potential.

*E. X. Albuquerque, S. S. Deshpande, and J. Garcia, unpublished data.

Albuquerque emphasized that the role of spinal motoneurons in the trophic regulation of fast and slow muscles has been clearly demonstrated in these experiments. The fast muscles are much more susceptible to central neural regulatory control of the muscle membrane than are slow muscles. Muscle activity alone, as induced by direct stimulation under conditions of 6-aminonicotinamide or batrachotoxin block, does not seem to be effective in reversing the electrophysiological changes in the muscle produced by the injections of these toxins into the subarachnoid space of the spinal cord.

Additional Evidence for Nontransmitter Trophic Effects

There are other data that further clarify the issue of the role of transmitters. First of all, Miledi and Slater (1970) have shown that ACh added to cultures of denervated muscle does not retard or prevent the development of supersensitivity. Secondly, as Fambrough (1970) has shown, the spread of sensitivity in denervated muscle can be prevented by the administration of ribonucleic acid (RNA) inhibitors to block protein synthesis. A somewhat different approach has been taken by Landmesser (1972) in her study of the contractile, electrical, and pharmacological responses of reinnervated muscle. In this experiment frog sartorius muscles were transplanted into the thorax and reinnervated by the gastric vagus nerve. Microelectrodes were used to measure electrical properties of the muscle fiber membrane, and histological studies of the sartorius and vagus nerves in reinnervated muscles were also carried out. It was found that the autonomic nerve fibers of the gastric vagus formed functional connections with the skeletal muscle fibers. Such vagus-innervated muscle fibers did not atrophy, and neither the contractile nor passive electrical properties of the muscle fibers were altered by vagal innervation. Synaptic transmission was quantal in nature and, like that at normal sartorial junctions, describable by a Poisson distribution. However, unlike normal sartorius junctions, the muscle fibers did show extensive multiple innervation. The vagal muscle junctions had a low quantal content and showed long-lasting facilitation. The properties of the vagus nerve fibers were not apparently altered by their synapsing with skeletal muscle fibers. They remained small in diameter and had a high threshold for electrical stimulation.

When the pharmacological properties of the nerve-muscle junctions of the vagus-innervated frog sartorius muscles were investigated, vagal evoked junctional potentials were found to be ten times more sensitive to hexamethonium than were the control end-plate potentials from muscles reinnervated with sartorius nerve. Hexamethonium did not affect passive electrical membrane properties or quantal content. On the other hand, sensitivity of vagus junctions to d-tubocurarine did not differ from that of the control. Furthermore, histologically detectable acetylcholinesterase activity was not demonstrable at the junctions. Although the vagus nerve was able to maintain the morphology and, to some extent, the electrical activity of the innervated sartorius, it could not, despite release of the same transmitter, maintain cholinesterase activity and thus a normal junction. This effect of a given nerve-fiber type on postsynaptic cholinesterase distribution is substantial evidence for a specific trophic factor that is unrelated to a transmitter.

The specificity of a nerve-fiber type for a muscle is, of course, not a new story. Buller, Eccles, and Eccles (1960a, b; see also review by Close, 1972; also Guth, 1974b) showed more than a decade ago that the nerve regulates the isometric contraction time of muscle and that this physiological property of muscle can be altered even during adult life. On reinnervating a fast muscle by a nerve that normally supplies a slow one and vice versa, they found that the isometric contraction time of the fast muscle became longer and that of the slow muscle became shorter. On the basis of this sort of data, it seemed likely that the basic properties of the myosin molecule are under neural control. This hypothesis was proved correct by biochemical studies by Samaha and co-workers (1970), and the interpretation has been verified by Bárány and Close (1971; see also Guth, 1974b). Thus, not only do we have evidence for specificity but also for the neural regulation of gene expression in the target cell.

Direct Stimulation, Use-Disuse Experiments, and the Influence of Exercise

Neurotrophism is not simply a matter of transmitter release; several factors are involved. What remains is to separate the activity and/or exercise factors (see Peter, 1971) from the molecular neurotrophic ones. Guth and Wells (1972) have denervated muscles antagonistic to the soleus and found physiological speeding of the soleus that was associated with increased adenosine triphosphatase (ATPase) activity (Jean et al., 1973). Thus, the lesson is quite clear: alterations in myofibrillary proteins can be brought about by procedures other than innervation per se. Putting these findings into perspective, Guth emphasized that the pattern of impulses delivered to a muscle cell is sufficient to alter the type of myosin synthesized by the cell.

The mechanism by which a pattern of impulses can alter genetic expression in the target cell is not clear. Might the effect simply be the result of rhythmic ion fluxes? An alternative solution is that axoplasmic transport changes in rate or qualitative or quantitative delivery of a crucial molecular factor. Barker and Ip (1966) have proposed that within muscle a continual breaking and remaking of synaptic contact occur; thus, a fiber within a given muscle may be converted from fast to slow or vice versa — a kind of internal cross-reinnervation experiment. In this case, it is obvious that maintenance of specificity of structure and function and neural specificity are crucial problems.

Recent studies have shown that direct stimulation of denervated muscle abolishes all ACh hypersensitivity at a rate that depends critically on the number or pattern of the stimuli (Lømo and Westgaard, 1975). If stimulation and denervation start simultaneously, a transient ACh hypersensitivity, attributed to nerve terminal degeneration, develops with a "slow" stimulus pattern (10 Hz trains) but not with a "fast" pattern (100 Hz trains), which is far more effective in suppressing ACh hypersensitivity (Lømo and Westgaard, 1976). Their results indicate that extrajunctional sensitivity to ACh normally responds solely to muscle activity per se, whereas the junctional sensitivity is under neural control.

Although elucidating such issues requires more study, the lesson is, however, quite clear. An experimental approach to so-called neurotrophic phenomena must incorporate into its design the control of multiple factors, such as time, activity, and transmitter release, if meaningful statements about the role of still other molecular factors are to be established.

Brain Extracts and Muscle Acetylcholinesterase Activity:
T. L. Lentz

Recognizing the various difficulties in analyzing neurotrophic phenomena and believing that the identification of trophic substances and mechanisms is critically dependent on the availability of a suitable bioassay system, Lentz (1971, 1974a,b) has developed an in vitro assay system utilizing the triceps muscle of *Triturus viridescens*. As shown in Figure 7, several assays are possible with this system. Although feasible for study, the state of histological differentiation of the muscle fiber and end-plate is not ideal because of the number of components involved. The effects of denervation on the distribution of ACh receptors have been studied extensively by electrophysiologists, and there is new data by Lϕmo (see above) in this regard. A third possible (quantifiable) assay is the use of a α-bungarotoxin to study neurotrophic influences on receptor metabolism, turnover, and localization. However, the model to which Lentz turned attempts to identify the trophic effects on muscle cholinesterase activity. The advantage of this model is that the cholinesterase (ChE) level is known to be dependent on innervation and can be easily measured.

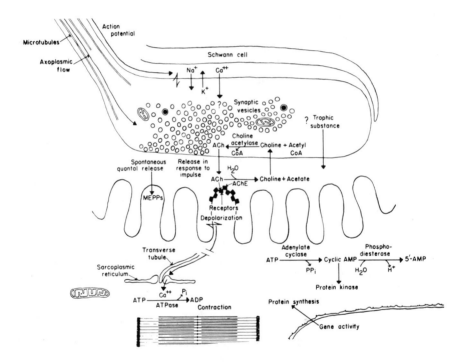

Figure 7. Diagram of the neuromuscular junction illustrating the types of interactions occurring at this region. Components thought to be trophically regulated include acetylcholine (ACh) receptors, acetylcholinesterase (AChE) activity, and the structural integrity of the end-plate and muscle fibers. Possible mechanisms of trophic regulation include muscle activity, ACh, and a hormonal trophic factor. ADP = adenosine diphosphate; 5-AMP = 5-adenosine monophosphate; ATP = adenosine triphosphate; ATPase = adenosine triphosphatase; CoA = coenzyme A; cyclic AMP = cyclic adenosine monophosphate; PP_i = pyrophosphate. [Lentz, 1974b]

Lentz used the cultured muscle system to study both the morphology of the motor end-plate and the ChE level. As a control, the muscle from the opposite limb was also cultured. Although cultured muscle ordinarily loses ChE activity as a result of denervation, Lentz found that nerve explants, including sensory ganglia and spinal cord and extracts of both newt and rat brain (Figures 8 and 9), maintained the ChE activity at levels higher than those in untreated controls. However, extracts of nonnervous tissue failed to do so. The same explants maintained normal end-plate morphology and ChE activity as well (Figure 10). Interestingly enough, the positive effect of the brain extracts is obtained only at certain concentrations in the culture medium. There are two peaks of activity, and concentrations above and

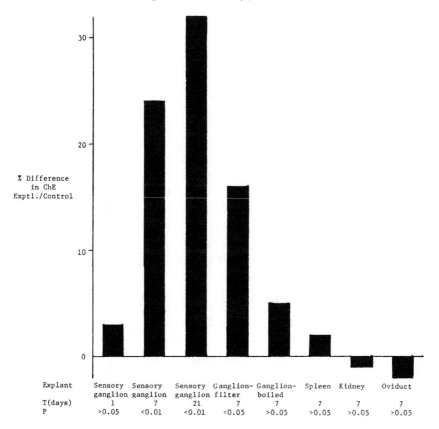

Figure 8. Effects of tissue explants on ChE activity of the triceps muscle of the newt in organ culture. Sensory ganglia prevent the decrease in ChE activity occurring in untreated muscle as a result of denervation. Other tissues and boiled ganglia are ineffective. [Lentz]

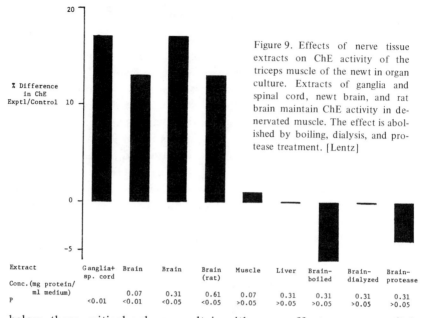

		Ganglia+ sp. cord	Brain	Brain	Brain (rat)	Muscle	Liver	Brain-boiled	Brain-dialyzed	Brain-protease
Extract										
Conc.(mg protein/ ml medium)			0.07	0.31	0.61	0.07	0.31	0.31	0.31	0.31
P		<0.01	<0.01	<0.05	<0.05	>0.05	>0.05	>0.05	>0.05	>0.05

Figure 9. Effects of nerve tissue extracts on ChE activity of the triceps muscle of the newt in organ culture. Extracts of ganglia and spinal cord, newt brain, and rat brain maintain ChE activity in denervated muscle. The effect is abolished by boiling, dialysis, and protease treatment. [Lentz]

below these critical values result in either no effect or even a slight depression of activity (Lentz, 1974a).

Of great importance is that Lentz has been able to characterize to some degree the agent responsible for this effect. When the ganglion is placed in a chamber, separated from the muscle by a Millipore filter, ChE activity is maintained at a higher level than it is in the controls. The effect can be abolished by boiling the ganglion for 1 min prior to placing it on the muscle and can also be inactivated by protease. On the basis of these findings, Lentz concluded that this substance is a small peptide. He is presently attempting further purification by passing the extracts through small-pore ultrafilters. Thus far, a fraction with components having a relatively low-molecular weight has been found to retain activity. Gel filtration analysis is also now in progress.

At this point, then, we have a peptide factor, specific to nerve and found across a wide phylogenetic range, that will maintain ChE at normal levels despite denervation. The next step is to look at the mechanism by which such trophic influences are exerted. Lentz, for example, has posed the following questions: How does the extract regulate the synthesis and proper arrangement of polypeptides that result in normal ChE levels? At what levels are the controls exerted — at the level of the gene, at the level of translation, or by increasing enzyme activity? Is a second messenger involved? These questions will be taken

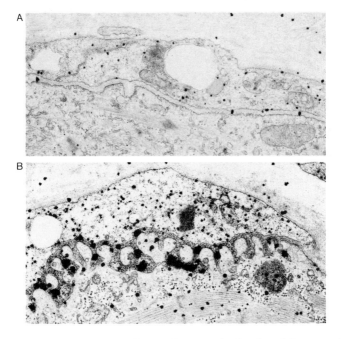

Figure 10. Neuromuscular junctions of newt triceps muscle after 1 week in organ culture and reacted for ChE activity. A. Muscle was untreated. B. Muscle was cultured in the presence of a nerve explant (sensory ganglion). The untreated muscle shows degeneration of the nerve terminal, regression of the motor end-plate, and loss of ChE activity. The treated muscle shows disappearance of the nerve terminal but maintenance of the motor end-plate and ChE activity. [Lentz, 1972a]

up in detail in Chapter VIII, which deals with mechanisms of neuron-target cell interactions. Suffice it to state for the present that cyclic adenosine monophosphate (cAMP) plus theophylline will mimic the effect of brain extracts which, themselves, alter cAMP levels.

Rathbone and co-workers (1973, 1975a,b) have not only confirmed the findings of Lentz, but have extended them further. They have also reported that denervated newt muscle loses ChE activity. Of the five species of acetylcholinesterase identified from newt muscle, two with sedimentation coefficients of 16S and 12S were selectively lost after denervation. The 16S form is associated with the motor end-plate region of muscle, and the 12S form is presumably extra-junctional. The changes in ChE activity in denervated muscles in culture are indistinguishable from those observed following denervation in vivo; therefore, the culture system may be used to study the effects of various treatments of postdenervation changes in muscle cholinesterase.

Rathbone found that the ChE level is maintained when the muscles are cultured in the presence of newt sensory ganglion (Figure 11). He also found that homogenates of 10-day-old chick embryo brain are a plentiful source of ChE-maintaining activity

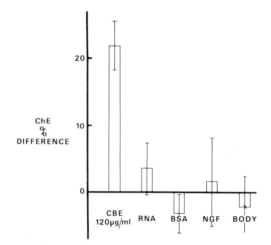

Figure 11. Effect of chick embryo brain extract (CBE) (120 μg of protein per ml), RNA obtained from chick brain, bovine serum albumin (BSA) (120 μg of protein per ml), nerve growth factor (NGF) (2.0 units per ml), or extract of chicken body (120 μg of protein per ml) on ChE activity of newt triceps muscle. Muscles were cultured for 1 week in the presence of these materials, and ChE activity of treated muscles was compared with ChE activity of untreated contralateral muscles. Mean values ± S.E.M. for 20 muscles. [Rathbone et al., 1975a]

(Figure 11). Furthermore, the ChE-maintaining effects of the chick brain extract are not due to a nonspecific enrichment of the culture medium. As for the analogous factor from newt brain characterized by Lentz, the active factor is heat-iabile, trypsin-digestible, and dialyzable (see Figure 12), and it has a molecular weight of less than 25,000. Dibutyryl cAMP and theophylline are able to mimic the effect of the extract by maintaining ChE activity in cultured muscles, but cyclic guanosine monophosphate (cGMP) is considerably less active (Figure 13). Although these results suggest that cAMP may mediate the neurotrophically controlled maintenance of muscle cholinesterase by acting as a second messenger, in further work Rathbone and co-workers have been able to dissociate cholinesterase maintenance from changes in intracellular cAMP levels (see Chapter VIII).

The work of Oh (1975) provides additional confirmation of the existence of a neurotrophic molecule. However, his data suggest that the crucial compound has a molecular weight of 300,000. At present, there seems to be no immediate resolution to this problem, although the possibility that Lentz and Rathbone are studying subunits has been raised.

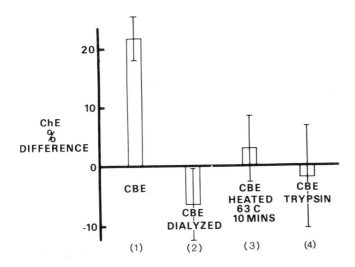

Figure 12. Effect of various treatments on ChE-maintaining activity of chick embryo brain extract (CBE): (1) untreated; (2) dialyzed for 16 hours at 4°C against 0.1 M phosphate buffer, pH 7.0; (3) heated for 10 min at 63°C, or (4) digested with trypsin. [Rathbone et al., 1975a]

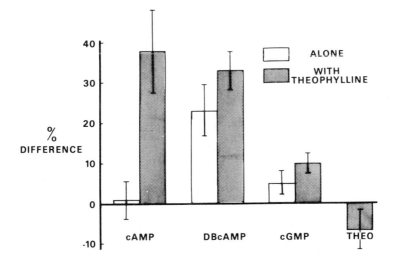

Figure 13. Effect of cyclic nucleotides (1 mM cAMP, 0.5 mM dibutyryl cAMP (DBcAMP), or 1 mM cGMP) alone (light bars) or in combination with theophylline (0.5 mM) (dark bars) on ChE activity of newt triceps muscles cultured for 7 days. Mean values ± S.E.M. of 20 observations in each experiment. [Rathbone et al., 1975a]

Spinal Cord Transplantation in Chick Embryos
of Different Genotypes

Another model* that meets the criteria needed for a system to establish neuron-target cell interactions is that of Rathbone and co-workers (1975b). In their studies, neural tubes from chicks of one genotype were transplanted to chicks of another (Figure 14). These investigations examined the question: "What phenotype develops in the muscles innervated by the transplanted neural tube?"

The inspiration for these experiments was derived from studies using muscle transplantation designed to test extramuscular influences on the progress of muscular dystrophy. These experiments had demonstrated that, when muscle from dystrophic embryos as young as 12 days was transplanted to normal chicks, the phenotypic expression of dystrophy in the donor muscle was unaltered. However, these experiments did not take into account the possibility that the defective gene might act extramuscularly at a much earlier stage of embryonic development, the muscle then being secondarily induced to express a dystrophic phenotype. In other words, they neglected the crucial factor of time. Attempts to look at either human or animal dystrophy without regard to time will almost certainly lead to different results and interpretations. If the nerve has an inductive effect on muscle, then later attempts to sort out the two factors developmentally will be hopelessly enmeshed in a bidirectionally abnormal situation in which the neurons may be acted upon by the muscle (see Chapters IV and VII) to produce further neuronal abnormality. If the circle is completed, the muscle, in turn, undergoes further pathological change. The current controversy as to whether the genetically determined defect lies within the muscle fibers themselves or whether it is an abnormality within the nervous system has been fueled by experiments where such factors cannot be distinguished.

With the factor of time in mind. Rathbone and his collaborators adopted a direct method for testing the role of the nervous system in the pathogenesis of hereditary muscular dystrophy, i.e., the transplantation of the nervous system from a dystrophic to a normal animal before the muscles have been influenced by nerves of their own genotype. They were careful to transplant the neural tube from dystrophic (as well as normal) to normal chickens during ontogeny but before the first known inductive neuronal influences are expressed in the development of cell lines and before muscle differentiation and innervation occur. To

*This model was presented by J. Diamond at the Work Session.

Donor Embryo   Host Embryo

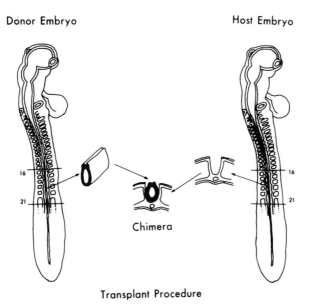

Chimera

Transplant Procedure

Figure 14. In the procedure used for transplanting neural tubes, the donor embryo was removed from the egg and washed in saline; the number of somites was then determined. The spinal cord between somites 16 to 21 was removed, washed in 0.25% trypsin to remove adherent mesenchyme, and subsequently washed in soybean trypsin inhibitor. It was then stored in Eagle's minimal essential medium buffered with N-2-hydroxyethylpiperazine-N'-2-ethanesulfonic acid (25 mM) while the host animal was being prepared. The host embryo was exposed by drilling a small window in the shell directly over the embryo, the vitelline membrane above the brachial region was removed, and the spinal cord was cut out with a fine-steel knife. Care was taken not to injure the somites or the underlying notochord. The donor cord was dropped in place from a Pasteur pipette and was oriented by means of a fine-tungsten needle under visual control both anteroposteriorly and dorsoventrally. The egg was sealed with sterile Parafilm and incubated with the window side up for a further 16 days. [Rathbone et al., 1975b]

accomplish this, they used the white fiber-fast twitch of superficial pectoral muscles; these muscles are innervated by the brachial plexus and show early and clear signs of muscular dystrophy in the chicken. Thymidine kinase activity of the muscles was chosen as a phenotypic expression of muscular dystrophy, since an increased thymidine kinase activity is the first enzyme change reported in dystrophic chicken muscles. It is even found before hatching.

Rathbone and co-workers (1975b) found that isotopic transplants of the brachial region of dystrophic neural tubes induced in genotypically normal host muscles a thymidine kinase activity characteristic of dystrophic muscle, whereas normal neural tubes did not (Figure 15). They propose that the neural tube has an early inductive effect on presumptive myoblasts that determines their subsequent course of development, whether it be normal or dystrophic. Once this interaction is complete, the muscle retains its induced characteristics even when placed in a different environment.

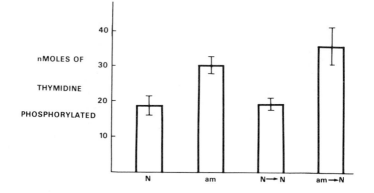

Figure 15. Thymidine kinase activity of experimental and control pectoral muscles of 18-day-old chicken embryos expressed as nanomoles of thymidine phosphorylated per gm (wet weight) of superficial pectoral muscle per 120 min. Mean values ± S.E.M. The values for N and N→N are not different (P>0.2)(Student's t-test), and the values for am and am→N are also not different (P>0.2). However, both am and am→N are significantly different from N and N→N (P<0.01). N = normal muscles from 8 unoperated embryos; am = dystrophic muscles from 10 unoperated embryos; N→N = normal muscles that had been innervated by neural tubes from 8 normal embryos; am→N = normal muscles that had been innervated by neural tubes from 6 dystrophic embryos. [Rathbone et al., 1975b]

Chimeric Mouse Studies in Genetic Dystrophy

An approach with great potential for the study of neuro-trophism is the work of Peterson (1974).* Like Rathbone, Peterson tackled the problem of sorting out neurotrophic from other factors in the case of murine muscular dystrophy. A useful method would be to study an adult animal in which either genetically dystrophic muscle was innervated by a normal nervous system or a genetically normal muscle was innervated by a dystrophic nervous system. The mouse chimera†

*Also, unpublished data reported by J. Diamond.
†Since the term "chimera" has been used in several different ways in the past, its usage here requires characterization. The mouse chimeras, which Peterson describes, are derived from the aggregation of two eight-cell embryos, each of differing genotypes. These mosaic embryos are cultured for 24 hours, develop into blastocysts, and are then transferred to the uterus of pseudopregnant females to complete development. The chimeras of particular interest here were derived from the aggregation of dystrophic and normal embryos.

offers such an opportunity without requiring any surgical manipulation that may complicate the issue.

Peterson's goal was to study the interaction between genetically defined muscle and the rest of the organism during development and in the mature state. If muscles of the identified dystrophic genotype were found to have normal characteristics, it would be unlikely that the disease could be due to a primary myopathy. In addition, if genetically normal muscles showed dystrophic characteristics, then this would support the inference that there was an extramuscular component of the disease. Conversely, a direct correlation between dystrophic genotype and dystrophic characteristics would support the original myogenic hypothesis.

Having set this goal, Peterson's principal requirement was an adequate genetic marker that would be clearly shown during the lifespan of an animal with the dystrophic genotype. For the experiment, seven chimeras of dystrophic $\leftrightarrow$ normal (C57Bℓ/6J dy^{2J}/ $dy^{2J} \leftrightarrow$ SWV) and two of normal $\leftrightarrow$ normal (C57Bℓ $\leftrightarrow$ SWV) composition were produced and proved suitable (all chimeras demonstrated coat color and hemoglobin mosaicism).

As the genetic marker, Peterson chose malic enzyme. The $Mod\text{-}1^b$ genotype is present in the C57Bℓ/6J mouse strain in which the dystrophic mutant gene is maintained. Normal embryos were obtained from SWV mice that have the $Mod\text{-}1^a$ genotype for the same enzyme. The goal was to obtain enough genotypically pure muscle of both normal and dystrophic composition (Figure 16) to assess the possibility of an extramuscular influence on the pathogenesis of the muscle disease.

Starch gel electrophoresis of malic enzyme revealed that the muscle could be 100% normal genotype and yet show abnormal morphology (Figure 17). On the other hand, the muscle could be 83% dystrophic genotype and show normal morphology. It could be argued that a small population of normal nuclei supporting synthesis of some postulated chemical deficient within the fibers of dystrophic muscles might prevent dystrophic pathology. This explanation seemed unlikely to Peterson, because muscles with a very high dystrophic genotype, including those with large populations of completely dystrophic fibers, appeared normal otherwise. Furthermore, genetically normal muscles showed pathological changes. The suggestion, then, is that, at least in the mosaic mouse, some entirely extramuscular factor is primarily responsible for the muscle degeneration. Unfortunately, this suggestion falls short of proving that it is the nerve that supplies the factor.

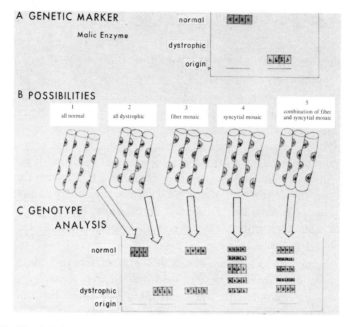

Figure 16. Theoretical use of electrophoretic variants of malic enzyme for analysis of functioning genotype within muscles from a chimera. [Peterson]

However, Peterson now has a nerve marker and expects to test this directly. He feels that chimeric or genetic mosaic techniques hold enormous, and as yet unrealized, potential for determining the interaction between neurons and their target cells.

Another important effort along these lines is that of LaVail and Mullen (1975, 1976; Mullen, 1975) who are studying mutants with abnormalities of the mammalian CNS to determine whether the gene in question is acting intrinsically or extrinsically. Using rat and mouse chimeras produced in the same way as those of Peterson, they have examined inherited retinal degeneration, which is characterized by progressive degeneration and loss of photoreceptor cells. The question to be resolved is whether the pigment epithelial cell, the photoreceptor cell, both, or neither is the site of mutant gene action.

In mouse chimeras, they found patches of normal photo-receptor cells interspersed with patches of degenerating cells. Since these patches were found underlying both mutant and normal pigment epithelium, the pigment epithelium is not the site of gene action resulting in retinal degeneration in the mouse.

Retinal degeneration in the rat is distinct from that in the mouse. In the rat chimeras, the degenerating patches of photoreceptor cells were found exclusively underlying mutant pigment epithelium, indicating that the pigment epithelial cells are the primary site of mutant gene action.

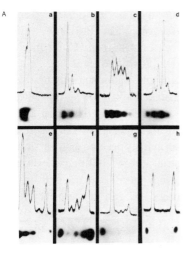

Figure 17. A. Electrophoretograms and corresponding densitometer traces of malic enzyme from chimera muscle. Origin is at right of each gel and the fastest moving band corresponds to the normal $Mod\text{-}I^a$ genotype. B. Left biceps femoris muscle in which 83% of functioning genotype was genetically dystrophic. There are no obvious features of dystrophic pathology. C. Left biceps femoris from another chimera. No functioning dystrophic genotype was detectable in this muscle. However, this section reveals fibers demonstrating several abnormalities, including a large variation in fiber size, coagulation necrosis, and central nuclei. [A and B, Peterson, 1974; C, Peterson]

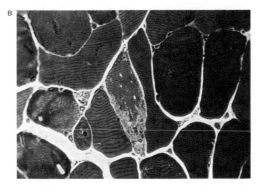

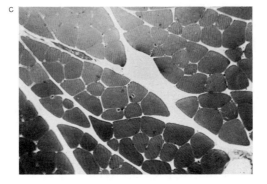

Mullen (1975) has recently examined mouse chimeras derived from an aggregation of embryos homozygous for Purkinje cell degeneration (*pcd*) with normal C57Bℓ/65 embryos. In *pcd/pcd* mice there was a loss of virtually all cerebellar Purkinje neurons. The *pcd/pcd* ↔ normal chimeras are the first example of mosaicism in the mammalian brain. The Purkinje cell mosaicism was extremely fine with some patches containing, perhaps, only a single cell. Using β-glucuronidase as an independent cell marker, Mullen has shown all of the surviving Purkinje cells to be of the normal genotype, suggesting that the Purkinje cell itself is the site of *pcd* gene action. β-Glucuronidase histochemistry on reeler (*rℓ*) chimeras showed patches of normal and abnormally positioned cortical cells containing *rℓ/rℓ* and +/+ genotypes. In other words, the positioning of cortical cells is determined by extrinsic factors in the local milieu. One might speculate that these factors are supplied by other neurons or, perhaps, by glia.

Establishing Neuron-Neuron Interactions

The chimeric experiments involving Purkinje cell loss raise the question of neuron-neuron interactions. Does one neuron send other than electrical transmission-related signals to its postsynaptic target neuron?

Kreutzberg and co-workers (see Chapter III) have shown that various amino acids and nucleosides are exchanged, in some cases rather specifically, between neurons. Although we can speculate as to the metabolic significance of such exchange, we do not as yet have data to support such speculation in systems studied by Kreutzberg and his associates.

Using a somewhat different approach, Black and collaborators (1971a,b,c,d, 1972a,b, 1974; Black and Geen, 1973, 1974; Black and Mytilineou, 1976) have been able to provide solid evidence for reciprocal regulatory relationships between cholinergic and adrenergic neurons at the synapse during development. As his model system, Black chose the neonatal mouse and rat superior cervical ganglion (SCG) (Figure 18) and employed two markers, tyrosine hydroxylase (TOH) in the postsynaptic adrenergic neuron and choline acetyltransferase (ChAc) in the presynaptic cholinergic cell. The normal development of enzyme activities and the number of synapses within the SCG are shown in Figures 19 and 20, respectively.

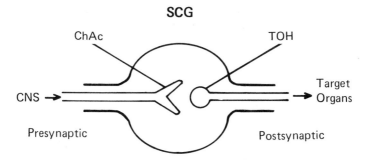

Figure 18. Schematic representation of the superior cervical ganglion (SCG). The enzymes choline acetyltransferase (ChAc) and tyrosine hydroxylase (TOH) are shown in their respective presynaptic and postsynaptic locations. [Black]

The maturation of postsynaptic neurons in SCG depends upon the presence of presynaptic cholinergic fibers. During maturation, postsynaptic TOH activity rises 6- to 8-fold, reflecting the developmental accumulation of enzyme molecules in each cell body (Black et al., 1974). The rise parallels the formation of ganglionic synapses (Figure 20). Moreover, transection of the preganglionic trunk prevents the normal development of TOH activity and the normal accumulation of enzyme molecules in each cell (Figure 21, A and B). Thus, presynaptic nerves regulate the maturation of neurons.

Of course, the question of the nature of the transsynaptic message involved in this regulation is of great interest. In principle, Black's results are strikingly similar to those obtained at the nerve-muscle junction. Administration of ganglionic blocking agents, such as chlorisondamine and pempidine, prevented the normal maturation of adrenergic enzyme activities, indicating (Figure 22, A and B) that acetylcholine plays a role. However, atropine, a muscarinic antagonist, did not affect TOH activity. Thus, nicotinic, but not muscarinic, receptor stimulation appears to regulate adrenergic ontogeny. However, the effects of decentralization cannot be entirely reversed with either acetylcholine or carbamylcholine. Therefore, as in the case of the nerve-muscle neurotrophic effects, we must conclude that acetylcholine, although necessary, may not be sufficient.

Nerve growth factor (NGF) would seem to be another likely candidate for consideration as the anterograde transsynaptic message. However, Black found that NGF cannot replace presynaptic terminals in the regulation of postsynaptic maturation. NGF cannot reverse the

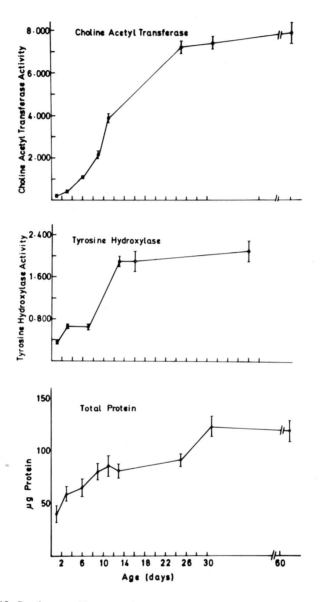

Figure 19. Developmental increases of transmitter enzyme activities and protein in mouse SCG. Groups of 6 mice were taken from litters of varying ages, and ganglion pairs from each animal were assayed for enzyme activities and total protein. ChAc activity (*upper graph*) is expressed as mean nmoles of product/ganglion pair/hour ± S.E.M. (vertical bars). TOH activity (*middle graph*) is expressed as 10^{-11} moles of product/ganglion pair/hour. Total protein (*lower graph*) is expressed as mean micrograms/ganglion pair ± S.E.M. [Black et al., 1971d]

effects of ganglion decentralization (Figure 23) and, thus, is not the "missing factor." Further research is required to determine the nature of the other factors involved.

The above studies define the anterograde transsynaptic regulation of adrenergic ontogeny. Black and co-workers (1972b) have also demonstrated that postsynaptic neurons regulate presynaptic development through a retrograde process. During the course of maturation, presynaptic ChAc activity increased 30- to 40-fold (Figure 19), and this rise paralleled the formation of ganglionic synapses (Figure 20). If postsynaptic adrenergic neurons in neonatal rats were chemically destroyed with 6-hydroxydopamine (Figure 24) or immunologically destroyed with antiserum to NGF (Figure 25), the normal development of presynaptic ChAc activity was prevented. These data, viewed in conjunction with the anterograde regulation studies, lead to the conclusion that there is a bidirectional flow of regulatory information at the synapse during development.

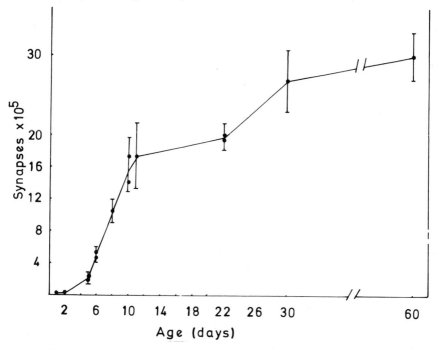

Figure 20. Development of ganglion synapses. Total synapses per ganglion were estimated in mice of different ages. Each point represents the estimated total synapses in a SCG from a single mouse. Vertical bars represent S.E. of determinations of synapse numbers in the 10 grid squares sampled for each ganglion. [Black et al., 1971d]

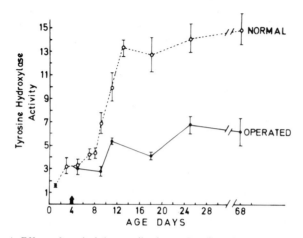

Figure 21. A. Effect of surgical decentralization at Day 4 on development of TOH activity in mouse SCG. Groups of 6 mice were killed at various times postoperatively, and TOH activity (pmoles/ganglion/hour) was measured in decentralized and contralateral control ganglia. The value obtained 1 day after surgery does not differ significantly from control value; all other values from decentralized ganglia are significantly lower than control values (P<0.01). [Black et al., 1972a]

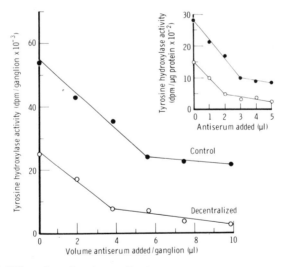

Figure 21 B. Effect of ganglion decentralization on immunotitration of ganglion TOH activity in neonatal mice. Ganglia were unilaterally decentralized in 4-day-old mice, and the animals were sacrificed at 2 weeks of age. Decentralized and contralateral control ganglia were homogenized in the same proportion of 16 ganglia per 200 μl of iced, distilled water. In the large diagram, results are expressed per single ganglion for comparative development purposes, and enzyme activity is expressed per 20-min assay incubation period. In the small diagram, enzyme activity is expressed per microgram of protein of homogenate supernatant fraction and per 20-min assay incubation period. Each point in each diagram represents the mean of duplicate determinations. [Black et al., 1974]

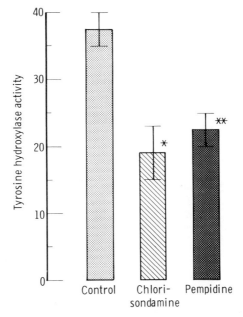

Figure 22. A. Effect of chlorisondamine and pempidine on development of ganglion TOH activity. Groups of neonatal animals were treated with chlorisondamine (5 μg/gm body weight) or pempidine (50 μg/gm body weight subcutaneously) every 12 hours beginning on Day 2 of life. Littermate controls were treated with saline at appropriate times. All animals were killed at 2 weeks of age. Each value represents the mean ± S.E.M. for 6 to 8 animals. TOH activity is expressed in pmoles/ganglion pair/hour. * differs from control at P<0.001. ** differs from control at P<0.001 but does not differ significantly from chlorisondamine. [Black and Geen, 1973]

Figure 22. B. Effect of chlorisodamine on development of ganglion TOH activity time course. Animals were treated with chlorisondamine (5 μg/gm subcutaneously) every 12 hours beginning on Day 2 of life (see arrow). Each value represents the mean ± S.E.M. (vertical bars) for 6 to 8 animals and is expressed as in Figure 22A. Control animals (solid line) were treated with saline at appropriate times. Each value of chlorisondamine-treated animals (dash line) differs from respective control at P<0.001. [Black and Geen, 1973]

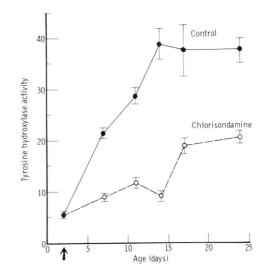

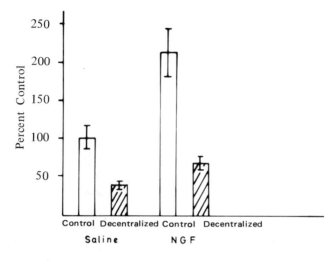

Figure 23. Effects of decentralization and NGF on development of TOH activity in mouse SCG. Mice were subjected to unilateral decentralization of the ganglion at 4 days of age, and one group of mice received 3 μg/gm of NGF daily for 10 days while the other received the saline. Values for enzyme activity are expressed as percent of saline-treated control, which was 12.7±0.9 pmoles/single ganglion/hour. The NGF values are significantly higher than the corresponding saline-treated controls (P<0.05), but the decentralized values are significantly lower than the corresponding controls (P<0.01). [Black]

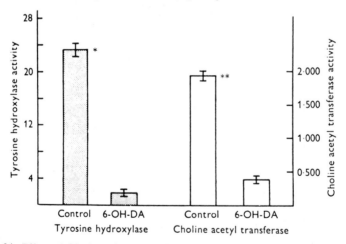

Figure 24. Effect of 6-hydroxydopamine (6-OH-DA) on developing ganglion. Six mice were injected with 6-hydroxydopamine in 0.2% ascorbic acid (150 mg/kg) and were killed on Day 13. Six littermate controls were treated with saline at appropriate times. Results are expressed as mean nmoles of product/ganglion pair/hour ± S.E.M. (vertical bars) for ChAc and as pmoles of product/pair/hour for TOH. * and ** controls differ from appropriately treated groups at P<0.001. [Black et al., 1972b]

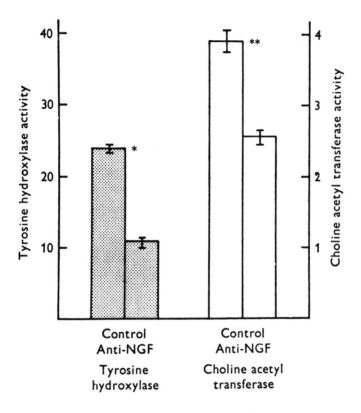

Figure 25. Effect of NGF antiserum on developing ganglia. Two-day-old mice were injected with NGF antiserum (0.05 ml. subcutaneously) and killed at 28 days of age. Littermate controls were treated with saline. Mice treated with anti-NGF are represented by the second bar in each pair. Results are expressed as mean nmoles of product/ganglion paid/hour ± S.E.M. (vertical bar) for ChAc and as pmoles of product/ganglion pair/hour for TOH. * and ** controls differ from appropriate anti-NGF groups at P<0.001. [Black et al., 1972b]

Other Evidence for the Functional Significance
of Neuron-Neuron Interactions

Can we look elsewhere for evidence of the importance of neuron-neuron interactions? We have already considered one pathological phenomenon — that of muscular dystrophy in the mouse and chick — and found that the neuron is an etiologic factor. There is a sizable body of animal and human pathological data that bears on the relations between neurons, which is discussed in detail in Chapter VII, "The Pathology of Neuron-Target Cell Interactions." For the present, it should be sufficient to state that both antero- and retrograde transneuronal degenerations have been known for many years. Although the potential of such studies has not been realized, the relatively gross data at hand again underscore the importance of the neuron in maintaining the health and even viability of both its pre- and postsynaptic partners.

What we must conclude, then, is that there is a bidirectional flow of information at the synapse between the presynaptic and postsynaptic neurons. In the case of anterograde regulation in the SCG, a transmitter is necessary but not sufficient. Other factors, molecular, developmental, and even activity-related, may modulate and/or control this inductive process. Most of these factors (all in the case of the retrograde regulation in the SCG) remain to be elucidated. What is clearly established is that there are molecular interactions between neurons that result in major changes in metabolism and/or gene expression. The findings confirm and/or parallel those obtained at the nerve-muscle junction.

Conclusion

The phenomenon of neurotrophism is well established, whether in terms of interactions between neurons and peripheral tissues or neurons themselves. Clearly, such effects involve much more than the nerve-muscle junction where so much of the debate on trophism has centered. Such interactions are, presumably, not the result of the exchange of a single trophic and nontransmitter molecule; rather, several factors, some of which are not actually trophic themselves, are operative, and, indeed, these same factors must be integrated in time to achieve the appropriate interactions. For example, a transmitter is necessary but not sufficient to maintain cell viability. Similarly, activity (impulse conduction and transmission) is important but, again, not sufficient. The identification of a proteinaceous and widely occurring trophic substance that maintains denervated muscle in culture is an important step forward, but it is unlikely that this factor operates independently of other physiological controls.

We know from the work of several investigators that a variety of materials are exchanged in neuron-target cell interactions. However, we cannot be sure that many of these materials represent part of an informational exchange process as opposed to representing nutritional conservation of substances, such as adenosine, which does not cross the blood-brain barrier (a sort of "garbage recycling" hypothesis). Undoubtedly, the list of trophic substances will grow.

The exact role of transmitters requires further clarification. At the 1968 NRP Work Session (Guth, 1969), the definition of neurotrophic effects excluded those of transmitters as such, but it is clear that these same transmitters have effects other than those related to the transfer of electrical activity from one cell to another (see Chapter VII below.) Some of these effects may not involve the usual receptors, whereas others may be secondary to a brief depolarization change that is coupled to long-term metabolic and membrane changes (see Chapter VIII).

Whereas many of the interactions are nonspecific and a common property of all nervous tissue, others are specific. The vagus nerve forms functional cholinergic synapses with muscle and yet will not maintain the same muscle's acetylcholinesterase. (This issue of specificity, a theme running through this entire *Bulletin,* is specifically dealt with in Chapter IX.)

The picture emerging from present studies is that of materials that are able to influence the metabolism, genetic expression, and even viability of target cells, whether they be other neurons or any other cell with which a neuron makes contact. The interrelations of such materials with other substances, such as hormones, and with a variety of physical factors, including time, form one of the most challenging areas of neurobiology today. Whether, indeed, these exchanges are part of higher neuronal and circuit functions, such as plasticity, learning, and memory, remains to be explored. Even more interesting, perhaps, than the identification of specific trophic molecules is the identification of the pathways by which they are exchanged and the mechanisms by which they exert their effects. These subjects are covered in ensuing chapters.

III. PATHWAYS OF INTRANEURONAL TRANSPORT AND TRANSNEURONAL EXCHANGE

Since the interactions between a neuron and its target cell are critical for the development, maturation, and viability of both cells and since these interactions involve, at least in part, a nontransmitter molecular exchange, then the routes by which the molecules travel from one cell to the other are of great importance. Again, the achievement of specificity is an issue. If satisfaction of nutritional requirements and the need for recycling certain compounds are the goal of such an exchange, then a nondirected "spray" of materials into the extracellular space with uptake by other neurons, glia, and vascular elements merely on the basis of proximity is sufficient. If, on the other hand, an exchange of metabolic or other information is to be targeted only for other neurons in the circuit, perhaps functionally yoked glia, or specific nonneural target tissues, then there must be structural specializations to ensure specific delivery.

Axonal and Dendritic Transport — Intracellular Pathways

Since the major part of neuronal synthetic activity resides in the soma, molecular signals, such as proteins and neurotransmitter enzyme systems, must be transported to the terminals for release. The phenomena of axoplasmic flow and transport are now well described, with flow occurring at a rate of 1 mm per day and transport at rates up to several hundred mm per day (see overview by Ochs, 1974). Most of the substances relevant to synaptic function and molecular exchange seem to be transported at fast rates (Miledi and Slater, 1970; Aguilar et al., 1973; Krygier-Brévart et al., 1974).

Over the past few years, increasing documentation of the existence not only of anterograde but also of retrograde transport has been obtained. Retrograde transport provides a route for signals from the periphery or postsynaptic cell to reach the neuronal soma. Such a message may indicate the functional state of the muscle or synaptic junction and provoke an appropriate action in the neuron. Like anterograde transport, retrograde transport can be very rapid and reach a rate of 13 mm per hour in the rat sensory neuron (Stöckel et al., 1975b).

Dendritic transport, like axoplasmic transport, is also bidirectional and rapid, e.g., at rates up to 250 mm per day (see Kreutzberg below; Lynch et al., 1975b). In other words, mechanisms exist for the movement of molecular signals to any part of the neuron for intracellular renewal or for release and exchange. Thus, the available rapidity of transport suggests a functionally dynamic system suited to intra- as well as intercellular communication.

In both axons and dendrities, the transport process is active (nondiffusional) and most likely dependent on the integrity of microtubules (Schmitt, 1970; for another view, cf. Droz et al., 1975). Thus, a logical approach to the study of the trophic influences of neurons would be the selective blockade of axonal transport with colchicine, which disrupts microtubule function.

Albuquerque and co-workers (1972, 1974b) were the first to test this approach when they applied colchicine to the sciatic nerve and found signs of denervation in the extensor digitorum longus or soleus muscle (see Chapter II for details). Their findings have been confirmed by some workers (see Fernandez and Ramirez, 1974), but others have cautioned against too quick an acceptance of such data because of the direct action of colchicine on muscle membrane (Lømo, 1974; Cangiano and Fried, 1976). When Aguilar and co-workers (1973) applied colchicine to peripheral nerves, they found that blockade of transport in one nerve resulted in the sprouting of adjacent nerves into the previously innervated fields. Their work suggests the existence of a neurally transported factor that may control innervated territory by preventing the sprouting of adjacent axonal bundles (see Chapter VI for further details).

Retrograde Transport in Axons: A Pathway for Target Cell-Neuron Interactions: H. Thoenen

Since the discovery of axonal retrograde transport, there has been speculation that it serves to convey information from the periphery to the neuron. For example, how can a neuron learn about the disruption of its axon and so develop a chromatolytic reaction if it were not for a signal from the site of injury to the cell soma? However, most of the substances used in the experiments to demonstrate retrograde transport are exogenous or even pathological, such as herpes virus, polio virus, tetanus toxin, Evans blue, labeled or iodinized albumin, and horseradish peroxidase. Thus, an important step in ascertaining the physiological significance of the process was the demonstration of retrograde transport of the biologically significant nerve growth factor by Thoenen and co-workers (Hendry et al., 1974; Stöckel et al., 1974, 1975a,b; Iversen et al., 1975; Paravicini et al., 1975; Stöckel and Thoenen, 1975a,b). According to Thoenen and co-workers, evidence from transplantation experiments and the fact that NGF is produced in organs innervated by adrenergic nerves argue in favor of NGF's acting as a messenger for the transfer of information from the effector organ to the innervating adrenergic neurons. The perikaryon receives this message from nerve terminals that pick up NGF specifically and transport it retrogradely. To test this hypothesis, Thoenen and co-workers (Hendry et al., 1974; Stöckel et al., 1974, 1975a,b; Iversen et al., 1975; Paravicini et al., 1975; Stöckel and Thoenen, 1975a,b) examined the role of retrograde transport of NGF, keeping in mind the following specific questions: (1) Is there evidence for retrograde *intraaxonal* transport of NGF? (2) Is retrograde transport of NGF specific? (3) Is the retrograde transport of NGF important for biological effects?

NGF Transport in Adrenergic Neurons

In looking for evidence of retrograde transport of NGF, Thoenen and collaborators (Hendry et al., 1974; Stöckel et al., 1974, 1975a; Iversen et al., 1975) injected ^{125}I-labeled NGF into the anterior chamber of the eye in mice and rats and examined the superior cervical ganglion for the presence of NGF. If retrograde transport occurs, then labeled NGF must be picked up by adrenergic nerve terminals in the pupillary dilator and ciliary muscles and transported back along the adrenergic axons, following the internal carotid artery to the cell bodies in the SCG. A large difference in radioactivity between the injected and noninjected sides of the eye was observed (Figure 26, A, B, and C), suggesting retrograde transport of NGF. This accumulation can be blocked by the injection of cold NGF and colchicine pretreatment of the NGF-injected eye. On electron microscope autoradiography, the NGF appeared to be contained within the axons and cell bodies of sympathetic postganglionic neurons.

The contralateral accumulation was due to escaped NGF being taken up by circulation, picked up by terminals, and transported retrogradely. If labeled NGF is injected intravenously, the radioactivity

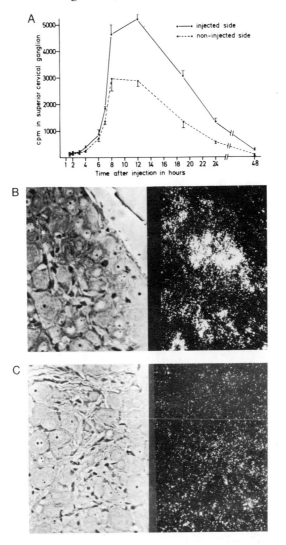

Figure 26. A. Time course of the accumulation of radioactivity in SCG after unilateral injection of 9 μCi of ^{125}I-NGF into the anterior eye chamber of a rat of 180-gm body weight. The SCG were removed 1.5 to 48 hours after the injection. The first significant difference between the injected and noninjected sides occurred after about 7 hours. This, calculated together with the distance between the site of injection and the SCG, gives a retrograde transport rate of about 2 to 3 mm/hour. B and C. Phase-contrast micrographs and dark-field autoradiograms of corresponding microscopic fields from mouse SCG on the injected (B) and noninjected (C) sides 12 hours after intraocular injection of ^{125}I-NGF. Note that on the injected side the label is concentrated over a few neuronal cells, whereas on the noninjected side the label is equally distributed over the whole area. [A, Stöckel et al., 1975a; B and C, Thoenen]

in the blood decreases rapidly (Figure 27); it drops to 10% after 4 hours, as shown by radioimmunoassay. The time course in the heart paralleled that in the blood. In SCG, a slight but distinct accumulation of ^{125}I-NGF was detected within the first hour. After this, the radioactivity level remained constant for about 4 hours; it then increased dramatically (7-fold) when the radioactivity in other tissues had declined to very low levels. These observations on the SCG are interpreted as follows: the initial small increase results from a direct accumulation of blood-borne ^{125}I-NGF by the cell bodies of the adrenergic neurons. The very marked increase occurring after 4 hours is caused by the moiety of ^{125}I-NGF reaching the ganglion by retrograde axonal transport. Further support for this interpretation comes from experimental findings obtained by transecting the postganglionic sympathetic nerve fibers. The time needed for NGF to appear in the postganglionic cell perikaryon correlates with the length of the remaining intact axon. Thus, as the distance from the cut end of the axon to the postganglionic cell body grows shorter, so does the time interval for the appearance of NGF in the perikarya of the post-ganglionic sympathetic neurons after systemic injection of NGF (Stöckel et al., 1976).

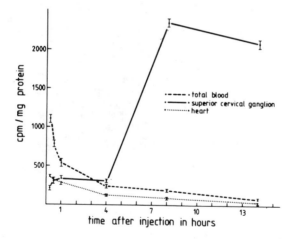

Figure 27. Time course of accumulation of radioactivity in blood, SCG, and heart, after intravenous injection of 5 μCi of ^{125}I-NGF into the tail vein of 120- to 150-gm female rats. At the given time points, the animals were killed, and the heart, SCG, and 100 μl of blood were removed. The radioactivity was counted directly in a γ-counter. Thereafter, the organs were homogenized in distilled water and the protein content was determined. Each point represents the mean ± S.E.M. of 5 animals. [Stöckel et al., 1976]

Specificity of NGF Transport

When a series of labeled proteins were injected into the eye, small amounts of radioactivity were detected in the SCG of the injected and noninjected sides (Figure 28; Stöckel et al., 1974). By contrast, NGF showed a much greater accumulation of radioactivity and a high ratio of ipsilateral to contralateral accumulation. Thoenen believes that specificity resides in the uptake mechanisms and that, if the extracellular material can get into the terminals, it will also be transported. No specific axonal transport system was found for NGF, i.e., NGF was transported at the same rate as tetanus toxin, which was found to be transported by adrenergic, sensory, and motor neurons without any specificity (Stöckel and Thoenen, 1975b).

The following questions are appropriate here: Is there specificity with respect to the neurons transporting NGF? To what extent does NGF act on nonsympathetic neurons? When ^{125}I-NGF is injected into the forepaw of adult rats, a marked increase in labeled NGF is seen

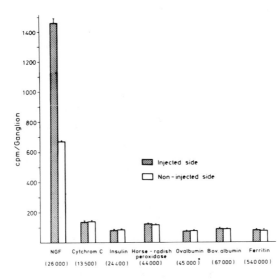

Figure 28. Comparison between the accumulation of radioactivity in SCG after unilateral intraocular injection of ^{125}I-labeled NGF and various other ^{125}I-labeled proteins. The isoelectric points are as follows: NGF, 9.3; cytochrome c, 9.8; insulin, 5.4; horseradish peroxidase, 9.7; ovalbumin, 4.6; bovine serum albumin, 4.8; ferritin, 4.6. The molecular weights of the injected proteins are given in parentheses. In each case the injected radioactivity amounted to 1 μCi. The labeled proteins were injected 14 hours before dissecting the ganglia. Each column represents the mean ± S.E.M. of 7 to 10 animals. [Stöckel et al., 1974]

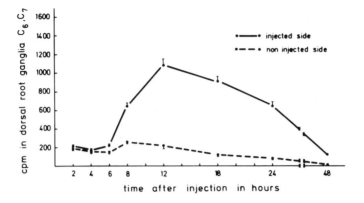

Figure 29. Time course of accumulation of radioactivity in dorsal root (C_6,C_7) ganglia after unilateral injection of 18 μCi of ^{125}I-NGF into the forepaw of albino rats (150 to 200 gm). The ganglia of the injected and noninjected sides were removed 2 to 48 hours after the injection and counted directly in a γ-counter at an efficiency of 50%. Each point represents the mean ± S.E.M. of 7 to 9 animals. [Stöckel et al., 1975b]

in the ipsilateral dorsal root ganglion cells (Figure 29). In contrast, injection of ^{125}I-NGF into the deltoid muscle does not result in a preferential accumulation of radioactivity in the corresponding spinal cord segments (C_6 to C_8), indicating that NGF is not retrogradely transported in motoneurons (Figure 30A) under experimental conditions that allow retrograde transport of tetanus toxin, as clearly demonstrated in Figure 30B. These experiments are especially interesting, since it is known that NGF stimulates sensory neurons only during a short episode in embryogenesis, e.g., at Days 5 (or earlier) to 16 in the chicken. Thus, it can be stated that sensory cell axons have not lost their specific ability to pick up and transport NGF retrogradely, although they no longer have a known in vivo or in vitro response to the molecule. The obvious question, then, is: What is NGF doing in these adult sensory perikarya? Does NGF have different functions during development and adulthood (see Stöckel et al., 1975b)?*

Effects of Retrogradely Transported NGF on the Perikaryon

In another study, following unilateral injection of NGF into the anterior eye chamber and submaxillary gland, the levels of TOH were measured in the SCG of the ipsilateral and contralateral sides at 48

*M. A. Bisby also reported differences in transport between motor and sensory neurons (see the next section).

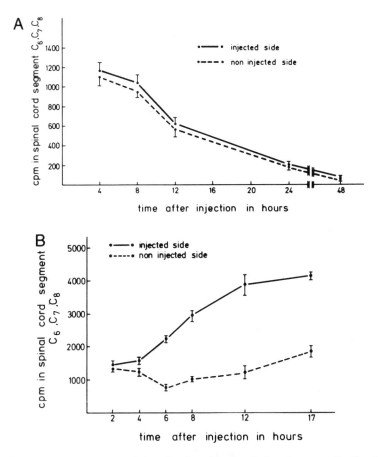

Figure 30. Time course of accumulation of radioactivity in spinal cord segment C_6-C_8 after unilateral injection of labeled NGF or labeled tetanus toxin into the deltoid muscle of albino rats (150 to 200 gm). A. 30 μCi of ^{125}I-NGF were injected unilaterally into the deltoid muscle. The spinal cord segments C_6-C_8 were removed 4 to 48 hours after the injection. B. 24 μCi of ^{125}I-labeled tetanus toxin were injected into the deltoid muscle. The spinal cord segments C_6-C_8 were removed 2 to 17 hours after the injection. In each case the spinal cord segments C_6-C_8 were separated along the mediosagittal plane and the right (injected) and left (noninjected) sides were counted separately in a γ-counter at an efficiency of 50%. Each point represents the mean ± S.E.M. of 5 to 7 animals. [Stöckel et al., 1975a]

hours. A clear difference was observed: the injected side contained twice as much TOH activity as the untreated controls and 1.5 times the contralateral (injected animals) side (Figure 31). After unilateral injection of similar amounts of cytochrome c, there was only a slight bilateral increase in TOH activity, reflecting transsynaptic induction due to the anesthesia and operation stress.

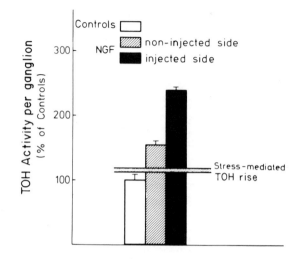

Figure 31. Effect of unilateral injection of NGF into the anterior eye chamber and submaxillary gland on TOH activity in the SCG. 2 μl of a 2 mg/ml solution of NGF were injected unilaterally into the anterior eye chamber, and 5 μl of same solution were injected into the submaxillary gland of adult mice weighing 20 to 30 gm. Forty-eight hours later TOH activity was determined separately in the ganglia of the left and right sides. In order to exclude a nonspecific effect, a further series of animals were injected with identical amounts of cytochrome c, a protein with a very similar molecular weight and isoelectric point as the monomer of the NGF β-subunit. The injection of cytochrome c resulted in a slight increase in TOH activity on both the injected and noninjected sides (indicated by the stippled thin cross bar labeled "stress-mediated TOH rise"). The results are expressed as percent of controls. Values are means ± S.E.M. for groups of 5 to 8 animals. [Stöckel and Thoenen, 1975b]

The significance of the retrograde transport of NGF can also be shown by transecting the postganglionic nerves in the SCG of newborn animals (Hendry, 1975a,b). This transection results in a permanent loss of TOH activity, closely paralleling a decrease in the number of neurons. If the axons of postganglionic sympathetic neurons are transected before Day 21, a decrease in the level of TOH activity is noted; also, the earlier the transection is performed, the more marked becomes the decrease. If these animals are treated with NGF prior to the observed fall in TOH, the reduction in TOH can be prevented. Furthermore, there is a block of cell death, and the SCG innervates its target organ effectively. These studies seem to suggest that transection of the postganglionic adrenergic nerve fibers interrupts the normal supply of NGF from the periphery, which, however, can be replaced by administration of high doses of NGF.

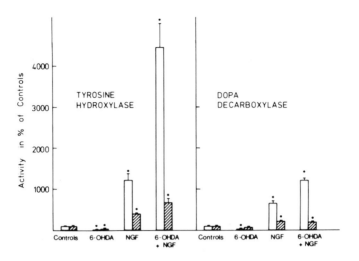

Figure 32. Effect of 6-hydroxydopamine (6-OHDA) and/or NGF treatment on TOH and dopa decarboxylase activity in rat SCG. Newborn rats were injected subcutaneously for 26 consecutive days with 6-OHDA (100 μg/gm of body weight) and/or NGF (10 μg/gm of body weight). The animals were killed 1 day after the last treatment. Enzyme activities are expressed as percent of controls either in terms of total activities (open bars) or specific activities (hatched bars). Total activities in controls were 0.564 ± 0.028 nmoles of dopa/ganglia pair/hour for TOH and 156 ± 17 nmoles of dopamine/ganglia pair/hour for dopa decarboxylase; specific activities were 2.03 ± 0.17 nmoles of dopa/mg of protein/hour for TOH and 536 ± 62 nmoles of dopamine/mg of protein/hour for dopa decarboxylase. Values represent means ± S.E.M. of at least 5 determinations. For bars with an asterisk (*), $P < 0.005$ as compared to controls. [Levi-Montalcini et al., 1975]

Similar conclusions can be drawn from recent experiments performed by Levi-Montalcini in collaboration with Thoenen and co-workers (Levi-Montalcini et al., 1975). In these experiments, the normal supply of NGF from the periphery was interrupted by destroying the adrenergic nerve terminals in neonate rats with 6-hydroxydopamine. This treatment normally causes the whole neuron to degenerate. However, the simultaneous administration of NGF not only abolished the effect of 6-hydroxydopamine on the adrenergic cell bodies but also, curiously, resulted in a potentiation of the inducing effect of NGF on TOH, possibly because of an enhanced retrograde transport of NGF (see Figure 32).*

*These experiments suggest that the amount of transported material that accumulates in cell bodies may respond to physiological demand (to injury here but perhaps to normal physiology as well). J. LaVail, pursuing an independent line of research with horseradish peroxidase as tracer, has confirmed these results (see Chapter IV; see also Bisby below).

It should be stressed that NGF acts not only intraneuronally but also on cell surface receptors (Herrup and Shooter, 1975). These authors, utilizing binding assays of ^{125}I-NGF to follow the development of embryonic chick sensory ganglia, have shown that the loss of biological responsiveness to NGF that occurs between 14 and 16 days corresponds to a 4- to 6-fold drop in the number of NGF receptors during this period.

Further Evidence Differentiating Transport Pathways in Motor and Sensory Neurons: M. A. Bisby

Bisby's main effort has been directed to the study of anterograde and retrograde transport of tritiated proteins in rat lumbosacral motor and sensory neurons. Given that little is known about the function of the labeled proteins reaching the axon terminals,* he has attempted to determine whether any of the labeled protein transported to the axon terminals was later returned to the cell body.

Utilizing nerve crushes† to detect accumulation of labeled material at various intervals after administration of ^{3}H-leucine in the vicinity of the spinal cord motoneurons, Bisby has identified a wave of labeled protein traveling down the sciatic nerve at a rate of 426 mm per day, in agreement with the earlier work of Ochs (1972). A delay of approximately 50 min occurred between the injection of precursor and the release of protein into the axon (Figure 33). By crushing the sciatic nerve at various intervals after injection of ^{3}H-leucine, Bisby could measure the accumulation of label at the crushes over a 3-hour period (Figure 34). Accumulation at the proximal side of a crush declined during the 9- to 99-hour period after precursor administration. In contrast, accumulation at the distal side of the crush was only 3% of the proximal accumulation 6 to 9 hours after administration, but it rose

*The volume of material leaving the soma by both flow and transport has been estimated by P. Weiss to be ten times the somal volume per day. Our lack of knowledge regarding the fate of the material has been a persistently embarrassing issue (see Barondes, 1967).

†The use of nerve crushes to accumulate usefully detectable levels of labeled materials has been rather widely employed and also criticized. As Bisby (1976) pointed out, the method has several disadvantages: First, it is not certain that crushing the nerve does not affect velocity or flux of transport (Bisby's results indicating a minimal contribution of blood-borne label, and the absence of local uptake or synthesis combined with a linear accumulation with time, mitigate against this possibility). Secondly, the actual accumulation of label will be greater than that measured because of retrograde transport. However, this accumulation will be small at most times of interest. Bisby does not feel that these considerations affect the conclusions of his experiments in any way.

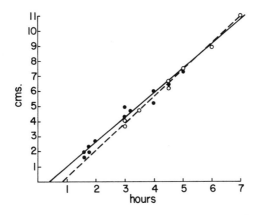

Figure 33. Velocity of wave front of fast transported protein in motor and sensory neurons. •, sensory neurons; velocity = 393 mm/day. ○, motor neurons; velocity = 428 mm/day. Note that in both cases there is an intercept on the time axis: for motor neurons this is 50 min; for sensory neurons, 26 min. Presumably, this represents the time necessary for synthesis and packaging of the protein before it is released into the axon. Lines fitted by method of least squares. [Bisby]

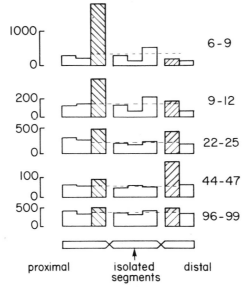

Figure 34. Profiles of protein activity in crushed nerves. Ordinate: activity of each segment in cpm per mm of nerve. The time interval in hours between injecting ^{3}H-leucine into the spinal cord and making the crush is shown by the left-hand number of the pair shown for each profile. The right-hand number is the time, 3 hours later, when the nerves were removed and analyzed. The horizontal dash line represents the mean activity of the isolated segments, and activity above this level in the accumulation segments (shaded areas) represents accumulation of transported activity. [Bisby]

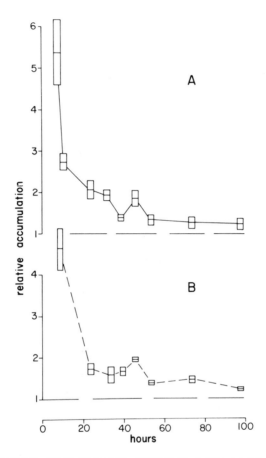

Figure 35. Accumulation of tritiated protein activity in the proximal crush made on a sciatic nerve. A. Motor axons after injection of ³H-leucine into ventral horn. B. Sensory axons after injection into dorsal root ganglia. Ordinate: accumulation relative to background activity in nerve. Abscissa: elapsed time since ³H-leucine injection. The rectangles have the vertical dimensions of mean ± S.E.M. of relative accumulation (n⩾10) and horizontal dimensions of the 3-hour time interval over which material accumulated at the crush. [Bisby]

until it became 192% of the proximal accumulation at 44 to 47 hours. These observations led Bisby to conclude that in motoneurons there is initially a wave of labeled protein that travels toward the axon terminals. About two-thirds of the transported material returns toward the cell body after spending about 30 hours in the terminals.

It is particularly interesting (see Figure 35B) that after injection of ³H-leucine into the lumbosacral dorsal root ganglia of anesthetized

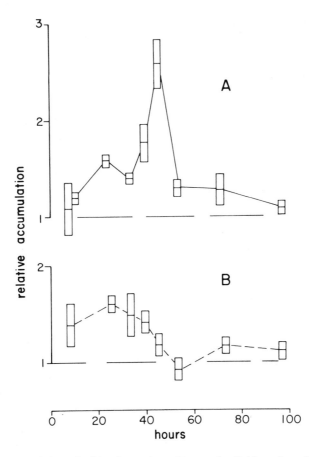

Figure 36. Accumulation of tritiated protein activity at the distal crush made on a sciatic nerve. A. Motor axons. B. Sensory axons. Note that the large accumulation, representing retrograde transport, observed in motor axons at 35 to 50 hours is absent from sensory axons. [Bisby]

rats, there was a similar anterograde transport in the sensory axons. However, the increase in retrograde transport that occurs in motor axons after 44 hours was absent in the sensory axons (Figure 36B) (Bisby, 1975b). Bisby suggests that the different patterns of protein transport in the two neuronal types may reflect functional differences. Alternatively, it may be that there are differences in the transport pathways or the materials transported. Bisby has tried to compare transport in the peripheral and central processes of sensory neurons expecting to find retrograde transport similar to that in motoneurons in the central process. Unfortunately, technical problems were such that the experiment was not feasible. However, it has been reported that smaller quantities of material are transported in central than in peripheral processes of sensory neurons (Lasek, 1968; Ochs, 1972; Smith, 1973) and that proteins of different molecular weight are transported in the two processes (Anderson and McClure, 1973).

Bisby's results may reflect differences in the turnover of transported endogenous protein in motor and sensory terminals rather than an absence of retrograde transport mechanisms in peripheral sensory axons. Both NGF (Stöckel and Thoenen, 1975a,b) and horseradish peroxidase (Furstman et al., 1975) are retrogradely transported by both motor and sensory axons. However, Abe and co-workers (1974), using a technique analogous to Bisby's, have shown that retrograde transport in frog sensory neurons does occur.

Role of Material in Synaptic Transmission

Bisby has hypothesized that the returning material in the motoneuron plays an essential role in synaptic transmission. As an example, he cited the work of Miledi and Slater (1970) who reported that, 36 hours after cutting the rat's sciatic nerve in the thigh, neuromuscular transmission failed in all leg muscles. If 3 hours are subtracted from the time the material travels from a cut in the thigh to the most distal motor terminals in the leg, then the lifespan of an essential factor in the transmission is 33 hours.

If such material does participate in synaptic transmission in some way, then a comparison of the material transported antero-gradely and retrogradely might be helpful. A preliminary study conducted with sodium dodecyl sulfate (SDS) gel electrophoresis showed that there is a difference in the material transported (Figure 37). The rapid return to the cell body of material that has participated in transmission may represent not only a recycling process, but also a means of providing feedback information about the functional state of the axon terminals. This may, in turn, be coupled to gene expression and/or control of the synthesis of proteins destined for the synaptic terminal.

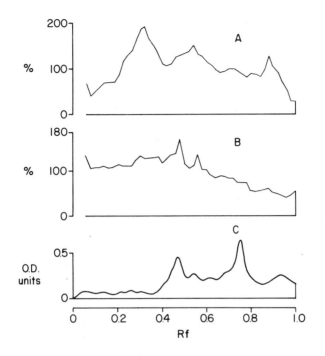

Figure 37. ³H activity (A and B) and protein content (C) of SDS-polyacrylamide gels. A. Material collected over 8 hours proximal to a crush made 2 hours after ³H-leucine injection into the ventral horn of the spinal cord. B. Material collected over 8 hours distal to a crush made 40 hours after ³H-leucine injection. C. Densitometer scan of a gel stained with Coomassie blue. Ordinate: A and B, ³H activity per gel slice as percent of mean activity per slice. The profiles are the means of 5 experiments. C, optical density units. Abscissa: Rf value (distance along gel as a fraction of distance travelled by wave front marker dye). [Bisby]

Transneuronal Transfer: Inter- and Extracellular Pathways

The Nerve-Muscle Junction and the Periphery

Having described the routes by which known and potential trophic substances can travel to and from the synthetic and regulatory machinery of the cell soma, we can now turn our attention to the characterization of the pathways of transneuronal transfer. This can be done in several ways. For nerve-muscle relationships, Korr and colleagues first described the delivery of neuronal proteins to muscle cells in 1967 (see also Korr and Appeltauer, 1974; Appeltauer and Korr, 1975). Unfortunately, these studies did not unequivocally demonstrate a transynaptic transfer of labeled protein, and, at present, resolution is inadequate to distinguish between labeled protein associated with nerve axons or with muscle cells. According to Bisby, the time course of terminal labeling is more easily followed in the superior cervical ganglion, and he suggests that this preparation might be a better model for the study of transneuronal transfer. Another preparation, in which transfer of material from efferent axons to effector cells has been detected, is the sensory epithelium of the vestibular system examined by Alvarez and Püschel (1972).

The release of proteins from stimulated nerve terminals has been well studied in the case of peripheral adrenergic terminals (Geffen et al., 1970; Gewirtz and Kopin, 1970; Smith et al., 1970). The released proteins, which are components of dense-core synaptic vesicles (Bisby et al., 1973), are involved in norepinephrine synthesis and amine storage complexes. Musick and Hubbard (1972), using an isolated preparation of mouse phrenic nerve-diaphragm, reported that protein is released concurrently with ACh at the neuromuscular junction. This protein may be derived from the soluble protein that exists in cholinergic synaptic vesicles (Whittaker et al., 1974). Adenosine triphosphate (ATP), another component of the vesicles, is also released by nerve stimulation (Silinsky and Hubbard, 1973). Hines and co-workers (1974) have claimed to be able to detect radioactively labeled proteins released from isolated nerves in conjunction with axonal transport. Whether such proteins can be released independently of nerve impulses and whether they can act as mediators of trophic influences remain unclear.

In contrast to the usual situation where studies of the neuromuscular junction have helped to clarify problems less easily resolved by attacking the CNS, the best present evidence regarding the pathways of transneuronal transfer comes from studies of the latter.

Transneuronal Transfer of Axonally Transported Material in the Visual System — Progress and Cautions: B. Grafstein

The transneuronal appearance of radioactive material in the CNS was first shown by Grafstein and co-workers (Grafstein, 1971; Grafstein and Laureno, 1973; Specht and Grafstein, 1973) after injection of radioactive amino acids (or sugars) into the eye bulb of the

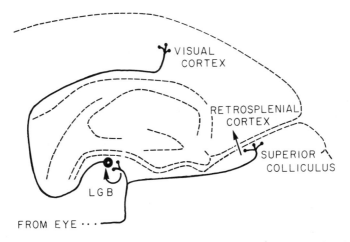

Figure 38. Diagram of mouse brain in parasagittal section showing terminations of optic fibers LGB and superior colliculus to which axonally transported material is conveyed. Arrows indicate sites of transneuronal transfer of radioactivity: (2) from presynaptic to postsynaptic elements in LGB, giving rise to material that is then conveyed by axonal transport to the geniculate axon terminations in the striate (visual) cortex; and (2) from superior colliculus to overlying retrosplenial cortex. [Grafstein]

mouse. Using relatively conservative amounts of labeled precursors (e.g., a few microcuries of ^{3}H-proline), they found that some of the radioactivity that was axonally transported in the optic axons to the lateral geniculate body (LGB) was transferred from the optic nerve terminals to the geniculate neurons; it subsequently appeared as labeled protein in the terminals of the geniculocortical axons in the striate cortex (Figure 38). The axonally transported material reached the optic terminals in two main waves, one arriving within 24 hours after the precursor injection and representing the so-called "fast component" of axonally transported protein, the other arriving at 6 to 10 days after the injection and representing the "slow component" of axonal transport (Figure 39A). Although the two components differed greatly in their composition (Grafstein, 1975), both contributed to the transferred material that appeared in the striate cortex (Figure 39B). However, the proportion of transferred material derived from the slow component was considerably greater than that derived from the fast component (Figure 39C). The reason for this could be either that the slow component contains a larger proportion of transferable material, or that the fast component has a shorter residence time in the nerve terminals (from which it is removed by metabolic breakdown or by retrograde transport); hence, the transferable material is available at the nerve terminals for a shorter period of time.

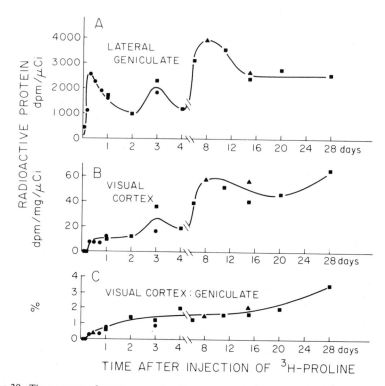

Figure 39. Time course of appearance of radioactive protein in (A) LGB body and (B) visual (striate) cortex after injection of ^{3}H-proline into contralateral eye. C. Radioactive protein accumulation in visual cortex as proportion of LGB radioactivity. Each point represents the mean of values obtained for 4 to 6 animals. Different symbols represent different experimental groups. [Grafstein and Laureno, 1973]

The amount of transferred radioactivity appears to be independent of the rate of physiological activity in the optic axons. This was determined by comparing the transneuronal transfer in normal mice and in mice subject to hereditary degeneration of the visual receptor cells (C57Bℓ/6J *le rd*), in which the level of electrical activity in the optic nerve is greatly reduced although the retinal ganglion cells are well preserved. The amount of axonally transported protein reaching the optic nerve terminals was reduced in the mutant mice, but the proportion of transferred radioactivity appearing in the visual cortex was not significantly different from that in normal mice (Figure 40). The absence of any relationship between the transferred radioactivity and physiological activity suggests that the transfer is not directly related to synaptic transmission mechanisms.

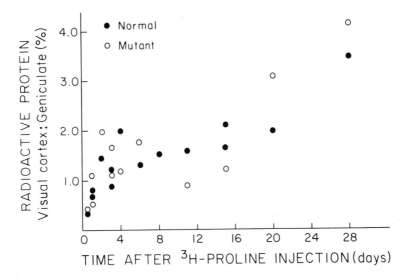

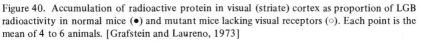

Figure 40. Accumulation of radioactive protein in visual (striate) cortex as proportion of LGB radioactivity in normal mice (●) and mutant mice lacking visual receptors (○). Each point is the mean of 4 to 6 animals. [Grafstein and Laureno, 1973]

A fundamental question to be considered is whether the transferred material consists of macromolecules directly derived from the axonally transported material and transferred without modification, or whether it consists of breakdown products of small molecular weight that are resynthesized into macromolecules in the cells to which they are transferred. Since the proportion of axonally transported radioactivity that may be transferred varies according to the precursors (Grafstein and Laureno, 1973), it is clear that only some of the transported constituents are susceptible to transfer. An extreme case is ^{35}S-methionine, which appears to give rise to very little, if any, transferred radioactivity.* This apparent specificity in the release process may be a function of the metabolic turnover mechanisms in the axon and its terminals and, therefore, does not provide any direct indications about the nature of the transferred material.

Another approach might be to consider the time relations involved in the transfer, specifically, whether sufficient time elapses during the transfer process to allow for breakdown and resynthesis. In the striate cortex, the initial appearance of transferred radioactivity lags about 5 to 8 hours behind the arrival of the transported protein in the LGB (Grafstein and Laureno, 1973). If the rate of transport in the

*U. C. Dräger, personal communication.

optic radiations is the same as that in the optic nerve, transport of the transferred material from the LGB to the cortex probably does not take more than 2 to 3 hours; thus, one may assume a "processing time" in the optic nerve terminals of at least 2 to 5 hours. In experiments with ^{3}H-fucose, Specht and Grafstein* found that some of the transferred radioactivity may not appear in the cortex until several days after its deposition in the terminals. These times are long enough to encompass various metabolic conversions.

Experiments with inhibitors of protein synthesis indicate that there may, indeed, be some transneuronal transfer of precursor molecules. Droz and collaborators (1973) have shown that, during axonal transport of labeled proteins in the presynaptic axons of the chicken ciliary ganglion, application of cycloheximide to the ganglion greatly reduces the amount of labeled protein appearing in the postsynaptic cell bodies. Heacock and Agranoff (1975) have reported similar results in the optic tectum of goldfish. However, by focusing on the cell bodies that are the site of protein synthesis, these studies would inevitably emphasize the contribution of the portion of transferred material that could serve as a precursor for postsynaptic synthesis. On the other hand, Specht and Grafstein (1973), who examined the transferred material appearing in the terminals of the geniculostriate fibers while protein synthesis was inhibited in the geniculate cell bodies, found that the reduction in transferred material was less than would be anticipated from the existing degree of inhibition. This suggests that a significant proportion of the transferred material was in macromolecular form and available for transport without further synthesis. Other indications that at least a portion of the transferred material is in the form of protein have been enumerated by Grafstein and Laureno (1973) and Specht and Grafstein (1973) (see also Miani, 1971).

The transneuronal transfer of radioactivity from optic axons to LGB cells has been useful in mapping the projections of the geniculate cells to the visual cortex (Dräger, 1974; Hubel, 1975; Wiesel et al., 1974). However, the transfer of radioactivity is not confined to neurons that are synaptically linked with the optic axons. This is evident from the finding that some of the radioactivity that is axonally transported to the optic nerve terminals in the superior colliculus is transferred to the retrosplenial cortex overlying the colliculus (Figure 38). Thus, areas that are merely contiguous with the labeled terminal field can also become labeled, a finding that again supports the idea that the process of transneuronal transfer is not necessarily connected with synaptic

*S. Specht and B. Grafstein, unpublished results.

mechanisms. It is possible that some of the transfer of radioactivity depends on a specific mechanism confined to the synapse, but at present there is no clear evidence for such a specific transsynaptic process. Instead, these experimental findings suggest that each nerve fiber discharges into its surround a considerable amount of material that then becomes incorporated into neighboring cells. This discharge is probably more prominent at the nerve terminals than along the course of the axon, because the terminals are the site of final disposition of much axonally transported material, and because they represent a large volume pool of this transported material. Cells closest to the discharging axon terminals would be in the best position to receive the discharged material. Thus, in the LGB, for example, the transfer of material from presynaptic axons to postsynaptic cells is effective not necessarily because of the special synaptic linkage between the elements but because of their proximity.

Could such a generalized discharge mechanism play a significant role in neurotrophic interactions? Generally, trophic effects are thought to be exercised between cells that have a specific functional relationship with each other, e.g., between a sensory nerve fiber and the sensory receptor cells it innervates. However, the trophic action of the nerve fiber can operate in the absence of functional innervation. For example, in connection with trophic effects on lateral line organs in amphibians, Jones and Singer (1969) suggested that the nerve produces its effect by generating "an aura of neurotrophic emanation." Nonetheless, it is reasonable to conclude that material discharged from the nerve in a relatively nonspecific way might come to have an important trophic influence on neighboring cells. This influence might appear to be selectively directed to a circumscribed group of cells if the discharged material happens to match the metabolic requirements of those cells at a particular time. Selective uptake mechanisms in the target cells yield specificity of transfer.

Dendritic Secretion and Transneuronal Transfer:
G. W. Kreutzberg

In their elucidation of the picture of intra- and transneuronal molecular traffic, Kreutzberg, Schubert, and collaborators have used a multidisciplinary approach that combines various techniques, i.e., microiontophoresis of radioactively labeled precursors of proteins, glycoproteins, lipids, and nucleotides, together with autoradiography, light and electron microscope histochemistry, and biochemical analysis (for a review, see Kreutzberg and Schubert, 1975).

Axonal Transport and Synaptic Maintenance

Fast axonal transport is a vehicle for the conveyance of neurotransmitter enzyme systems and other materials required for the maintenance of the presynaptic terminal. A study of the anterograde axonal transport of ^{3}H-leucine-labeled proteins from the striate cortex to the lateral geniculate nucleus in the rabbit revealed that, by far, the highest incorporation of radioactive proteins was in fractions containing external synaptosomal membranes (Krygier-Brévart et al., 1974).

Anterograde axonal transport is not only involved in maintaining the presynaptic terminal, but also carries materials for release from the terminal and for transneuronal transfer. A specific transfer, as observed for adenosine, guanosine, and uridine derivatives, may provide a means for tracing activity in neuronal circuits and suggests possible metabolic coupling between the two neurons involved (see also Schubert's discussion in Chapter VIII). Other substances released from the presynaptic terminal include amino acids, possibly peptides and proteins (see Grafstein above; Ingoglia et al., 1974).

Intradendritic Transport and Dendritic Secretion

Intradendritic transport and dendritic release of various compounds have been studied by Kreutzberg and collaborators (for a review, see Schubert and Kreutzberg, 1975a,b,c). In demonstrating intradendritic transport, they used ^{3}H-glycine as the microiontophoretically applied precursor, since it remains strictly confined to the injected neuron, with the neighboring nerve cells and neuropil elements remaining essentially free of silver grains (Globus et al., 1968; Schubert et al., 1971). Within 15 min after iontophoresis in cat spinal motoneurons, radioactive material reached the limits of the dendritic tree and could be traced as far as 1000 μ from the soma (Figure 41). Using the data obtained, Kreutzberg and collaborators have been able to determine that dendritic transport is an active and not a diffusional process that can be blocked by colchicine in a manner similar to the blocking of axonal transport (Schubert et al., 1972; Schubert and Kreutzberg, 1975b,c). Moreover, it involves the conveyance of glyco-

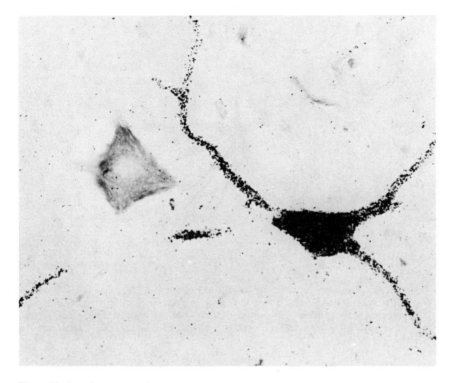

Figure 41. Protein transport in the dendrites of a cat spinal motoneuron 30 min after injection of ^{3}H-glycine into the cell body. Labeling is restricted to the injected neuron. The neighboring cell shows no radioactivity. [Kreutzberg]

proteins and acid mucopolysaccharides (Kreutzberg et al., 1973, 1975a), acetylcholinesterase (Kreutzberg et al., 1975b), and nucleoside derivatives (Kreutzberg and Schubert, 1975). As in axonal transport, dendritic transport is bidirectional, thus providing a means for communication to and from the soma. Utilizing horseradish peroxidase injected into rat hippocampal pyramidal cells, Lynch and co-workers (1975b) confirmed these findings.

Kreutzberg and collaborators have also described the release of various materials from dendrites – a process they call "dendritic secretion." In the process, ^{3}H-glycine, as a metabolite, a free amino acid, or as part of a peptide, is released from the spinal motoneuron and transferred to one or two other neurons (Globus et al., 1968), probably via dendrodendritic pathways (Kreutzberg and Schubert, 1975; Kreutzberg et al., 1975a) (see Figure 42, A and B). Glycoproteins or

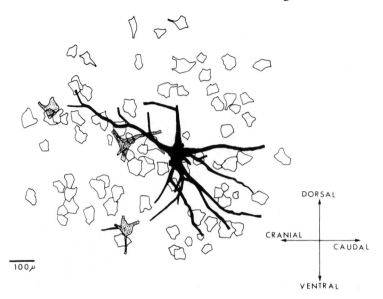

Figure 42. A. The neuron in the center (solid) was injected with ³H-glycine and reconstructed from a series of autoradiographs. Three other neurons in the vicinity (dotted) also show a light label, suggesting a transfer of radioactive material from the injected neuron to a selected number of neighboring neurons. No radioactivity is detected in all the other neurons (open) of the area. [Kreutzberg]

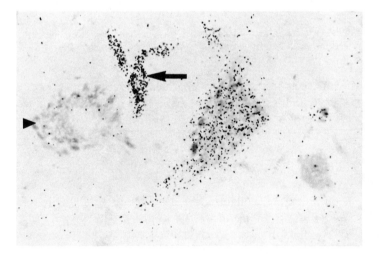

Figure 42. B. Noninjected neuron revealing a distinct labeling. It is found close to a more heavily labeled dendrite (←) of the injected neuron that has received ³H-glycine about 5 hours before sacrifice. Only single silver grains are seen over the neighboring nerve cell (▶). Autoradiography; stained with toluidene blue. ×850. [Kreutzberg et al., 1975a]

precursors are also released from the dendrites and accumulate in an organized fashion in the extracellular space. These findings suggest that the dendrite has control over its own local environment (Kreutzberg and Schubert, 1975; Schubert and Kreutzberg, 1975b,c).

Recent data from Thoenen's laboratory also show a release of macromolecular material from neurons (Schwab and Thoenen, 1976). Radioactive tetanus toxin was shown to travel in axons of motoneurons in a retrograde direction. After reaching the cell bodies, the toxin was released; later on it was demonstrated in presynaptic terminals impinging on the soma and in dendrites of the motoneurons.

Acetylcholinesterase (AChE), which is synthesized in the neuronal soma, is transported in dendrites in association with tubular and vesicular structures resembling the cisternae of smooth endoplasmic reticulum (Figure 43). These large cisternae typically approach the

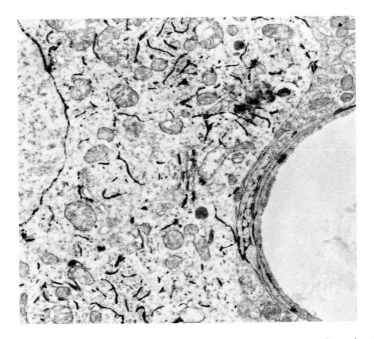

Figure 43. Facial motoneuron of the rat, 36 hours after diisopropyl fluorophosphate treatment, demonstrating the postulated transport route from neurons to the vasculature. Observe the normal AChE activity in the cisternae of the rough endoplasmic reticulum and decreased activity in the cellular envelope. Activity is prominent in the extracellular spaces between the neuron and the capillary and in the basement membrane of the capillary. ×18,000. [Kreutzberg and Schubert, 1975]

dendritic membrane where the enzyme is released to become incorporated in the dendritic membrane. From the dendritic membrane, the enzyme is released into the extracellular space. This secretion is especially enhanced in chromatolytic neurons and in the recovery phase after diisopropyl fluorophosphate intoxication. In these cases, the dendritic membrane almost loses its capability to retain AChE. The enzyme appears in the extracellular clefts and is concentrated in the basement membranes of the capillaries. The capillary endothelial cells apparently cannot synthesize AChE, but they can take up pinocytotic vesicles from the basement lamina containing activity of the neuronal enzyme (Figure 44, A and B) (Kreutzberg and Kaiya, 1974; Kreutzberg

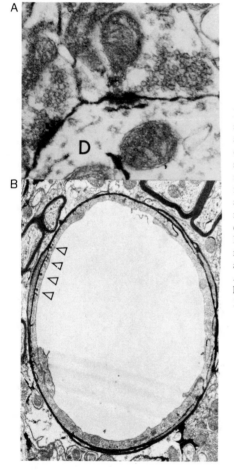

Figure 44. A. Two axon terminals making synaptic contacts on a dendrite (D). AChE activity is demonstrated by the electron-dense reaction product in tubulocisternal structures inside the dendrite and in the synaptic cleft. ×43000. B. Capillary in the facial nucleus of guinea pig. Two to 3 weeks after facial nerve transection, the basement membranes show increasing AChE activity, demonstrated by the solid reaction product. No activity is seen in the endoplasmic reticulum of the endothelial cells, suggesting a nonvascular origin of the enzyme. Note AChE-containing pinocytotic vesicles (arrow heads). ×12000. [Kreutzberg and Tóth, 1974]

et al., 1975b). AChE may not, of course, be the only substance that follows this route from the neuron to the vasculature. Conceivably, such substances regulate capillary permeability, thus allowing the neuron still further control over its local environment. It is interesting that both glycoproteins and AChE are released and yet are not taken up by neighboring neurons, whereas horseradish peroxidase and nerve growth factor are taken up. Thoenen (see above) suggests that the answer may lie in the specificity of neuronal uptake mechanisms.

If molecular exchange is involved in the actual transfer of information between neurons of a given circuit, and perhaps in the development of particular circuit connections, then the means by which the specificity of neuron-to-neuron transfer is achieved assumes importance. From the data of Kreutzberg and co-workers, it is clear that dendritic secretion, in a narrow sense, is a selective process and that there can be a highly directed cellular transfer of only certain molecules. Specificity of transfer could also result from geometrical parameters that could include proximity, synaptic contact, and dendritic bundling. The highest degree of specificity, however, might be more reliably achieved by a true structural specialization, and the gap (or electrotonic) junction, which occurs between some neurons, could be such a device.

Gap Junctions and Directed Exchange

With the above observations in mind, Rieske and collaborators (1975; see also Globus et al., 1973) examined transneuronal transfer in electrotonically coupled Retzius cells (Rc's) of the segmental ganglia of the leech nerve cord (Figure 45). Intracellular application of fucose, glucosamine, glycine, leucine, orotic acid, and uridine was carried out by means of microiontophoresis. Within several minutes, the precursors were incorporated into macromolecules and distributed in a specific pattern over the cell somata and then released into the nerve processes. There was labeling not only of the injected Rc but also of the electrically coupled but noninjected cell, indicating a specific inter-neuronal transfer (Figure 46). The other ganglionic compartments showed no or little labeling. Intracellular injection of one Rc with puromycin, followed by injection of amino acids or fucose into the same Rc or into the coupled Rc, resulted in an inhibition of precursor

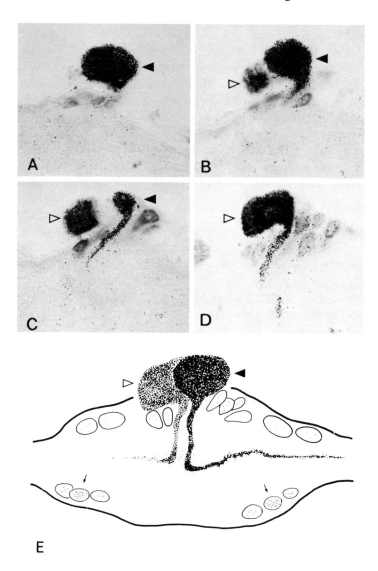

Figure 45. Transneuronal transfer of radioactive material 2 hours after intracellular injection of ³H-glycine into one Rc. A–D. Autoradiographs of serial transverse sections through a leech ganglion reveal incorporation of amino acid not only in the injected Rc (solid arrows) but also in the electrically coupled noninjected Rc (open arrows). ×376. E. Schematic reconstruction made by superimposing tracings of serial radioautographs. Radioactive proteins are released down the Rc main process at an estimated transport rate of 5 to 6 mm/day. Compared to the other nerve cells, small distinctive neurons of two dorsal compartments (small arrows) show increased label, indicating a special relationship to the Retzius cells. [Rieske et al., 1975]

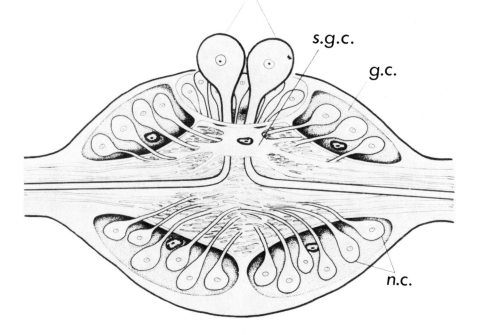

Figure 46. Semidiagrammatic representation of a transverse section through a segmental leech ganglion with its ventral side at the top (modified slightly after Coggeshall and Fawcett, 1964). Within each of the peripheral compartments, the nerve cells (n.c.) and their proximal processes are surrounded by a single large glial cell (g.c.). Nearly all nerve cells send their main process with its fine branches into the dense mass of the central neuropil, which contains two large stellate glial cells (s.g.c.); only one of them is represented here. The ventral central compartment contains the two electrically coupled giant nerve cells (R.c.), which send their processes out of the ipsilateral ganglionic roots. To provide a clear demonstration of the course of the R.c. processes, their ramifying dendrites are not shown. After an incision is made through the sheath enveloping the ganglion, the glial cytoplasm of this compartment streams out and the two R.c.'s protrude out of the incision. Histological section (see top, toluidine blue and eosin, ×403) shows no somatic contact between the R.c.'s. [Rieske et al., 1975]

incorporation within the puromycin-injected Rc and an exclusive labeling of the coupled Rc, thus indicating that the precursors themselves were transferred. The transfer of relatively low-molecular weight (<1000) substances is in accord with findings on other systems where gap junctions have been demonstrated by electrophysiological and morphological techniques (Payton et al., 1969; Bennett and Dunham, 1970; Bennett and Goodenough, 1976). Furthermore, uncoupling the two Retzius cells by Ca^{2+} deprivation blocks the transneuronal transfer of material.

Hermann and co-workers (1975) have also examined the transjunctional flux of radioactive precursors across electrotonic junctions between lateral giant axons (LGA's) of the crayfish. The segmented LGA's, one on each side of the ventral nerve cord, join each other at intraganglionic septa in which nonrectifying electrical synapses are located. In addition, each LGA joins with its contralateral counterpart in a presumably nonrectifying electrical synapse at the commissural junction, and there is also a rectifying synapse with the motor giant axon. Knowledge of this anatomy enabled the investigators to ask questions about the permeability of electrotonic junctions with different electrical properties, the transfer of material via successive electrically coupled neurons and neuronal segments, and the presence of orthograde and retrograde transport processes in single identified axons.

After injecting ^{3}H-glycine and ^{3}H-glucosamine into the LGA just anterior to the septum of the third abdominal ganglion isolated from the crayfish, *Astacus fluviatilis,* Hermann and colleagues (1975) found a selective transjunctional movement of label across the nonrectifying electrotonic junctions of the septum and the commissural connection (Figure 47). No material passed the rectifying junction between the LGA and the giant motor axon. As in the leech Retzius cells, it appears that glycine and glucosamine, themselves, are transferred.

Although both leech Retzius cells and crayfish LGA segments show evidence of low-resistance coupling and selective transfer of materials of low molecular weight, the actual morphological demonstration of the gap junction has not been made. Also, the morphological basis for the specific transfer of materials between cat spinal motoneuron dendrites is not known.

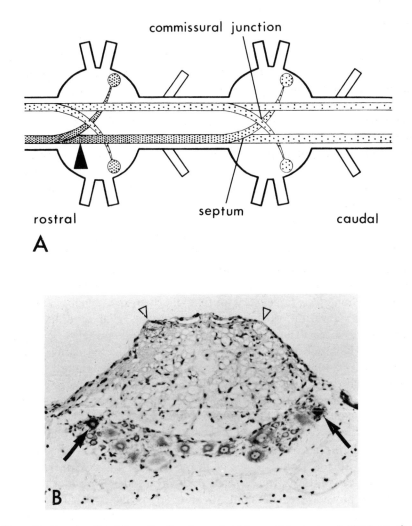

Figure 47. Transjunctional flux of radioactive material in crayfish nerve cord. Five hours after injection of ^{3}H-glycine in the LGA just posterior to the septum (solid arrow head in A), the nerve cord was fixed with glutaraldehyde. To facilitate LGA penetration by electrodes, the dorsal part of the connective tissue sheath has been removed. A. Schematic reconstruction from serial sections. Silver grains, which represent newly synthesized proteins and their soluble precursors, are found exclusively in the coupled LGA's at the ipsilateral and contralateral sites, indicating a selective material transfer across the electrotonic synapses at the septum and the commissural junction. B. Autoradiograph of a cross section through the third ganglion. Open arrow heads point to labeled LGA's; solid arrows to labeled LGA soma. ×95. [Hermann et al., 1975]

Conclusions

The picture that is now emerging is one of active bidirectional transsynaptic and transcellular exchange between neurons as well as between neurons and their peripheral target cells. This molecular exchange is critical for the maintenance of the health, pattern of innervation (see Chapter VI), and even the viability of the cells involved. Intraneuronally, there is a busy two-way "traffic" of intra-, extra-, and transcellularly channeled molecules; hence, information received at one point ultimately influences the entire developing or mature neuron, as well as its relations to other cells in the same structural and functional domain.

Much about the extra- and transcellular pathways, as well as about what substances are transferred, remains to be determined. The specific transfer of molecules involved in intercellular communication may require structural specializations, and one potential device is the gap junction. Other factors in this specificity of transfer include dendritic geometry, target cell uptake mechanisms, synaptic mechanisms, regionalization of release, and, perhaps, glial modulation of extracellular space. There may be other structural specializations that remain to be discovered. Where there is a nondirected spray and/or leakage of materials into the extracellular space with uptake by other neurons, glia, and vascular elements, then proximity and target cell uptake mechanisms may be sufficient to explain the process.

To complete the discussion of the pathways of neuron-target cell interactions, four other issues need to be considered in some detail:

1. If the molecular exchange is as important a part of neuronal and target cell function as it seems to be, then we might expect to find responsiveness of the intraneuronal pathways and release mechanisms to changed physiological demands. Is there any evidence for this?

2. Are all the pathways local; i.e., do they involve interactions between neighboring cells? What are the pathways for the circulating hormones that provide communication between the target cell and neuron separated by many centimeters?

3. The control of neuronal death by the peripheral target cell is a well-known phenomenon. What is the signal for neuronal death and how is it sent to the neuron? How does this phenomenon add to our understanding of the relations between neurons and target cells?

4. What is the role of glia in transneuronal exchange? Do they represent another pathway?

The first three issues comprise much of the excitement of the rapidly growing field of target cell-neuron interactions, which is discussed in Chapter IV. The participation of glia in transcellular exchange pathways, as well as their interactions with neurons in general, is taken up in Chapter V.

IV. TARGET CELL-NEURON INTERACTIONS

The fact that the peripheral target cell can influence central neurons is now well established. In 1909 Shorey showed that the removal of a limb from a chick embryo resulted in hypoplasia of the ventral horn. Hamburger (1934, 1948, 1958), Bueker (1943), Barron (1946), Hughes and Tschumi (1958), Hughes (1961), and Prestige (1967b, 1970) have confirmed these findings, and others have extended them to the (1) chick ciliary ganglion (Landmesser and Pilar, 1974a,b), including the preganglionic fibers (Cowan and Wenger, 1968); (2) chick and amphibian spinal ganglia (Levi-Montalcini and Levi, 1943; Prestige, 1965, 1967a); and (3) avian mesencephalic nucleus (Rogers and Cowan, 1973). All these studies demonstrated the existence of critical periods in embryonic development, during which time neurons lacking a periphery die in large numbers.

It is also well known that the influence of the periphery on the central nervous system is important for the mature as well as the developing organism. As discussed in Chapter III, Stöckel and co-workers (1975a,b) have shown that nerve growth factor continues to be transported retrogradely by adult neurons, and Hendry and Iversen (1973) have demonstrated that reduced tyrosine hydroxylase activity in sympathetic ganglia correlates with a drop in plasma and tissue NGF concentrations after surgical removal of the submaxillary glands of adult mice. Similarly, metabolic alterations for the developing organism need not be so drastic as to lead to cell death. Giller and co-workers (1973) have found that the activity of choline acetyltransferase is more than 10-fold greater in combined cultures of spinal cord and muscle cells than in cultures of spinal cord cells alone. Furthermore, the increase in ChAc activity is associated with the formation of a functional neuromuscular junction. Also, as already alluded to in Chapter II, Black and co-workers (1972b) have elegantly defined the retrograde transsynaptic regulation of ChAc in preganglionic sympathetic nerves by postganglionic neurons.

All such interactions require a means for getting a signal from the target cell to the neuronal soma (see the discussion on retrograde transport in Chapter II). A crucial question, however, is whether the retrograde transport mechanism is functionally responsive (as we might expect it to be) if it is involved in the dynamic metabolic balance between the target cell and neuron. Contact between the neuron and target cell is not always direct, and not all molecular signals (particularly the peripherally produced hormones) travel to the cell soma by way of intraaxonal retrograde transport mechanisms. In view of the profound effects such signals exert on the development and mature function of neurons, the pathways by which they act should be delineated.

Having discussed the molecular signals and the pathways and mechanisms by which they travel to and from the neuronal metabolic and biosynthetic control centers in Chapters II and III, we will attempt in this chapter to elucidate phenomena such as the peripheral control of cell death. The central issues are as follows: (1) What is the nature of the peripheral control of neuronal death? Can the signal be identified? (2) Is the retrograde transport mechanism responsive to changes in physiological demands? (3) What are the indirect pathways by which peripherally produced substances can act on their target neurons and what is their relative importance compared to the intraaxonal pathway of retrograde transport?

The Role of the Periphery in Cell Death:
L. T. Landmesser

Utilizing the chick ciliary ganglion (Figure 48), Landmesser and Pilar (1972, 1974a,b; Pilar and Landmesser, 1975, 1976) have investigated not only the way in which the peripheral target organ of a nerve cell influences the developing nervous system but also the role that cell death plays in the process. The chick ciliary ganglion, which is normally situated just distal to where the oculomotor nerve sends medial and lateral branches to the extraocular muscles, contains two cell types, the choroid and the ciliary. Each of the choroid cells is characterized by multiple innervation by two to three preganglionic fibers, whereas each of the ciliary cells is innervated by a single preganglionic fiber.* The ciliary nerves, consisting of axons of the larger, myelinated ciliary cells, emerge from the ganglion and immediately penetrate through the sclera to run within the optic cup to the striated iris and ciliary muscles. Medial to the ciliary nerves, a second group of two to three finer nerves from the smaller choroid cells emerges from the ganglion. These nerves

---

*Each preganglionic fiber, however, innervates more than one ciliary cell (G. Pilar and L. T. Landmesser, unpublished observations).

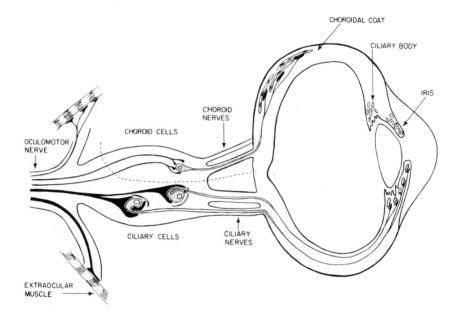

Figure 48. Anatomical relationship of the ciliary ganglion to its peripheral targets. The large ciliary cells, which receive single calyciform synapses, send their axons out the ciliary nerves to the iris. The smaller choroid cells, which receive multiple bouton terminals, send axons out the choroid nerves to innervate vascular smooth muscle. The optic cup is drawn much reduced with respect to the ganglion. [Landmesser and Pilar, 1974a]

pierce the sclera and branch profusely in the vascular choroid tissue where they innervate smooth muscle.

In essence, Landmesser and Pilar have found that peripherally deprived ganglionic neurons (i.e., with an excised optic vesicle) differentiate in normal numbers and send functional axons to the postganglionic nerve. Both calyciform and bouton synapses form on these neurons and remain functionally and ultrastructurally normal until Stage 34. However, from Stages 35 to 38 most cells die; thus, only 8% of the original cells remain (Figure 49). The fact that this cell death occurs nearly synchronously with the establishment of peripheral connections by ganglion cells (at least for the ciliary cell population) suggests that those cells that die do so because they have failed to form adequate peripheral contacts. Shortly before the period of cell death, there is a failure of transmission in approximately half of the cells, and there is some evidence to suggest that this is preganglionic in origin. Landmesser believes that the death of the preganglionic fibers is also

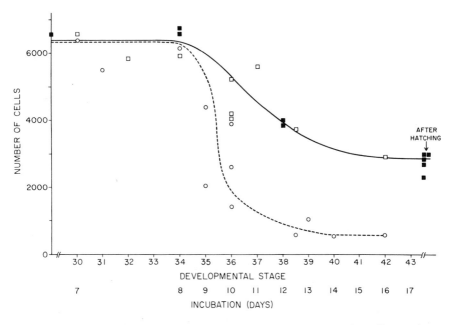

Figure 49. The number of neurons in peripherally deprived and control ganglia at various developmental states (indicated in both days and stages according to Hamburger and Hamilton. The number of ganglion cells in unoperated controls (■) and from the contralateral control ganglia of operated animals (□) decreases to about 50% between Stages 34 to 38. The cell number in peripherally deprived ganglia (○) decreases to about 10% during the same time period. [Landmesser and Pilar, 1974a]

due to a failure of the cells to form synapses and finds no evidence of centrally programmed cell death.*

    During normal embryonic development of the chick, cell death occurs during Stages 35 to 39, thus reducing the number of ganglion cells by half, i.e., from 6500 to 3200 cells. At the ultrastructural level, Pilar and Landmesser (1975, 1976; Landmesser and Pilar, 1976) have compared this normally occurring neuronal death to that brought about by removal of the peripheral target. Since both processes presumably have as their basis a lack of peripheral connections, Pilar and Landmesser (1976) expected the ultrastructural changes to be the

---

*Pilar and Landmesser cited a number of studies documenting that neuronal death is not genetically determined. These include the studies of Piatt (1946), Levi-Montalcini (1950), Shieh (1951), Hamburger (1958, 1975), Hughes (1961), and Prestige (1967a,b). One must be careful, however, in that genes may be indirectly involved in cell death, as one of many factors producing an observed developmental pattern.

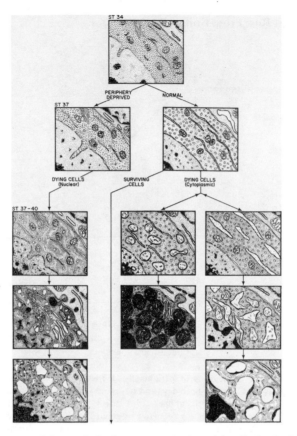

Figure 50. Summary of the cytologic changes occurring in peripherally deprived (left side) and normal (right side) ganglia during ganglion cell differentiation and death. Arrows indicate probable sequence of ultrastructural change. Some of the early changes in normal cell death may be reversible as indicated. All pictures show a section through a typical ganglion cell with the nucleus located at the lower left corner. An adjoining satellite cell is shown in the upper right corner. [Pilar and Landmesser, 1976]

same; however, they found rather striking differences between the two types of cell death. Prior to the period of cell death, all neurons in the normal ganglion developed a well-organized rough endoplasmic reticulum (ER). None of the peripherally deprived neurons underwent this change, indicating that some interaction with the periphery triggered the secretory state. Death of the latter cells was signalled by nuclear changes and followed by a freeing of the ribosomes from polysomes and rough ER, and, presumably, a cessation of protein synthesis. In contrast, normal cell death followed dilatation of the rough ER with eventual cytoplasmic disruption. Nuclear changes appeared only secondarily. (See Figure 50 for a summary of these events.)

298

The following suggestion emerged from the above study: cells that die in the course of normal development may have formed some synapses before degenerating and that there ensued a competition for postsynaptic sites. To check this hypothesis, Landmesser and Pilar (1976) attempted to determine more directly whether, prior to cell death, neurons (1) sent axons to the periphery, (2) reached the proper target organs, and (3) established synaptic connections with them. They found suggestive evidence that, after sending out initial axons, ciliary cells sprout numerous collaterals at the time of peripheral synapse formation. Subsequently, a large loss of axons from nerves occurs just after the onset of ganglion cell death, as well as a later loss of collaterals that is accompanied by no change in the number of cells (Figure 51).

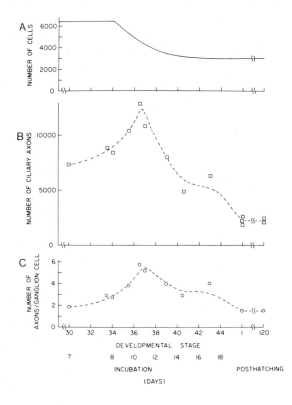

Figure 51. Decline in ganglion cell number during normal development (A) compared with the number of axons in the ciliary nerves over the same developmental stages. This is expressed both as total number of axons per ciliary nerve (B) and axons per ciliary cell (C). [Landmesser and Pilar, 1976]

Measurements of conduction velocity and axon diameters indicated that all ganglion cell axons grew in the proper pathways from the start and formed synapses with preganglionic fibers. An interesting difference between normal and peripherally deprived neurons was that, although the latter sent out initial axons, the collateral sprouting shown by the neurons with a target was not present.

Although it was not possible to determine whether all such axons had formed synapses peripherally, it could be shown that preganglionic fibers synapse selectively with all ganglion cells prior to cell death. The preganglionic fibers made unmistakable calyciform synapses on both degenerating and nondegenerating cells. Some of these preganglionic terminals on both normal and degenerating ganglion cells also degenerated, suggesting both transneuronal degeneration and that one synaptic connection is not enough to maintain a preganglionic cell. After this degeneration, the remaining healthy fibers sprouted collaterals; following this event, the second wave of fiber loss occurred. The latter was not associated with further loss of cell numbers.

Several conclusions (Figure 52) about the influence of the periphery on cell death can be drawn from such experiments: (1) Initial

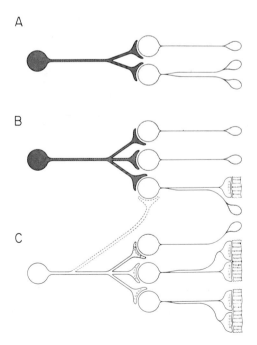

A

B

C

Figure 52. Summary of anatomical changes that occur in the ciliary ganglion during and following the period of cell death. A. Ganglion cells, which fail to make contact with the iris, degenerate (light stippling) with subsequent degeneration of the preganglionic cell ending on them (dark stippling). B. The preganglionic cell also degenerates because it has not formed synapses with a sufficient number of surviving ganglion cells, and thereby leaves the one ganglion cell transiently denervated. This cell is later reinnervated by a collateral axon of a surviving preganglionic cell. C. This preganglionic cell survives by virtue of synapsing with a sufficient number of surviving ganglion cells. Excess axon collaterals, both pre- and postganglionic (shown in B and C), which failed to make synapses or have synapsed with degenerating cells, are also lost. [Landmesser and Pilar, 1976]

nerve differentiation does not require the target organ because peripherally deprived ganglion cells migrate, send out functional axons, and differentiate normally. Furthermore, these cells form functional synapses with preganglionic fibers at the proper time. Although the ganglion cells do migrate, two ganglia may be formed, indicating that peripheral cues play some role. (2) The periphery triggers increased protein synthesis in the ganglionic neurons, and the presence or absence of this stimulus results in the different types of cell death shown by normal and peripherally deprived neurons. (3) Axonal sprouting is under the influence of the periphery and will not occur in its absence. (4) The preganglionic cell's synapse on the ganglion cell does not save it from death if it has not made an adequate number of peripheral connections. In turn, preganglionic cells seem to be dependent on their target cells for their own viability. Central programs do not seem to be a factor in the neuronal death pattern observed. (5) There is a quantitative requirement for synapse formation, since one synapse is not sufficient to maintain one preganglionic neuron. If a molecular signal is involved, it must be delivered in sufficient amount to maintain the presynaptic neuron. (6) Neuronal death does not seem to operate to achieve synaptic specificity, at least in this system; rather, specificity seems to reside in the initial outgrowth and synapse formation. The neuronal death process is concerned with the quantitative matching of neurons and target cells. Thus, the initial overproduction of neurons observed in so many systems need not be regarded as inefficient, since a mechanism whereby groups of synaptically related cells are quantitatively matched can function with very little genetic information. (7) A molecular signal seems implicated in all of these relations, and its identification remains an exciting challenge.

Dynamics of Retrograde Transport and Accumulation of Horseradish Peroxidase by Injured Neurons: J. H. LaVail

If the peripheral target cell sends a molecular signal to its neuronal partner via the synapse, then a mechanism to convey the messenger, or at least the message, to the neuronal soma must exist. The available evidence indicates that the mechanism is retrograde transport. Not only the marked changes in qualitative and quantitative physiological demands during neuronal development but also the varying levels of activity in the mature neuron suggest that the retrograde transport system should be functionally responsive. Evidence both for and against this proposition was discussed in the preceding chapter (see the sections by Bisby and Thoenen). Hence, a more critical examination of the available evidence is in order, and the experiments of LaVail and Bisby provide a useful starting point.

The sequence of morphological changes that occurs in neuronal cell bodies after axotomy has been carefully studied, but the mechanisms by which the cell body recognizes the fact of axonal transection remain obscure. Kristensson and Olsson (1975) have found that the rate of retrograde transport is sufficiently rapid to carry material from the cut axon to the cell body before chromatolysis can be detected. Halperin and LaVail (1975) have also studied the characteristics of retrograde transport in injured and intact neurons in an attempt to determine whether retrograde transport mechanisms might be involved in the signal for chromatolysis. As a model, LaVail and co-workers have used the chick isthmooptic nucleus (ION), whose neurons are located in the midbrain and project their axons to the opposite retina where they terminate in the inner nuclear layer (Figure 53). From earlier work (LaVail and LaVail, 1974), it was

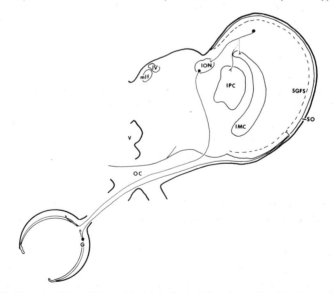

Figure 53. Diagram of the chick centripetal (retinotectal) and centrifugal (isthmoopticoretinal) pathways. Neurons of the ION project their axons topographically to the contralateral retina. IV = trochlear nucleus; G = ganglion cell layer of retina; IMC = isthmimagnocellularis nucleus; IPC = isthmiparvocellularis nucleus; mlf = medial longitudinal fasciculus; OC = optic chiasm; SGFS = stratum griseum et fibrosum superficiale; SO = stratum opticum; V = third ventricle. [LaVail]

determined that 3.5 hours after horseradish peroxidase (HRP) is injected into the vitreous of a chick eye, it can be identified in neuronal cell bodies of the contralateral ION following its retrograde transport (Figure 54A).

The ION pathway is useful for studies of transport in injured neurons for several reasons. Diffusion of HRP out of the eye is limited; hence, extracellular spread of.the marker to the ION is not a problem.

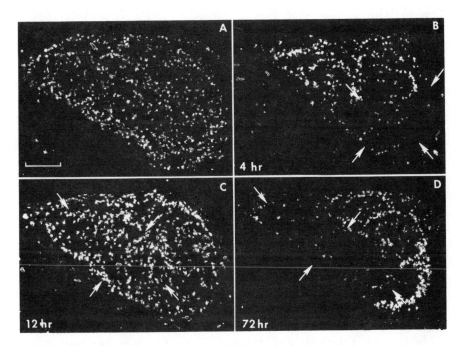

Figure 54. Comparable sagittal sections of ION photographed in dark-field microscopy at different intervals after injection of HRP into the vitreous of the contralateral eye. The ION neuronal cell bodies that are filled with HRP-positive granules appear clear. A. The ION of a chick in which HRP was injected 7 hours before fixation. The retina was not lesioned. B and C. Coincident with the HRP injection, the retina was deliberately injured in a region approximately along the horizontal meridian. The arrows in each case indicate that part of the nucleus that projects to the injured part of the retina. B. 4 hours after injection. Very little HRP has accumulated in cell bodies within the region corresponding to the retinal lesion. C. 12 hours after injection. Neuron cell bodies in the experimental portion of the nucleus have accumulated more HRP in general than the control neurons in remaining regions, although some of the neurons at the upper and lower right margins also contain more HRP. D. The contralateral retina was injured 72 hours before fixation, and the HRP was injected into the vitreous 48 hours after injury. The portion of the ION corresponding to the lesion (arrows) contains cell bodies with less HRP than those cells of the remaining portions of the nucleus. [Halperin and LaVail, 1975]

Furthermore, the neurons send their axons topographically to the contralateral retina. Therefore, by introducing a needle through the sclera of the eye, one portion of the retina, including the ION terminals and the axons that pass through this region, can be selectively lesioned, and the cells that project to that area can be identified. The neurons in the remaining portions of the same nucleus can serve as controls. Lastly, the intravitreal injection presumably exposes all axon terminals of the nucleus within the retina to approximately the same concentration of HRP at the same time. Since all of the ION neurons must transport the HRP approximately the same distance (about 14 mm), the accumulation in neurons whose axons have been cut may be compared with that of adjacent neurons that have not been directly injured.

The qualitative appearance of HRP labeling in the regions of the ION corresponding to the retinal lesion differed from the rest of the nucleus at various times after injury and injection of the HRP. A reduced intensity of labeling was seen consistently in the experimental portion of the ION in chicks fixed between 3.5 and 6 hours after injury (Figure 54B). After a time lapse of 6 to 20 hours, the cells in the experimental portion accumulated more HRP than other neurons (Figure 54C). If more than 20 hours lapse between the time of retinal injury and fixation, the cells in the experimental portion are again less heavily labeled than the remaining control neurons (Figure 54D).

Quantitative estimations of the level of labeling in ION cells were also made by counting the number of HRP-positive granules visible per cell. At 4 hours there were 28% fewer granules in cells whose axons had been damaged than in the controls, but by 12 hours the experimental cells showed 38% more granules than the controls. By 72 hours the situation was reversed, and the cells in the region corresponding to the retinal lesion contained almost 50% fewer granules.

In order to test whether the early decrease in the accumulation of HRP was due to a change in the rate of transport or in the rate of uptake of HRP by the axon stump, additional experiments were done. The marker was injected into the vitreous; 1 hour later a needle was introduced through the same point in the sclera, and the retina was lesioned. If the injury altered the rate of transport, an early difference might be revealed in the labeling pattern of the ION, such as a decrease in the intensity of label in cells in the area corresponding to the lesion if the rate of transport were decreased. No obvious difference in either the qualitative intensity of labeling or in the quantitative number of

HRP-positive granules per cell was found. Thus, at least initially, the rate of retrograde transport was not altered by axotomy.

Although experiments to determine the rate of inactivation of HRP in ION cells are still in progress, Halperin and LaVail feel that the explanation for their findings resides in changes in uptake at the terminal and not in the rate of retrograde axonal transport or of inactivation of HRP.* For example, it may take the axon terminal up to 1 hour postinjury to repair itself. After this, the rate of uptake at least approaches the normal rate and, perhaps, increases. Thus, the amount of HRP accumulating in the soma could increase. The fall-off in accumulation from 20 to 72 hours is probably more apparent than real, reflecting the physiological state of the cells that are degenerating.

In support of this concept of increased uptake following axotomy, Thoenen and Levi-Montalcini† (as noted in Chapter III) conducted studies showing potentiation of NGF effects (i.e., increased TOH levels) by 6-hydroxydopamine (6-OHDA). Since 6-OHDA is known to destroy sympathetic nerve terminals in the adult, Thoenen has hypothesized that this injury leads to increased uptake and more transport of NGF to the neuronal soma; hence, the metabolic effects of the same environmental concentration of NGF are more pronounced in the case of 6-OHDA injury than in the case of control experiments.

Monoamine Oxidase Inhibitors and Axoplasmic Transport: M. A. Bisby

At least in the case of axonal and axon terminal injuries by mechanical or pharmacological means, it is the uptake mechanisms of the terminal that are functionally responsive. If materials, such as the transmitter enzyme system, that are involved in the metabolism of the synaptic terminal (but not released) are returned in altered states to the soma as messages regulating somal biosynthesis and, perhaps, anterograde transport, we might expect to find alterations in the rate of retrograde and anterograde transport of such materials. Increased synaptic input to a given cell might also increase protein synthesis and axoplasmic transport in that cell.

*Lysosomal enzyme activity may actually be unchanged at the early time intervals involved in these studies. The increase in lysosomal activity occurs generally after 20 or more hours (Holtzman et al., 1967; Matthews and Raisman, 1972). The possibility that the increased rate of inactivation of HRP contributes to the increased accumulation between 6 and 12 hours in the experiments of Halperin and LaVail seem unlikely.

†H. Thoenen and R. Levi-Montalcini, unpublished data.

Bisby drew attention to the work of Boegman and colleagues, who have studied the effects of a variety of procedures on axoplasmic transport in rat lumbosacral motor neurons. Administration of pargyline (a monoamine oxidase inhibitor) produced a dose-dependent increase in the velocity of axonal transport (Table 3). Another monoamine oxidase inhibitor, phenelzine, produced similar results, suggesting that an increase in monoamine levels was involved in altering the velocity of transport (Boegman et al., 1975). Administration of serotonin also increased transport (Boegman and Wood, 1975). Changes in amine levels do not affect axonal transport generally, for Bisby* has found that pargyline treatment has no effect on transport of sensory axons.

TABLE 3

Pargyline-Induced Increase in Fast Axoplasmic Transport of ^{3}H-Labeled Material in the Rat Sciatic Nerve [Boegman et al., 1975]

Pargyline, 75 mg kg^{-1}			Pargyline, 25 mg kg^{-1}		NaCl control
1 day	3 days	7 days	3 days	7 days	7 days
552 ± 9	1,262 ± 117	1,996 ± 270	877 ± 45	1,428 ± 35	390 ± 13
n = 4	n = 7	n = 8	n = 3	n = 4	n = 5

The figures are in mm per 24 hrs ± S.D. n = number of rats.

According to Boegman and collaborators, these effects arise from an activation of the inhibitory response in the central nervous system, leading to a depression of motor neurons in the spinal cord and decreased muscle activity. With such an alteration in the balance of activity and specific neurotrophic control, the factor responsible for the latter would be required in greater quantity by the muscle. Thus, the transport mechanism would be required to supply more of the factor, and an increased transport rate would be a means of supplying it. The signal the muscle sends to the nerve to indicate its requirement is not included in this hypothesis, but it may not be unreasonable to postulate a retrograde molecular message. An increase in the velocity of axoplasmic transport was also produced by ligation of the abdominal aorta, perhaps as a result of partial spinal cord ischemia that destroys

*Unpublished results.

interneurons and alters the pattern of activity of spinal motoneurons (Wood and Boegman, 1975a).

Bisby pointed out that pargyline treatment not only increases the velocity of the wave front, but also decreases its amplitude. At the Work Session, Wurtman suggested that pargyline acts by decreasing protein synthesis. An increase in the rate of protein transport would tend to compensate for this reduction and to ensure the delivery of a constant quantity of vital materials to nerve terminals and, perhaps, to target organs. That catecholamines and serotonin influence brain protein synthesis has been shown by Roel and co-workers (1974) and Moskowitz and co-workers (1975) in Wurtman's laboratory. Supportive of Wurtman's suggestion is the finding of Wood and Boegman (1975a) that aortic ligation, which accelerates transport, did reduce by 26% the incorporation of amino acid into spinal cord protein.

Though increasing monoamine levels increased transport velocity, reducing monoamine levels by administering reserpine,* or a specific inhibitor of serotonin synthesis (Boegman and Wood, 1975), did not have the opposite effect. It is possible that the transport of only a small fraction of proteins is modulated by amine levels, and it may be difficult to identify retardation of this component in the large-amplitude "wave front" of labeled protein traveling at a normal velocity. More research will be required to clarify the dimensions and basis of this effect.

At this point, then, the potential for the functional responsiveness of transport seems to exist. Kerkut and co-workers (1967) provided evidence that glutamate transport in invertebrate neurons was increased by electrical stimulation and was interfered with by local anesthesia of the axons. However, it is known that local anesthetics (Byers et al., 1973; Edström et al., 1973; Bisby, 1975a) have a direct effect on transport that is separate from their influence on electrical activity. Geffen and Rush (1968), Jankowska and co-workers (1969), Lux and collaborators (1970), Ochs and Smith (1971), as well as Grafstein and co-workers (1972), have seen no change in the rate of transport with alterations in activity. If the terminal pool of transmitter is large compared to that being delivered to the terminal,† then it is not

*M.A. Bisby, unpublished data.
†Dahlström and Häggendal (1967) and Geffen and Rush (1968) have calculated that the amount of norepinephrine that accumulated in 24 hours at a nerve constriction was only 1% of that stored in the terminals; thus, local synthesis and uptake would seem to be relatively more important than transport.

surprising that transport is unaffected by functional demands. On the other hand, the recent data of Boegman and co-workers (1975) suggest that, under certain conditions that may relate to either changed electrical or metabolic activity, at least the rate of anterograde transport can be dramatically altered. If the difference in retrograde transport between motor and sensory nerves is substantiated (Bisby, 1975b), this will add to the evidence for such functional responsiveness.

Regeneration is another situation where axoplasmic transport might be altered. After axotomy, there is an initial decrease in the fast axonal transport of protein, while transport of glycoproteins is increased (Frizell and Sjöstrand, 1974). At later times, during the period of reinnervation, fast transport of proteins is increased (Kreutzberg and Schubert, 1975). Grafstein and Murray (1969) found a two-fold increase in fast transport in goldfish optic nerve 2 weeks after reinnervation, as well as a three-fold increase in velocity of slow transport. The amount of retrograde-transported material may also be increased in regenerating nerves (Sjöstrand and Frizell, 1975). O'Brien (1975) has evidence that there may actually be decreased transport of choline acetyltransferase and acetylcholinesterase during regeneration of rabbit peroneal nerve. These findings suggest that caution must be exercised in interpreting altered transport rates. The marker used in any given set of physiological circumstances must be specified. In the case of mechanical or pharmacological injury to nerve terminals, the evidence of Halperin and LaVail (1975) suggests that the rate of uptake or of innervation may be altered, but the rate of retrograde transport is not increased. It is obvious that more work will have to be done to clarify the conditions under which one or another mechanism is operative.

Hormonal Effects on Neurons: G. Raisman

Not all target cells are in direct contact with, or even in close proximity to, the neurons on which they exert profound structural and functional effects. This is particularly true of the various endocrine cells. While it is possible that some hormonal signals find their way to the neuronal soma via retrograde axonal transport, they may also act directly on the soma via hematogenous routes. Such indirect target cell-neuron interactions are exceedingly important and pervasive. At the Work Session, Raisman brought this issue into focus with his discussion of the control of neuronal sexual differentiation by gonadal steroids.

As their model system, Raisman and Field (1973b) studied the development and control of cyclic ovulation and mating behavior in the female albino rat. In the system (see Figure 55), the CNS initiates the production of hormones; these act back on the CNS, which, in turn, affects the secretion of luteinizing hormone (LH) and mating behavior. In the presence of functioning ovaries, the female shows cyclicity of release of pituitary gonadotrophins and the male does not. Taleisnik and co-workers (1971) have demonstrated a biochemical difference between the male and female rat brain by showing that progesterone causes a massive release of LH in estrogen-primed gonadectomized females, but it is without effect in males (Figure 56).

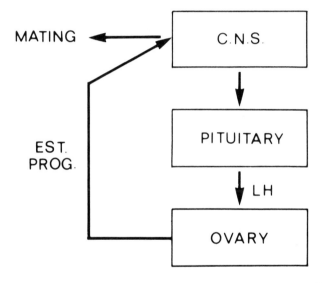

Figure 55. A schematic representation of the reciprocal relationship between the CNS and the ovary. LH = luteinizing hormone; EST = estrogen; PROG = progesterone. [Raisman]

By investigating the structure of those areas of the brain concerned with reproduction, Raisman and Field have attempted to establish an anatomical basis for this functional difference. Thus, they turned their attention to the preoptic area since previous experiments involving lesions and electrical stimulation or recording (Everett, 1964; Harris and Campbell, 1966) had indicated that this area was involved in the triggering of the release of pituitary gonadotrophins preceding ovulation, and probably in mating behavior as well (Lisk, 1967). Both 3H-estrogen-binding studies (Stumpf and Sar, 1971; Pfaff and Keiner, 1973) and stimulation experiments (Velasco and Taleisnik, 1969)

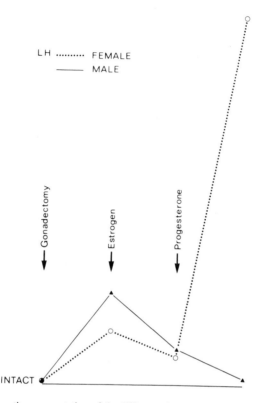

Figure 56. A schematic representation of the difference between the control of LH secretion in male and female rats. In response to a single injection of progesterone in the gonadectomized, estrogen-primed rat, the female shows a surge of LH secretion and the male does not. [Adapted from Brown-Grant, 1972]

showed that the amygdala is also involved. These techniques point to a system composed of the amygdala, preoptic area, hypothalamus, and pituitary, in which the amygdaloid projections through the stria terminalis to the medial preoptic area (POA) and the ventromedial hypothalamic nuclei (VMH) could have an important role. Following the observations of Heimer and Nauta (1969), Raisman and Field utilized the technique of anterograde degeneration at the electron microscope level to make a qualitative assessment of the mode of termination of the stria terminalis in the neuropil of the dorsal part of the preoptic area (see Figure 57) and in the relatively cell-free region lying between the ventromedial and arcuate nuclei of the hypothalamus (Field, 1972; Raisman and Field, 1973b).

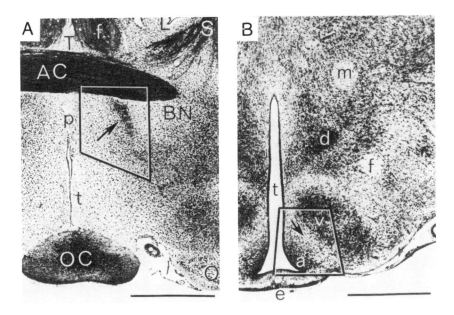

Figure 57. A. A light photomicrograph of a coronal section through the preoptic area. The box in the center shows the location of the area taken for ultrathin sections. Arrow = strial part of the preoptic area, AC = anterior commissure; BN = bed nucleus of the stria terminals; f = fornix; L = ventral tip of the lateral ventricle; O = olfactory tubercle; OC = optic chiasm; p = periventricular part of the preoptic area; S = main part of the stria terminalis; t = third ventricle; T = triangular septal nucleus (note the commissural component of the stria terminalis just ventral to this on the dorsal aspect of the anterior commissure). Bodian stain. Scale bar = 1 mm. B. A light photomicrograph of a coronal section through the mediobasal part of the tuberal hypothalamus showing the cell-free zone (arrow) lying between the arcuate nucleus (a) and the ventromedial nucleus (v). The box outlines the region sampled for electron microscopy. d = dorsomedial nucleus; e = median eminence; f = fornix, m = mammillothalamic tract; t = third ventricle. Nissl stain. Scale bar = 1 mm. [Raisman and Field, 1973b]

In both the VMH and the POA, synapses are largely axodendritic. Synapses on dendritic shafts outnumber those on dendritic spines in the VMH, and to an even greater extent in the POA. In both VMH and POA, strial axons terminate on both dendritic spines and shafts, and approximately half of the spine synapses are of strial origin. Two days after a lesion of the stria terminalis, the reaction of electron-dense degeneration was used to identify the terminals belonging to axons running in the stria terminalis. Axon terminals were divided into four classes: (1) Strial (i.e., degenerating) terminals on dendritic spines, (2) strial terminals on shafts, (3) nonstrial terminals on spines, and (4) nonstrial terminals on shafts. It was found that nonstrial

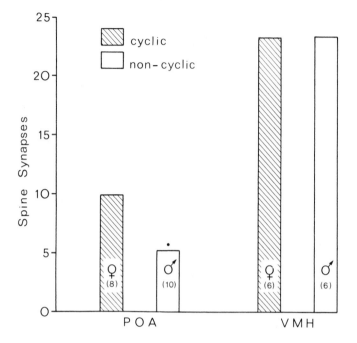

Figure 58. The number of nondegenerating spine synapses per unit area (one grid square of approximately 1800 μ^2) in the preoptic areas (POA) in 8 female and 10 male rats, and in the ventromedial hypothalamic nuclei (VMH) of 6 female and 6 male rats. There are roughly twice as many nonamygdaloid spine synapses per unit area in the females as in the males. No such difference occurs in the ventromedial nuclei. The number of rats in each group is shown in parentheses. Scatter is indicated by the standard error of the mean (dots above bars), although because of the distribution of the data, nonparametric (ranking) tests were used to assess the significance of differences. Hatched bars are used to designate animals with a cyclic (female) pattern of gonadotrophin release. [Raisman, 1974]

synapses on spines were twice as common in the POA of the female as in the male rat. There was no such difference in the incidence of shaft synapses or of any of the synapses of strial origin in the POA. No difference between the sexes in any category of synapses was found in the VMH (Figure 58). It is suggested that this sexual dimorphism in the connections of the POA, taken in conjunction with the evidence from the effects of lesions, electrical stimulation, recording, estrogen binding, etc., might be correlated with the ability of the female rat to maintain a cyclic triggering of gonadotrophin release and/or behavioral estrus.

Following the lead of Harris (1970) and introducing the developmental time dimension into their studies, Raisman and Field (1973b) carried out various hormonal manipulations of genetically male and female rats during the critical postnatal period for the development

TABLE 4

Adult Pattern of Gonadotropin Secretion (Cyclic or Noncyclic) in Rats
Subjected to Neonatal Endocrine Manipulations [Raisman]

Genetic sex	Age				Adult function
	Day 1	Day 4	Day 7	Day 16	
Female		Untreated		Untreated	Cyclic
		1.25 mg of TP			Noncyclic
				1.25 mg of TP	Cyclic
Male	Untreated		Untreated		Noncyclic
	Castrated				Cyclic
			Castrated		Noncyclic

Six groups of rats were subjected to the neonatal endocrine manipulations mentioned in the text. Genetic females were either untreated or treated with a single subcutaneous dose of 1.25 mg of testosterone propionate (TP) either on the 4th day of life (during the critical period for neonatal differentiation) or on the 16th day of life (after the critical period). Males were either intact or castrated on either the 1st or 7th day of life.

of cyclicity (the first 10 days of life) and checked for synaptic count differences in the adult. Castration of the genetic male within 12 hours of birth (but not at 7 days of age) caused an increase in the number of nonstrial spine synapses in the POA to a level equivalent to that of the normal female; it also permitted the functional development of a cyclic (i.e., feminine) pattern of gonadotrophin release, as well as the ability to show a progesterone-facilitated release of LH and an increase in receptivity after gonadectomy and estrogen priming. Conversely, females treated on Day 4 (but not on Day 16) with 1.25 mg of testosterone propionate developed a smaller number of nonstrial spine synapses in the POA, i.e., in the range found in males; this treatment abolished the cyclic pattern of gonadotrophin release and the pro-gesterone-facilitated release of LH and increase in receptivity (androgen "sterilization"). The data (see Table 4 and Figure 59) further substantiate the idea that these nonstrial synapses* are important in cyclicity and mating behavior.

There is some evidence that the critical hormone in development may be estrogen. Androgen is present during the neonatal period in male rats, but the neonatal limbic system has an aromatizing enzyme that converts it into estrogen (Naftolin et al., 1972). Raisman specu-

*Although the source of these synapses is not known, Raisman suggests that they could be of hypothalamic origin.

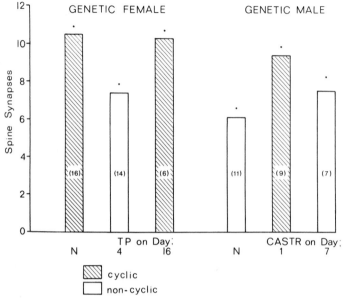

Figure 59. The number of nonamygdaloid spine synapses per unit in the preoptic area of the 6 groups of rats (see Table 4). The genetic females were either normal (N) or treated with testosterone propionate (TP) on either the 4th or the 16th day of life. Genetic males were either normal (N) or castrated (CASTR) on either the 1st or the 7th day of life. The number of animals in each group is shown in parentheses. Hatched bars indicate groups of rats with a cyclic (female) pattern of gonadotrophin release as adults. Dots indicate one standard error of the mean (see legend to Figure 58). A high incidence of nonamygdaloid spine synapses is associated with a cyclic adult pattern of gonadotrophin release, regardless of the genetic sex of the animal. Conversely, a low incidence is associated with a noncyclic release pattern, regardless of genetic sex. [Raisman, 1974]

lates that the preoptic neurons could be sensitive to estrogen; hence, estrogen acting during development could cause an alteration in the quantitative aspects of synapse formation, perhaps by changing the timing of synaptogenesis.* The neurons may not lose their responsiveness to estrogen, but in the adult they may express their sensitivity as a positive feedback response to progesterone (as prevously shown in Figure 56) and not as synaptic changes.†

The findings of Raisman and Field, though quantitatively subtle, are, nonetheless, of great importance: Circulating hormones, in

*Altered cell death patterns could be an alternative explanation.
†The differential action of trophic agents in development and maturity is probably very common. Note the discussion by Thoenen (see Chapter III) on the role of NGF and sensory neurons in this regard.

relatively small or even minute amounts, control neuronal development; thus, a genetic male or female can be transformed to the functionally and behaviorally opposite sex by the presence or absence of such hormones during critical periods. The extent and variety of these indirect interactions between neurons and their target cells not only in developing but also in the mature animal are only beginning to be appreciated.

Glucocorticoids and Neural Control of Enzyme Induction in Target Cells: H. Thoenen

Thoenen and his collaborators (see Goodman et al., 1975; Otten and Thoenen, 1975) have recently used the rat adrenal medulla as a model system for the study of transsynaptic enzyme induction. Their aim was to develop organ culture conditions representative of an in vivo situation. The processes responsible for transsynaptic enzyme induction, initiated in vivo by injecting 5 mg per kg of reserpine 2 hours prior to the removal of the adrenal medulla, continued in this culture system, and the final levels of TOH were comparable to those observed in vivo (Figure 60). The finding that transection of the splanchnic fibers supplying the adrenal medulla prior to reserpine administration

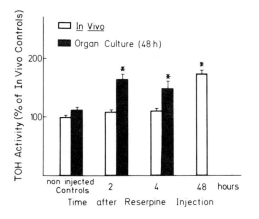

Figure 60. Adrenal medullary TOH response in organ culture to reserpine administered in vivo. Male rats weighing 120 to 130 gm were given a single intraperitoneal dose of 5 mg/kg of reserpine. The adrenal medullae were removed 2, 4, and 48 hours later and assayed for TOH activity immediately (☐) or after a further 48 hours in organ culture (▮). The changes in enzyme specific activity were expressed as a percent of uninjected in vivo controls. The specific activity of TOH in control adrenal medulla was 8.81 nmoles of DOPA/ hour per mg of protein. Values given represent the mean   S.E.M. of 8 adrenal medullae. Bars with an asterisk (*) are significantly higher than in vivo controls   (P<0.005). [Goodman et al., 1975]

abolished the rise in TOH activity, not only in vivo but also in culture, also supports the premise that these culture conditions are representative of the in vivo induction process. Actinomycin D injected prior to reserpine blocked the induction of TOH in vivo and in organ culture. In addition, the investigators found that high concentrations (0.29 mM) of corticosterone in the culture medium inhibited the increase in TOH activity caused by reserpine. According to Thoenen and co-workers, this suggests that glucocorticoids act as modulatory agents in transsynaptic enzyme induction.

In the initial study (Goodman et al., 1975), such steroidal inhibition was exhibited only when corticosterone was added at the initiation of the culture period. If it was added 2 or 4 hours later, there was little or no effect on the subsequent increase of TOH. The modulating role of glucocorticoids is demonstrated by the transsynaptic induction of TOH in the adrenal medulla and sympathetic ganglia, as effected by short-term (1 to 2 hours) cold stress at 4° C*; this induction exhibited a circadian rhythm causally related to the diurnal changes in adrenal glucocorticoid synthesis (Otten and Thoenen, 1975). In the adrenal medulla the initiation of TOH induction was maximal during the morning hours, when plasma corticoid concentrations (reflecting corticoid synthesis in the adrenal cortex) are minimal, whereas in the sympathetic ganglia, TOH induction was possible only in the afternoon. Thus, TOH inducibility in the adrenal medulla seems to be optimal during periods of low corticoid synthesis, whereas in the sympathetic ganglion, induction is only possible during the period of high plasma corticoid concentrations. This assumption is supported by the investigators' observation that in the first postnatal weeks, when the pituitary adrenocortical system is not yet operating and plasma corticoid concentrations are low, the initiation of TOH induction in the adrenal medulla is possible at any time of the day, whereas in sympathetic ganglion it is not possible at all. If glucocorticoids are administered to newborn animals or adults in the morning hours, then TOH induction in sympathetic ganglia is possible. The observation that, in cultured sympathetic ganglia, induction of TOH by cholinomimetics is possible to a normal extent only when glucocorticoids are added to the culture medium reinforces the notion of steroidal modulation of

*It has been shown that a prolonged increase in preganglionic neuron activity leads to an induction of TOH. Cold stress of 1 to 2 hours duration is sufficient to initiate TOH induction (Guidotti et al., 1973b; Otten et al., 1973a) and so provides a useful model for transsynaptic inductive effects.

transsynaptic induction processes (Otten and Thoenen, 1976). Neuro-trophic factors and/or influences do not act in isolation but rather in a matrix of interacting processes. The target cell may modulate the neuron's influence on itself, or a cell may regulate the interactions of a distant, unrelated neuron-target cell pair.

Other Peripherally Produced Substances Involved in Target Cell-Neuron Interactions

Substances, including hormones, that are produced peripherally and act directly on neurons and/or modulate neuron-target cell interactions will undoubtedly grow not only in numbers but also in functional significance in the next few years. The effects of too-little or too-much thyroid hormone on the developing animal, as well as in the adult, have been known for many years, particularly in the clinical literature. In their study of synaptogenesis in the rat cerebellum, Nicholson and Altman (1972) found that the number of synapses in the molecular layer of the rat cerebellum was reduced by both early hypo- and hyperthyroidism. Hypothyroidism retarded synaptogenesis after 10 days, whereas hyperthyroidism accelerated synaptic genesis initially but, by 21 days, resulted in a reduction in the number of synapses. Under conditions of hyperthyroidism, the cells of the external granular layer have been shown to cease proliferation early, producing fewer stem cells from which basket, granular, and stellate cells are formed. This premature termination is associated with an early initiation of cell differentiation. Although the same end result occurs in hypothy-roidism, the mechanism seems to be a general retardation of the differentiation of cerebellar neurons.

In the adult, hypo- and hyperthyroidism have profound neurological effects that are not only different from those in the developing animal but probably are the result of different mechanisms. Williams* has shown that triiodothyronine may enhance regeneration of neurons in adult rats. Such an effect may represent a general metabolic "tune-up," but it is also possible that triiodothyronine has other, more specific influences on sprouting.

Curiously, thyroid-binding sites have been described throughout the brain. Guillemin and collaborators at the Salk Institute (see Brazeau

---

*T. Williams' data were reported by Guth (1974a). They substantiate previous findings that thyroid hormone enhances peripheral and central nervous regeneration (see Harvey and Srebnik, 1967; Fertig et al., 1971; Kiernan and Rawcliffe, 1971; Cockett and Kiernan, 1973).

and Guillemin, 1974; Vale et al., 1974; Brown and Vale, 1975) have found a rather ubiquitous brain distribution of certain peptide inhibitors of the releasing factors involved in neurohypophysial secretion. In the study by Vale and co-workers (1974), rat brains were divided into five general regions, extracted with acidic acid, and defatted with ether. The extracts were tested for their effects on the spontaneous secretion of growth hormone and prolactin in cultures of dissociated rat pituitary cells. It was found that somatostatin* activity and prolactin-release-inhibiting activity occur throughout the brain. Although the hypothalamus contains the highest concentrations, the cerebral cortex, thalamus, midbrain, and brainstem contain significant amounts (about half the concentration of that in the hypothalamus). The concentration in the cerebellum was smaller by a factor of ten. The regions that contained somatostatin activity also contained prolactin-release-inhibiting activity. This prolactin-release-inhibiting activity of the cerebral cortex was not inhibited by treatment of the pituitary cells with perphenazine or phenoxybenzamine.† Thus, the cortical prolactin-inhibiting action is probably not due to catecholamines, since perphenazine and phenoxybenzamine block the dopamine- and norepinephrine-induced inhibition of prolactin secretion. Furthermore, the effect is a specific one, since neither the cortical nor hypothalamic extracts inhibit the secretion of LH and follicle-stimulating hormone (FSH).‡

The functional significance of the widespread distribution of such peptides is not clear at present. There is, however, increasing evidence of the role of peptides as both neurohormones and neurotransmitters in the nervous system (Bloom, 1972). Somatostatin, for example, has been localized to nerve terminals (Hökfelt et al., 1974; Pelletier et al., 1974). Studies on the systemic injection of thyrotropin-releasing hormone (TRH), which is also widely found in the CNS (Burt and Snyder, 1975), indicate that TRH is a CNS stimulant, while somatostatin seems to be a CNS depressant. The effects of both peptides are independent of the hypothalamic-pituitary axis action (Brown and Vale, 1975). Many investigators, including the above, believe that these behavioral actions are consistent with a direct influence of these peptides on neuronal activity.

Renaud and co-workers (1975) have recently looked at both extracellular and intracellular single-unit activity in the hypothalamic

---

*Growth hormone-release inhibiting hormone.
†Also true for the hypothalamus.
‡The extracts, however, do suppress the release of thyroid-stimulating hormone by thyrotropin-releasing factor.

ventromedial nucleus, the cuneate nucleus of the brainstem, and the cerebellar and cerebral cortex, after microiontophoretic application of luteinizing hormone-releasing hormone (LH-RH), TRH, and somatostatin. In each area of the CNS examined, only a certain population of neurons responded to the application of individual peptides. In responsive neurons, all three peptides depressed discharge frequency, often with an associated increase in spike amplitude, suggestive of membrane hypopolarization. The characteristics of this response in sensitive cells were similar for each peptide; i.e., rapid onset after application of current, rapid recovery after cessation of the injection current, graded decrease in excitability with increased current, reproducibility with successive application, and lack of similar responses during application of positive sodium control currents. The discharge frequency of insensitive neurons showed no consistent change even when peptides were applied with currents as high as 100 to 160 nA.

Twelve of fourteen peptide-sensitive neurons (six in the cerebellar cortex, four in the cerebral cortex, and four in the hypothalamus) were sensitive to both TRH and LH-RH, and the two remaining neurons were responsive to LH-RH only. Although TRH-sensitive neurons were more frequent in the hypothalamus than elsewhere in the brain, they were also found in the cerebellar cortex, despite the fact that this area has a low content of TRH and lacks high-affinity TRH-binding sites. A varying TRH responsiveness for neurons in any one area in the CNS has been reported (Renaud and Martin, 1975). Similarly, a substantial number of neurons were responsive to LH-RH and somatostatin, even in areas where these peptides have either not been detected or are found in low concentration.

Such observations indicating that peptide-responsive neurons are not restricted to the hypothalamus gain broad support from microiontophoretic studies of substance P, which has a predominantly excitatory action when applied to extrahypothalamic neurons (Konishi and Otsuka, 1974; Phillis and Limacher, 1974). Otsuka and co-workers (1975) proposed that hypothalamic substance P is an excitatory transmitter of primary afferent neurons.* Hökfelt and collaborators (1976) have localized substance P to dorsal root primary afferent

*In their elegant study, Otsuka and co-workers used pharmacological, chemical, and immunological methods to show that the active peptide isolated from the dorsal root of bovine spinal nerve is identical to an undecapeptide, substance P, isolated from bovine hypothalamus. The structure of hypothalamic substance P is Arg-Pro-Lys-Pro-Gln-Gln-Phe-Phe-Gly-Leu-Met-NH$_2$. Its potency relative to L-glutamate is 200:1.

terminals as well. Angiotensin II has also been reported to excite central neurons (Nicoll and Barker, 1971a). Recently, a peptide known as morphinelike factor or "enkephalin" has also been identified and sequenced; it is thought to be a transmitter (Hughes et al., 1975).

It is tempting to speculate that such peptides reflect the neurosecretory heritage of the neuron. The idea that they can act both as neurohormones and neurotransmitters has been proposed for vasopressin (Nicoll and Barker, 1971b; see also Bloom's review, 1972). In minute amounts, these peptides (and others yet to be identified) can initiate profound electrical and metabolic effects, and thus have a role in neurotrophism. It is possible that they contain information reflecting a given neuron's "experience."

Other substances that ought to be considered for target cell-neuron interactions include the prostaglandins. For example, Hedqvist (1973) showed that three different and unrelated inhibitors of prostaglandin synthesis increased the release of noradrenaline from the stimulated vas deferens. He has hypothesized that locally formed prostaglandins of the E type have the capacity to modulate noradrenaline release from sympathetic nerve terminals. Moreover, there is good reason to believe that prostaglandin E acts in this respect by restricting the neuronal influx of calcium necessary for the release of the transmitter into the junctional cleft. Since prostaglandins can alter intracellular calcium concentration and interact with cyclic nucleotide mechanisms, it is possible that they may ultimately cause major metabolic changes in neurons.

Conclusions

While the influence of neurons on target cells has received much recent attention, the influence of target cells on neurons, which can be very powerful, also needs to be emphasized. In many cases, it is the peripheral target organ that determines whether a neuron will make the proper connections and function normally or, for that matter, even survive. The signals responsible for mediating these influences may reach the neuronal soma either (1) by the direct route of retrograde intraaxonal transport or (2) by indirect routes, particularly where the affected neuron itself is not in direct contact with the active peripheral cell, such as hematogenous delivery. Identification of the molecular identity of the signals has only begun. Examples include nerve growth factor, the prostaglandins, glucocorticoids, and several peptides, some of which have both neurohormone and neurotransmitter actions. It is clear that neurotrophic factors do not act in isolation. It may not even be possible for them to achieve their effects if other elements of the system, such as testosterone for taste bud formation and glucocorticoids for tyrosine hydroxylase induction in the adrenal medulla, are not present. Neurotrophic factors and influences exist in a matrix of multiple interacting variables, where the delicate check-and-balance system is crucial to development, maturation, and adult function.

V. NEURON-GLIA INTERACTIONS

Most of the current hypotheses concerning glial function originated from nineteenth century anatomical studies by investigators such as Golgi and Virchow. According to the majority of these hypotheses, the glial cell-neuron relationship is regarded as that of a slave to master, with glial cells providing mechanical support, nurture, environmental control, and electrical insulation. However, recent data challenge these ideas. Nutrients destined for neuronal metabolism probably travel directly to the neuron via extracellular pathways, and, as has been frequently pointed out (e.g., Orkand, 1975), the suggestion that glial cell cytoplasm is the extracellular environment of neurons is untenable, because the intracellular potassium concentration of these cells is too high to sustain neuronal spike activity. Brightman and Reese (1969) showed that the blood-brain barrier to large molecules in mammals is not comprised of astrocytic footplates but rather resides in the capillary endothelial cell.

The concept now emerging is that of a complex interdependency between neurons and glia in which mutual regulatory controls and influences are exerted. Although the symbiosis of neurons and glia was suggested a number of years ago (Galambos, 1961, 1967; Hydén, 1967), the true dimensions of this interdependency are only now becoming clear. Glia function in the uptake, excretion, and metabolism of putative transmitters (Henn et al., 1974; Schrier and Thompson, 1974; Miledi, 1975); they modulate and, perhaps, redistribute potassium ions, transmitters, and other molecules (Orkand, 1975); and they influence neuronal transmitter and enzyme synthesis (Giller et al., 1973; O'Lague et al., 1974, 1976; Patterson and Chun, 1974; Patterson et al., 1974, 1976). Glia also appear yoked to their adjacent neurons (Orkand et al., 1966; Kelly and Van Essen, 1974) and respond to ions and transmitters with sustained depolarization and increased cAMP (Gilman and Nirenberg, 1971a,b; Gilman and Schrier, 1972). Because glia form an electrical syncytium (they are interconnected by gap junctions), they may be able to modulate the electrical activity of an entire neuronal circuit (Somjen, 1975). Additionally, they may guide neuronal development (Sidman and Rakic, 1973; Henrikson and Vaughn, 1974), be involved in neuronal sprouting and regeneration (Lynch et al., 1975a), and remove nonfunctional synapses (Blinzinger and Kreutzberg, 1968). On the other hand, neurons seem to control glial mitosis (Illis, 1973b). Glia may supply trophic factors such as

(1) NGF, which affects cell development, maturation, and maintenance (Varon, 1975a); (2) amino acids (Globus et al., 1973); and (3) unidentified proteins, as in squid giant axons (Lasek et al., 1974). As Kreutzberg, Schubert, and collaborators (see Chapter II) have shown, amino acids and nucleotides also travel from neurons to glia.

A longer list of the complex interrelationships between neurons and glia could be presented, but it would not serve the purposes of the present discussion.* Although glia are not ordinarily regarded as target cells for neurons, they can be considered so in the broad context of our comments. In the following sections, "The Influence of Nonneuronal Cells on Transmitter Synthesis in Sympathetic Neuron Cultures" and "Glial Control of Neuronal Sprouting," examples of the neuron as the target cell of nonneuronal or glial cells are given.

The Influence of Nonneuronal Cells on Transmitter Synthesis in Sympathetic Neuron Cultures: P. Patterson

The analytical separation of glia from neurons has been a difficult task. Although various methods have been proposed, adequate biochemical markers to distinguish the two cells have not yet been developed. For this reason, pure cell cultures of both primary neurons and glia, as well as cloned cell lines, have been valuable tools, particularly in studies of interactions between neurons and glia (see Burnham et al., 1972; Varon and Raiborn, 1972). Mains and Patterson (1973a,b,c) have documented some of the basic biochemical properties of dissociated sympathetic neurons in culture. Their method is as follows: neonatal rat sympathetic ganglia are disrupted by mechanical agitation to yield dissociated primary neurons. These neurons are then grown with or without (virtual absence) nonneuronal cells simply by the addition or deletion of bicarbonate during growth in culture. If the ganglionic cells are grown in a modified Leibovitz medium in an air atmosphere, nonneuronal cells will not survive; thus, a pure neuron culture is obtained (Figure 61A). The addition of bicarbonate leads to a mixed culture of neurons and ganglionic nonneuronal cells (Figure 61B). If the cells are kept in Leibovitz medium plus CO_2 and no NGF is added, the neurons die, and a culture of nonneuronal cells, probably including satellite cells as well as fibroblasts, is obtained.

---

*Recent excellent reviews of the subject have been provided by Watson (1974), Somjen (1975), and Varon (1975a,b). The reader is referred to these reports for further information.

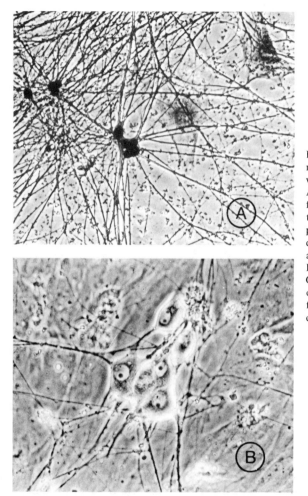

Figure 61. Morphology of neurons grown with or without nonneuronal cells. A. Leibovitz-air culture fixed and stained with toluidine blue. Neuronal processes and somas stain darkly, and two fibroblasts are seen in the background. B. Unstained Leibovitz-CO_2 culture with neurons on a monolayer of cardiac fibroblasts. [Patterson et al., 1976]

By this technique, Mains and Patterson have been able to determine some of the kinetic parameters, nutritional requirements, and developmental time course of catecholamine synthesis and accumulation. Such neuronal cultures are capable of synthesis and accumulation of both radioactive dopamine and norepinephrine after addition of ^{3}H-tyrosine to the medium and show no evidence of synthesis of radioactive γ-aminobutyric acid, 5-hydroxytryptamine, or histamine from their respective labeled precursors. The cultured neurons show a steady increase in RNA, lipid, and protein after plating, and older cultures show both more rapid production and turnover of the catecholamines than younger cultures, suggesting maturation in culture. Mains and Patterson have also noted the synthesis of very small amounts of acetylcholine in the older neuronal cultures.

On the other hand, O'Lague and co-workers (1974; Nurse and O'Lague, 1975) have found electrophysiological and pharmacological evidence for functional excitatory cholinergic synapses between the sympathetic neurons themselves and between the neurons and skeletal myotubes. Concomitant with synapse formation is the synthesis of large amounts of ACh (Patterson and Chun, 1974). It has been shown that the induction of such synthesis requires nonneuronal cells. When nonneuronal cells derived from sympathetic ganglia are added to neuronal cultures, ACh synthesis from labeled choline is increased 100- to 1000-fold. This effect does not seem to be due to an increased plating efficiency of neurons, since the numbers of surviving neurons are not greatly increased by nonneuronal cells, and, furthermore, the nonneuronal cells are capable of increasing ACh synthesis after only 48 hours of contact with neurons previously grown in isolation for 2 weeks. Direct cell-cell contact is not required for the effect, because nonneuronal-cell-conditioned medium* acting directly on pure neuronal populations can produce the increase (Patterson et al., 1976). Furthermore, the nonneuronal cells themselves do not synthesize detectable ACh under these conditions.

In investigating this finding further, Patterson and Chun (1974) tested several types of nonneuronal cells for their effectiveness in promoting ACh synthesis. Nonneuronal cells from the sympathetic ganglia showed a large effect, the increase they produced being roughly dependent on the number of ganglionic nonneuronal cells present. Rat C6 glioma cells also stimulated ACh synthesis, as did cells from newborn rat cardiac and skeletal muscles; but 3T3 mouse fibroblast and BHK cells stimulated little or no synthesis. Thus, a nonspecific conditioning effect† from any kind of added cell can be ruled out.

---

*In this case, conditioned medium is a cell culture in which nonneuronal cells have been grown and then removed prior to the addition of the medium to a neuronal culture. Presumably, the nonneuronal cells secrete a factor (or factors) into the medium that can increase ACh synthesis in neurons.

†Schrier, Nelson, and co-workers (see Giller et al., 1973; Nelson, 1976) have shown a 4-fold increase in choline acetyltransferase activity in combined spinal cord-skeletal muscle cultures over combined spinal cord-fibroblast cultures and a 10-fold increase over spinal cord cultures alone. Again, there is some specificity, but muscle and other peripheral cells, in addition to glia, will have to be considered in such effects. The issue of specificity in neuron-target cell interactions is an important one and is taken up again in Chapter IX.

Further indication of specificity is that the effect is restricted to ACh production with little change in catecholamine synthesis and accumulation.

The nature of this powerful effect of nonneuronal cells has not been ascertained. One question is whether the observed phenomena represent changes in differentiation or survival and growth of a new population of neurons in the cultures. There is evidence to support the notion that cellular environment can influence differentiation as expressed by transmitter synthesis. Le Douarin and co-workers (1975) have shown that neural crest tissue, which normally gives rise to sympathetic neurons, when transplanted to a presumptive parasympathetic region, will give rise to cholinergic parasympathetic neurons. Conversely, a transplant from a presumptive cholinergic region of the crest to a presumptive adrenergic region will yield catecholamine-containing cells (Cohen, 1972; Norr, 1973). Thus, in the cultures of Patterson and Chun, the nonneuronal cells may be inducing presumptive adrenergic neurons to produce ACh.

One might, of course, argue that the cells in culture possess completely disrupted control mechanisms and that their behavior bears no resemblance to any in vivo developmental phenomena. However, according to Patterson, when grown in the virtual absence of other cell types (which might seem the least natural environment), neurons do not behave in a bizarre fasion. They develop the capacity for taking up, synthesizing, storing, and releasing catecholamines along the expected time course (Patterson et al., 1976). They also possess many of the expected electrophysiological properties (O'Lague et al., 1976). It is in the presence of the nonneural cells that the neurons synthesize ACh and form cholinergic synapses.

It is possible that two populations of cells, adrenergic and cholinergic, exist in the dissociated ganglia preparation and that the cholinergic population is active only in the presence of nonneuronal cells or a conditioned medium.* This possibility is being investigated by use of histochemical means, as well as by biochemical analysis of single neurons.

Just as the nature of the transmitter synthesis effect is not clearly understood, so the characterization of the factor (or factors) responsible for it remains to be accomplished. Thoenen reported that

---

*Evidence for a minority population of cholinergic neurons in some sympathetic ganglia has been provided by Sjöqvist (1963), Aiken and Reit (1969), and Yamauchi and co-workers (1973).

Monard and co-workers (1973) have begun to characterize a factor produced by C6 glioma cells that increases process formation by neuroblastoma cells. According to Monard, the factor is a protein with a molecular weight of about 80,000. Observations that this glial factor, in contrast to NGF, does not produce sprouting in either chicken dorsal root ganglia or dissociated rat sympathetic ganglia indicate that it is not identical to NGF. On the other hand, NGF does not induce process formation in neuroblastoma cells, and the process formation produced in these cells by the glial factor is not impaired by NGF antibodies (Monard et al., 1975).

More glial and/or nonneuronal cell-line factors will probably be reported. Some of these may be specific to certain glial populations, while others may be produced by many nonneuronal cell lines. For example, a number of cell lines, including L and 3T3 fibroblasts, mouse salivary gland cells, and neuroblastoma cells, can produce NGF (Young et al., 1975). At the Work Session, Arnason reported finding NGF by radioactive iodine and radioimmunoassay in C6 glioma cultures. However, the material isolated from the supernatants of these cultures did not have the typical effects of NGF on dorsal root or sympathetic ganglia. Arnason suggests that there may be a molecular inhibitor of NGF's effects in this case, but more data are needed to clarify this.

Glial Control of Neuronal Sprouting: G. Lynch

Using a different system and marker to determine the effects of glia on neurons, Lynch and his associates (1975a; for a review see Lynch and Cotman, 1975) have examined axonal sprouting and regeneration in the immature and adult rat brain. It is known that, at least in some brain regions, partial deafferentation is followed by sprouting and reestablishment of function in the afferents remaining in that region (Raisman, 1969). The nature of this sprouting process and the factors controlling it, as well as the anatomical and biochemical changes underlying it, are only dimly understood at present. With these facts in mind, Lynch, in collaboration with Cotman, turned to the hippocampus to establish the temporal sequence in which the multiple constituents of the neuropil respond to partial deafferentation. The hippocampus and, particularly, the dentate gyrus offer a number of important advantages as experimental preparations. First, the hippocampus has a relatively simple anatomy, consisting of a row of granule cells whose dendrites radiate outward into a reasonable homogeneous and almost neuron-free molecular layer (Figure 62). Secondly, the afferents to the dentate gyrus are rigidly laminated: the supragranular zone contains septal inputs; the inner molecular layer contains commissural and associational afferents; and the middle and outer molecular layers receive a massive input from the entorhinal cortex, as well as very small septal and contralateral entorhinal inputs (Figure 62). Such an anatomical arrangement, with virtually no "overlap" of zones, permits deafferentation of a part of the dendritic tree and quantitative, anatomical, histochemical, and neurophysiological measurements of axonal regrowth and synapse formation.

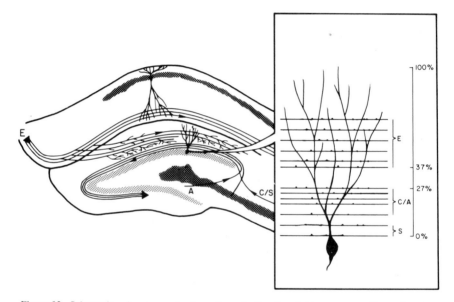

Figure 62. Schematic of a coronal plane through the dorsal hippocampus illustrating the location of the major cell types and the distribution of the four main afferent fiber systems. (1) The associational system (A) originates in the CA3-CA4 region of the hippocampus and projects into the molecular layer, terminating on the inner portion of the granule cell dendrites. (2) The commissural fibers (C) arise in regio inferior of the contralateral hippocampus, enter the ipsilateral hippocampus via the fimbria, and terminate in the same zone of the molecular layer as is occupied by the associational system. (3) A discrete projection from the septum (S) also enters via the fimbria, terminating at the base of the granule cell dendrites. (4) The afferent fibers from both the ipsilateral and contralateral entorhinal cortices enter the hippocampus through the angular bundle (E) and course laterally. The ipsilateral projections innervate the apical tips of the pyramidal cells and the outer three-fourths of the granule cell dendrites; the crossed fibers are restricted to regio superior except for the rostral end of the hippocampus where recent work suggests they contribute a small projection to the dentate gyrus. The inset at right summarizes measurements of the location and percentage occupancy of the fiber plexuses generated by the various afferents. The zone between 27 and 37% is innervated by fine axons and terminals of entorhinal origin. [Lynch et al., 1975a]

Following lesions of the entorhinal cortex, a sequence of striking morphological changes in the dentate gyrus occurred. Terminal degeneration, detectable in the electron microscope within 24 hours of the lesion, was fully developed by 72 hours (Figure 63). Concomitant with the appearance of degeneration products, the astroglia of the ipsilateral hippocampus hypertrophied (but did not divide) and aligned themselves in rows, with their processes oriented toward the cortical surface (Lynch et al., 1975a; Rose et al., 1976) (Figure 64). By the

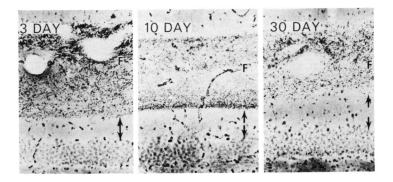

Figure 63. Photomicrographs of degeneration products (Fink-Heimer method) in the dorsal leaf molecular layer of the dentate gyrus from rats with three different postlesion survival times. Note that the degeneration-free zone (arrows) above the granule cells expands with time (initial magnification ×100). F indicates location of hippocampal fissure. [Lynch et al., 1975a]

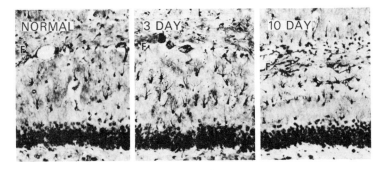

Figure 64. Photomicrographs of the dentate gyrus at various times following a lesion of the ipsilateral entorhinal cortex stained with Cajal's gold sublimate method for astrocytes. Note the apparent hypertrophy of the cells at 3 days postlesion without an increase in actual cell number (initial magnification ×100). F indicates location of hippocampal fissure. [Lynch et al., 1975a]

third postlesion day, a gradual decline in the number of astrocytes in the inner molecular layer began, a process which was accompanied by a corresponding increase in astrocytes in the outer molecular layer. These results suggest that astrocytes in the inner dendritic zone migrate into the outer deafferented molecular layer.

Although the astrocytes did not divide, the microglia proliferated. Forty-eight to 60 hours after lesioning the entorhinal cortex, there was a local (ipsilateral) rise in the number of microglia; the rise continued more slowly for 12 days and then declined. A smaller rise was noted in the contralateral hippocampus control (Lynch et al., 1975a). If ^{3}H-thymidine was injected into the ventricular system 20 to 80 hours after the lesion, large numbers of microglia incorporated the label. Before or beyond this time interval, only a few cells were labeled, suggesting that the initial rapid rise was due to cell division whereas the slower phase was related to cell migration into the dentate gyrus. This conclusion was strongly supported by experiments using groups of rats injected at a single postlesion time point but allowed varying postinjection survival times. At 6 hours, labeled cells were distributed throughout both hippocampal hemispheres, but by 4 days, and markedly by 8 days, they were clustered in the zones of degeneration. On the basis of these findings, Lynch concluded that the lesion induces a diffuse proliferation of microglia that then migrate to the sites of degeneration or deafferentation.

Studies in which a variety of neuroanatomical techniques (Lynch et al., 1973a,b, 1976) were used reveal that the commissural and associational fibers, which are normally restricted to the inner molecular layer (Figure 62), extend outward into the deafferented middle molecular layer. Recent work with both fiber stains and the electron microscope indicates that this effect occurs 5 to 7 days after lesioning the entorhinal cortex in adults. Of particular interest is the observation that in immature rats these remaining fibers will sprout to cover almost the entire dendritic tree (Lynch et al., 1973a,b; Zimmer, 1973, 1974), whereas the effect is much more limited in the adult. Lynch suggests that this difference may be related, in part, to the speed of removal of degenerating axonal elements, since degeneration products are removed rapidly in neonatal animals while they persist for months in adults. There is also evidence that the sparse septal (Lynch et al., 1972) and crossed entorhinal (Stewart et al., 1974) inputs, which are normally located in the outer molecular layer, undergo reactive changes, possibly including sprouting, when the dendritic zone is denervated by lesions of the ipsilateral entorhinal cortex (see Figure 65).

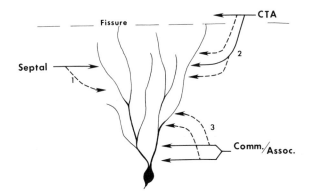

Figure 65. Summary of changes in the afferents remaining to the dentate gyrus following a lesion of the ipsilateral entorhinal cortex. The outward movement of the commissural and associational systems (3) has been observed with several anatomical techniques, whereas the "sprouting" of septal projections (1) is inferred from increased AChE activity. An increase in the size of the crossed entorhinal projections is indicated by anatomical and physiological analysis (2). Two routes by which this increase could be accomplished are illustrated: proliferation of existing projections to the dentate gyrus, or development of new branches that cross the fissure from the pyramidal cell field. CTA = crossed temporoammonic tract. [Lynch et al., 1975a]

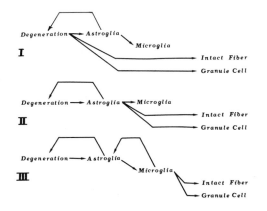

Figure 66. Schematics illustrating some possible interactions between the various elements showing pronounced changes after deafferentation. The length of the arrows indicates the extent of the postlesion interval. [Lynch et al., 1975a]

What defines an innervation field or, more specifically, how one neuron or class of neurons specifies its territory and controls an invasion by neighboring sprouts is, of course, a vital question. This problem will be taken up in more detail in Chapter VI, "Target Cell Innervation."

Lynch has proposed three possible models of axonal growth and synaptic reoccupancy in which glia play a prominent role (Figure 66).

According to Model I, most of the morphological developments that follow deafferentation are initiated directly by the degeneration products or by the loss of something released by the normal fibers. The early stages of degeneration induce hypertrophy in the astroglia, which then begin to phagocytize the degeneration products. The links between the degeneration products and other elements depicted, i.e., microglia, intact fibers, and the granule cells themselves, are not specified. If such direct links exist, then different times or requirements for initiation and mobilization of responses of these elements must be involved.

In Model II, the astroglia play a much more central role, with degeneration initiating only one event, i.e., astrocytic hypertrophy. The astroglia induce further changes either by removing degeneration products (thus making space available) or by a direct action on other elements.

Model III introduces two further thoughts: (1) degeneration induces a direct response in some but not all of the cellular elements (in both glial types here), and (2) the microglia have, primarily, a regulatory and not a phagocytic role as is most often supposed. The point emphasized in each of these models is that the timing of morphological changes in the deafferented dentate gyrus suggests that the glial cells play a regulatory role in the sprouting phenomenon; i.e., these cells undergo profound transformations well in advance of any sign of axonal growth or synaptic reoccupancy. Lynch thinks that it is reasonable to hypothesize that this temporal precedence indicates a causal linkage. It should also be noted that the problem is not only one of analyzing glial-neuronal interactions but glial-glial (i.e., microglia-astroglia) relationships as well. As Lynch pointed out at the Work Session, establishing causal relations for these events will require more precision in our understanding of time courses, as well as a means to isolate, identify, and manipulate the various components of the total response selectively.

Just as experimental strategy is important in the elucidation of trophic effects at the nerve-muscle junction (see Chapter II), so it is a crucial issue here. Lynch and co-workers (1975b), using a technique similar to that of Yamamoto (1972), have recently maintained 0.5-mm-thick slices of adult hippocampus alive in vitro for 40 hours (Figure 67, A and B). In preliminary studies, they collected the medium from slices obtained from both "normal" and denervated hippocampi, and, by means of polyacrylamide gel, found evidence for differences in

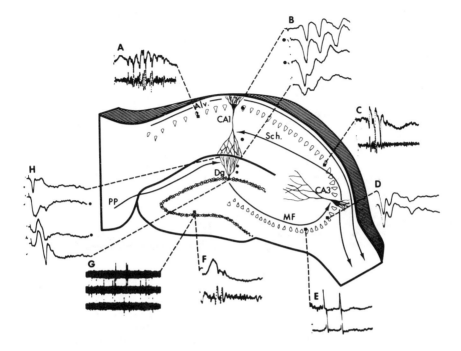

Figure 67. A. Extracellular potentials recorded during stimulation of three separate fiber systems of a single hippocampal explant. A. Unitary discharges from CA1 cell layer to stimulation of Schaeffer collaterals; upper trace is unfiltered record, lower is after high pass (500 Hz to 10 kHz) filtering. Stimulus at onset of trace. Amplitude of units is 500 μV; sweep duration is 50 msec. In this and all other traces, negativity is down and positivity is up. B. Field potential profile from CA1 region to Schaeffer collateral stimulation. Dash lines indicate potentials recorded from tip of apical and basilar dendrites. Solid dots represent maximal negative (synaptic) potential (lower) and cell layer responses (upper). Largest peak negativity is 4.0 mV; sweep duration is 20 msec. C. Driven unitary activity recorded from the CA3 region from stimulation of the mossy fiber pathway. Calibration same as in A. D. Higher intensity stimulation of mossy fibers elicits short-latency negative potentials in CA3. Calibration same as in B. E. Spontaneously firing CA3 unit well isolated by microelectrode (unfiltered recording). Amplitude is 2 mV; sweep duration is 20 msec. F. Driven dentate granule cell unitary discharge (lower trace) and field potential (upper trace) and low-intensity stimulation of perforant path axons. Calibration same as in A and C. G. Spontaneous activity of dentate units. Spike amplitude 100 μV; sweep duration is 500 msec. H. Field potential profile from dentate molecular and cell layers. Dash lines indicate potentials recorded at the obliterated hippocampal fissure (upper) and within the dentate cell layer (lower). Alv. = alveus containing axons of CA1 cells exiting the hippocampus; DG = dentate gyrus (granule cell layer); MF = mossy fiber axons of the granule cells innervating the inner molecular layer of CA3 cells; PP = perforant path containing axons originating in cells of the entorhinal cortex and terminating in dentate gyrus and CA1 outer molecular layers; Sch = Schaeffer collaterals of CA3 axons terminating in middle dendritic zone of CA1 cells. Calibration, peak negativity is 2.5 mV; sweep duration is 20 msec. [Lynch et al., 1975b]

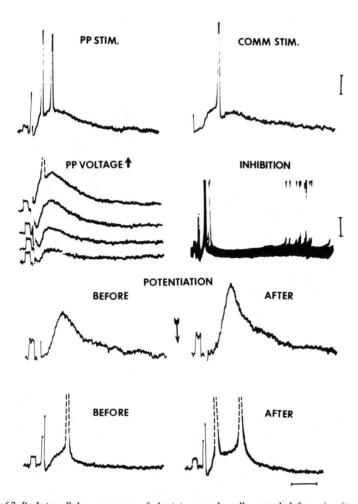

Figure 67. B. Intracellular responses of dentate granule cells recorded from *in vitro* hippocampal explants. PP stim: response of a granule cell to stimulation of perforant path axons. Note double discharge. Calibration pulse is 4 mV followed by stimulus artifact. Spike amplitude is approximately 55 mV; EPSP, 12 mV; total sweep duration, 50 msec. Comm stim: response of a different granule cell to stimulation of commissural axons. Spike amplitude is 60 mV; excitatory postsynaptic potentials, 15 mV. Calibration is 15 mV; sweep duration, 40 msec. PP voltage: response of another granule cell to increases in stimulus voltages; bottom to top stimulus voltages were 15, 25, 40, and 70 V applied to perforant path axons. Calibration pulse is 4.0 mV; sweep duration, 50 msec. Inhibition: inhibitory period (60 msec) following initial excitation by perforant path stimulation. Sweep duration is approximately 125 msec; calibration, 15 mV; spike amplitude, 50 mV. Seventeen superimposed sweeps. Potentiation: sub- and suprathreshold responses of two granule cells (upper and lower traces) to 1.5/sec perforant path stimulation before and after a 15-sec train of 15/sec pulses. Calibration pulse is 2.0 mV in the upper traces and 5.0 mV in the lower traces; total sweep is 50 msec in all cases. Calibration bar is 10 msec. [Lynch et al., 1975b]

the profiles of proteins released into the medium from the two kinds of slices. If these findings are substantiated, then it may eventually be possible to ascertain whether or not a molecular factor, perhaps glial in origin, is responsible for controlling sprouting and, if so, identify it.

Summary

Our understanding of neuron-glia relations and interactions is changing rapidly. The outlines of a complex interdependency in which neurons and glia exert mutual regulatory controls and influences are emerging. Whereas neurons may dominate in some functions, glia seem to be the controlling factor in others. While glia may not be regarded as active information processors at this time, it is clear that, by guiding circuit formation as well as ongoing electrical activity and metabolism in mature neurons, they have the potential to modulate neuronal information transactions. The further elucidation of neuron-glia interactions offers great promise of significant conceptual advance in the neurosciences.

VI. TARGET CELL INNERVATION

The study of the relationships between neurons and their innervation field is important for what it can tell us about the end products of multiple neuron-target cell interactions as expressed at the levels of gross circuits, patterns of peripheral innervation, and, ultimately, function. Obviously, much of the molecular, receptor, single-cell, and neuronal culture work discussed in the preceding chapters is implicitly concerned with these relationships. Explicit concern with the entire innervation field is part of Landmesser's studies of the chick ciliary ganglion (Chapter IV), Raisman's data on sexual dimorphism and preoptic area synapses (Chapter IV), and Lynch's studies on regeneration and sprouting (Chapter V). That the area of innervation determines the development of the innervating neurons was shown in the classical experiments of Hamburger in 1934.

In his discussion of NGF at the Work Session, Thoenen referred to the work of Olson and Malmfors (1970) and Björklund and collaborators (1974) on the transplantation of adrenergic tissue into the anterior chamber of the eye or hypothalamus. Whether it is in the anterior chamber or hypothalamus, the adrenergic tissue develops its normal innervation pattern. Moreover, Björklund and co-workers (1974, 1975) noted that bathing the adrenergic tissue to be transplanted with NGF markedly increased the density of innervation. Conversely, bathing the tissue with antibody to NGF reduced the density of innervation. These observations, together with the finding that organs with adrenergic innervation can synthesize NGF, indicate that NGF is acting as a messenger for the transfer of information from effector organ to the innervating adrenergic neurons. It was on the basis of such data that Thoenen and his collaborators investigated the retrograde transport of NGF (see Chapter III).

In this chapter, we will attempt to bring these several threads together so that the relationship between neurons and their innervation field may be more clearly stated. To do this, we will examine three studies: (1) the work of Diamond and co-workers on sprouting, regeneration, and competition among nerves in the salamander; (2) that of Raisman and co-workers on the process of reinnervation in the superior cervical ganglion and the septal nuclei of rats; and (3) that of Black on the transsynaptic regulation of target organ innervation in the rat iris and pineal.

Sprouting, Regeneration, and Competition in Salamander Skin Innervation: J. Diamond

Sprouting is an important neuronal phenomenon that occurs in both the central and peripheral nervous system of vertebrates. Although it has generally been regarded as compensation for neuronal damage, degeneration of other neuronal fibers has been shown by Diamond and collaborators (Aguilar et al., 1973; Diamond et al., 1976) to be unnecessary for sprouting to occur. Diamond and co-workers proposed that the mechanisms involved in the sprouting phenomenon are important in determining how shared target territory is divided among the nerves supplying it, even in the mature organism. In consonance with the idea of Thoenen, and perhaps of Lynch as well (see above and Chapter V), they postulate that the target tissue continually releases a signal (e.g., it could be NGF) for the neuron to sprout. At the same time, however, individual axons transport and release a factor that neutralizes the effects of this signal, by essentially "telling" both themselves and adjacent axons not to sprout.

The symmetry of the nerve fields of the right and left hindlimbs of the salamander (*Amblystoma tigrinum*) provides a unique opportunity to investigate questions of sprouting and antisprouting factors, regeneration, and competition in the development of innervated fields. Evidence for the hypothesized antisprouting factor was obtained when Aguilar and co-workers (1973) compared the effects of partial denervation with those of colchicine-induced block of axoplasmic flow on the peripheral fields of nerves innervating the hindlimb. Acute application of colchicine solution (0.03 to 0.10 M) to spinal nerve 16 resulted in a dose-dependent increase in skin and muscle fields of the adjacent nerves 15 and 17. In contrast to the situation with nerve section, sprouting of adjacent nerves occurred after colchicine applications without loss of impulse conduction, functional deficit, or subsequent degeneration of the treated nerves.

As discussed in Chapter II, the use of colchicine is not without hazards. Diamond and collaborators were specifically concerned to exclude the possibility (1) that an undetected scattered degeneration of nerve terminals might have occurred *within* the field of the treated nerve and so produce products of degeneration, and (2) that colchicine may have been accumulating in the skin to cause nonneural local effects. They were able to rule out the first concern by physiologically measuring the actual number of mechanosensory endings; this involved determining the threshold stimulus required to evoke an afferent impulse at each of a large number of points in the fields of normal, cut, and colchicine-treated nerves (Cooper et al., 1976). They were able to determine that touch receptors are uniformly distributed (150 to 250 μ apart) and that a single axon can provide from six to one hundred receptors. Eighty percent of the receptors no longer responded 7 days after nerve section, whereas, after colchicine application, the threshold pattern was normal even at 14 days (when adjacent sprouting was well established). In other words, the number of mechanosensory endings of the colchicine-treated nerve was unchanged when the newly sprouted ones from the adjacent nerves were fully functional (Figure 68).* By using tracer experiments they were also able to show that the small amount of ^{3}H-colchicine, which did circulate systemically, accumulated symmetrically in the skin of the control and experimental hindlimb and, thus, did not cause sprouting by direct action on the skin.

According to the hypothesis of Diamond and co-workers, nerve fibers adjacent to the colchicine-treated or severed axons sprout because there is no longer an adequate supply of axonally transported factor(s) to neutralize the sprouting stimulus of the target organ.† These workers also found that after partial denervation a new functional mechanosensory ending appeared in the skin for every one that was lost by nerve section, the final number of receptors being determined by the equilibrium between the antisprouting factor and the tissue stimulus. In this regard, it is interesting that colchicine application actually produced a hyperinnervation, which in one experiment resulted in a virtual doubling of the total receptor population (Figure 69).

---

*At the Work Session Lynch raised another concern: that an early reversible form of degeneration was actually being produced and, hence, that the blockade of transport of an antisprouting factor had not been unequivocably established. The contention of Diamond and co-workers is that reduction of neuronal transport is, indeed, likely to be the earliest change during degeneration. Moreover, if this reduction leads to adjacent sprouting, then the real question is: "Is neuronal transport under physiological control?" If it *is*, then it provides a "nondegenerative" means of influencing sprouting. If it is not, then neuronal transport may be an all-or-nothing mechanism that only changes during degeneration. Furthermore, in many experiments the colchicine treatment did not raise the threshold of the receptors belonging to the treated nerve at the time when adjacent nerves were sprouting. Threshold changes in these mechanoreceptors are very sensitive indicators of otherwise undetectable adverse effects on the endings.

†Diamond and co-workers have not excluded the possibility that colchicine blocks the uptake and retrograde transport of the target tissue growth factor, thus allowing it to become available to neighboring terminals and cause them to sprout. However, they think that this explanation is unlikely.

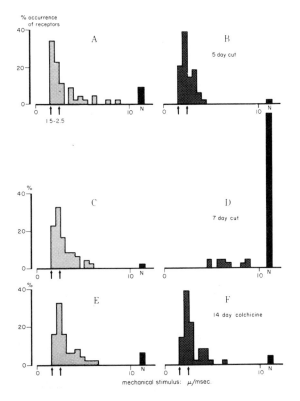

Figure 68. Density of touch receptors indicated by distribution of "threshold stimuli." Mechanosensory impulses were recorded from the 16th spinal nerve in response to mechanical stimulation of the skin with a probe 10 μ in diameter, attached to a voltage-driven piezoelectric crystal. The probe was aligned vertical to the skin and just touched it. Each histogram represents the results of stimulating 75 random points on the skin. At each point repetitive stimuli were delivered: the rate of rise of each mechanical pulse was progressively increased until an impulse was evoked repeatedly in successive tests at a constant latency from the onset of the stimulus. Abscissa: rate of rise of stimulus, binned in increments of 0.5 μ/msec. The arrows show the range of the first 2 bins (1.5 to 2.5 μ/msec). Ordinate: the percent occurrence of thresholds in each bin. The solid bin (N) on the extreme right of each abscissa indicates "failures," i.e., points that were insensitive to mechanical stimulation over the range used. The paired histograms AB, CD, and EF refer to the control and treated limbs, respectively, of each of 3 animals. In B the 16th nerve had been cut 5 days, and in D 7 days, before the skin was tested; the recording was made from the nerve distal to the point of section. In F the nerve trunk had been exposed for 30 min to a 100-mM solution of colchicine 14 days previously. Colchicine-treated nerves tested at periods of 1 to 21 days gave similar results. Sprouting can be detected 5 days after adjacent nerves are treated or sectioned and is completed by 10 days. The variations between A and B, and E and F, are within the normal limits between right and left sides. Therefore colchicine (and nerve section up to 5 days) did not cause any detectable signs of degeneration of the mechanosensory endings. Clearly, in D only a few receptors were still functional, and these were of high threshold. The skin mechanoreceptors are all rapidly adapting, and, although salamander nerve axons frequently can conduct impulses for up to 10 days or more after they are sectioned, receptor function is usually impaired earlier. [Diamond]

339

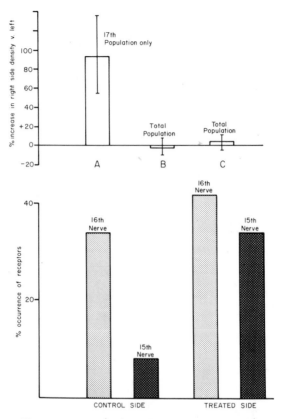

Figure 69. *Upper histograms:* quantitative sprouting after partial denervation. The percent occurrence (the density) of the "low-threshold" receptors feeding into the 16th and 17th nerves from a shared region of the skin was measured and the values between right and left limbs were compared. Column A refers to a group of animals in which the right 16th nerve had been sectioned 3 weeks previously and shows the right-left percent difference for the 17th nerve touch-receptor population only. Column B shows, for the same group of animals, the right-left difference for the total receptor population (i.e., 17th nerve on the treated side, 16th and 17th nerves on the control). Column C shows right-left difference in total population of touch receptors in a control group of animals, with 16th and 17th nerves intact on both sides. There is no significant difference between Columns B and C, indicating that the increase in 17th nerve receptors on the right side of the experimental group had quantitatively made up the loss due to section of nerve 16 (vertical bars = S.E.M.). *Lower histograms:* sprouting after colchicine treatment of adjacent nerve. Results from a single animal showing touch-receptor density in a region of skin shared by the 15th and 16th nerves. The number of touch receptors associated with the 15th nerve was only a small proportion of the total. There was no loss in the population of receptors feeding into the right colchicine-treated 16th nerve compared to the left (the slight increase is within the normal variation). However, on the right side the 15th nerve supplied an extra population of receptors almost equal to the number associated with the 16th nerve. [Diamond]

However, sprouting is not simply a matter of filling any vacated nerve field. The salamander hindlimb is normally shared between spinal nerves 15, 16, and 17. The 16th nerve innervates most of the dorsal surface, and, when it is cut or treated with colchicine, fields 15 and 17 enlarge (see Figure 70). This enlargement continues only until these two fields meet; they never overlap. In many animals, fields 15 and 17 already share a common frontier, and in these cases there is no territorial enlargement when nerve 16 is cut, although the intact nerves sprout within their own territory. Surprisingly, neither nerve 15 nor 17

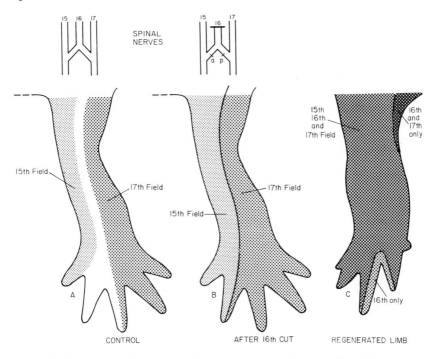

Figure 70. Nerve territories in dorsal skin of salamander hindlimb. Because of the symmetry between right- and left-limb nerve fields in normal animals, the control limb indicates the preoperative state of the experimental limb fields. Areas of mechanosensitivity were mapped by recording impulses from the three spinal nerves while the skin was lightly stroked with a fine bristle. The control (A) and experimental (B) limbs of a single animal were mapped 3 weeks after the 16th nerve was sectioned in the experimental side (as indicated in the inset above B). The 16th nerve field included the whole of the skin, and the boundary (not shown) between the fields of its anterior (a) and posterior (p) branches was identical in location to the boundary between the enlarged 15th and 17th fields in the experimental limb (B). Hindlimb (C) had regenerated for 4 months after amputation at the level where the limb emerges from the trunk. Its control fields were similar to those of the limb in A (see the text). [Diamond]

will initially invade the other's territory, even when that territory is totally denervated. Experiments in progress show that after longer periods, e.g., 1 to 2 months, nerve 17, but, interestingly, not nerve 15, does achieve a limited incursion into the other's territory.

Perhaps the simplest explanation is that there is a physical barrier preventing the mutual invasion of the territories of nerves 15 and 17. This possibility was eliminated by a fortuitous finding. Diamond and co-workers noted that nerve 16 has one anterior and one posterior branch; these branches join the trunks of nerves 15 and 17, respectively, and it is to the frontier between the two subfields of nerve 16 that nerves 15 and 17 will grow. If nerves 15 and 16 anterior or nerves 17 and 16 posterior are cut together, then the remaining branch of nerve 16 often invades the denervated region beyond the frontier that stops nerves 15 and 17. In other words, there cannot be a physical barrier. Furthermore, the results cannot be due to a limited capacity of nerves to enlarge their territories, because there can be extensive sprouting of fibers within their own territory but never more than a fractional distance across this invisible frontier.

The above findings imply the possibility of a neuron recognizing either its territory or the territorial specificity of the sprouting stimulus of the target tissue. It would seem reasonable to hypothesize that position along the neuraxis is crucial and that the nerves impose an appropriate matching specificity on the periphery they innervate. However, when one adult hindlimb was amputated and allowed to regenerate along with its original nerves, there was often no selectivity of innervation, and all three spinal nerves could overlap everywhere in the limb. This was particularly so when one spinal nerve was given an opportunity to innervate the blastema in advance of the other two (Figure 70). In such virgin territories, then, the peripheral stimulus did not discriminate between nerves to the degree that it did in the normal adult. One might argue that such territories had not yet "learned" anything from the innervating nerves. If so, why are the normal nerve fields so sharply defined and without such intermingling?

Another approach to the question as to whether specificity resides in the sprouting stimulus of the target cell or in the nerve is to guide the regenerating fibers along the distal stump of another cut nerve. Under these circumstances, fibers that were guided to foreign skin formed normal mechanosensory endings (see Johnston et al., 1975). However, the regeneration "drive" was effective only up to the limits of the presumed mechanical guidance provided by the distal trunk of nerve 16 (Figure 71). From this evidence it seems that

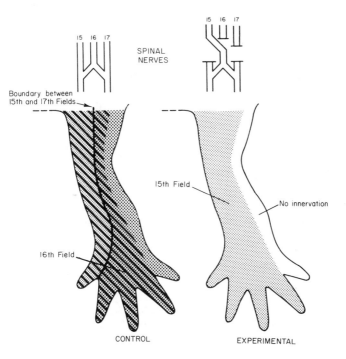

Figure 71. Redirection of regenerating nerves. Nerve fields were mapped as in Figure 70. In the control limb the continuous line marks the division between the 15th and 17th fields, and the hatching indicates the field of the 16th nerve, which in this animal did not include the whole of the dorsal skin. In the experimental limb all the nerves had been cut, and the central end of nerve 15 was redirected to permit regeneration into the distal end of nerve 16, as shown in the inset above. The limb was mapped 10 weeks later, and only nerve 15 fibers were present. The field of the regenerated 15th nerve is identical with the original field of the 16th nerve. The completely denervated region of the lateral border of the experimental limb was that which was occupied only by nerve 17 fibers in the control. [Diamond]

regenerating nerves retain certain characteristics, and the abnormal innervation pattern in the regenerated limbs is unlikely to result from changes in the nerves.*

In one final series of experiments, which gave important clues to what might be responsible for the apparent selectivity, Diamond and co-workers examined the question of the positional specification of

*These findings indicate that caution must be exercised in using regeneration experiments in studies designed to elucidate how innervation develops normally. The results from the salamander indicate that normal developmental processes may be quite different from regeneration. Another difference is that in winter (particularly from December to February), salamander nerves will often not sprout collaterals after the cutting of adjacent nerves, but the cut nerves, themselves, always regenerate normally and form the usual mechanosensory endings in the skin. Diamond and co-workers conclude that the target organ-sprouting stimulus may well be deficient or absent in winter.

nerve fields. When areas of hindlimb skin (up to 100 mm^2) were rotated 180°, their reinnervation patterns (Figure 72) were unexpected. The ingrowing nerve 15 fibers ignored the rotated frontier of nerves 15 to 17 in the skin and, instead, created a new one, coincident with the original position of the frontier on the limb (as though no skin rotation had occurred). This creation of a new frontier was not simply dependent on the location of the surviving central nerve stumps beneath the rotated skin flap. In preliminary experiments in which the limb was partially denervated, in addition to rotating the skin, the uncut branch of nerve 16 was frequently observed to grow across the implant, as it often does in unrotated skin. The remaining nerve 15, however, seemed to be confined to the newly created frontier, even when this frontier straddled a region that was originally part of the

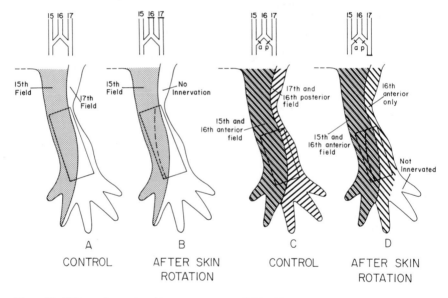

Figure 72. Effects of rotating skin areas on nerve fields. The results of two experiments are shown, each with a control and experimental side (A and B; C and D). A and B refer to an experiment in which the rectangle of skin shown in A was rotated by 180° in B. In addition, both the 16th and 17th nerves in limb B had been cut. The dash line in B shows the original boundary between the 15th and 17th nerve fields in the skin (before rotation). The new 15-17 nerve boundary in B is in the identical position in body space to that in the preoperative condition, as can be seen from A. The experiment in C and D was different in that the 16th anterior nerve was left intact along with the 15th nerve. As before, the 15th nerve field took up its original position in body space; however the 16th anterior nerve sprouted across as shown in D. The dotted line in D shows the original boundary between the 15th and 17th nerve fields (before rotation). The 15-17 nerve boundary in the control (C) corresponded exactly to the boundary between the 16th anterior (a) and 16th posterior nerve fields (p). [Diamond]

territory of nerve 15 (Figure 72). Nerve 17, however, as was frequently observed in other kinds of experiments, tended to spread over the transplant, along with its corresponding (posterior) branch of nerve 16. This spread was almost certainly a function of the regenerating nerve 17 fibers and not a sprouting of nerve 17 fibers that had not been cut in the making of the skin transplant.

Diamond and collaborators concluded that nerve territory is not defined by *skin* fields, but by a coordinate system that relates to the body; they call it "body space." For nerve 15, this coordinate system determines where the nerve will sprout, i.e., where its nerve field occurs. They pointed out that nerves are capable of sprouting in response to the stimulus provided from skin, even "foreign" skin, provided that the skin is within the "body space" territory of the nerve. However, the stringency with which different nerves conform to the territorial limitation of this body space is variable, and, thus, the position of origin of the nerve along the neuraxis may be significant. Moreover, there is a time dependency, in that nerve 17 conformed to the body-space control for about a month, whereas nerve 15 was strictly confined to its own territory for at least 4 months.

Conclusion

The findings of Diamond and co-workers indicate that there are active mechanisms for regulating nerve fields in the adult salamander. These workers suggest that body territories become established during primary development by unknown mechanisms that could involve chemical gradients. Thereafter, the target tissue is involved in determining the relative density and appropriateness of the innervation. The finding that undamaged sympathetic nerves sprout to innervate a nerve-free piece of iris transplanted into the anterior chamber of the eye (Olson and Malmfors, 1970) is consistent with the hypothesis of Diamond and collaborators that production of an innervation field is the result of an interaction between sprouting and antisprouting factors. Also explained is the sprouting of axons to maintain a constant level of innervation of a growing organ.

Similar mechanisms may be operative in the central nervous system, although this has not yet been proven. The finding that cortical projections of the lateral geniculate neurons connected to one eye enlarge their territories following enucleation of the other eye (Wiesel and Hubel, 1974) supports this hypothesis. It is interesting that a similar territorial enlargement can result from mere lid suture (Hubel et al., 1975), suggesting that reduced or abnormal neural activity, perhaps correlated with changes in neuronal transport, may be involved in causing such a redistribution of terminal fields. Diamond and co-workers are now examining this possibility in the salamander nerve-skin system.

At the Work Session, Lynch voiced concern about imposing peripheral models, such as that presented here, on the phenomena of sprouting, regeneration, and competition in the brain. Furthermore, since the model of Diamond and collaborators may not account for all central regeneration phenomena, other mechanisms should also be considered. Guth commented that such a competition model poses problems in terms of the selectivity and specificity of neural connections. Perhaps more difficult to explain is the known displacement of inappropriate connections by correct ones – a process occurring over months.*

Isolation and identification of the sprouting and antisprouting factors involved in the salamander model would be an important step forward, as would the clarification of the role of activity and the establishment of body-space territories. Perhaps the next section, in which a rather different model system is discussed, will help to clarify the extent to which peripheral and central target cell innervation processes are comparable.

Regeneration and Sprouting in Sympathetic Ganglia and Septal Nuclei: G. Raisman

In an attempt to compare target cell innervation directly in both central and peripheral sites, Raisman has examined regeneration and sprouting in both the superior cervical ganglia and the septal nuclei. In their quantitative investigations of the development of collateral reinnervation after partial deafferentation of the septal nuclei, Raisman and Field (1973a) noted, first, that there was a fixed number of postsynaptic sites that persisted during the process of degeneration of the presynaptic elements. Secondly, these denervated sites were reinnervated by existing local axon terminals in their immediate vicinity. Raisman and Field refer to this process as "collateral reinnervation," by analogy with the process of collateral sprouting first

---

*Four months is the longest time a preparation has been followed by Diamond and co-workers. They are now designing experiments to investigate possible reversions of enlarged, adjacent, or overlapping fields when axoplasmic transport is restored in nerves whose fields have been invaded.

described in the peripheral nervous system. Collateral reinnervation is very rapid and efficient and results in a reoccupation of virtually all the deafferented sites. In this process, there is a reciprocal relationship between nondegenerating and degenerating terminals. Since the cut fimbrial axons do not regenerate across the lesion, they do not reestablish their original connections with the septal neurons, a finding that is consistent with the hypotheses of Diamond and his collaborators presented above.

After deafferentation of the sympathetic ganglion, synapses disappeared (95% loss), but the postsynaptic sites could be recognized by vacated synaptic thickenings (Raisman et al., 1974). In contrast to the situation in the septal nuclei (Figure 73), degenerating terminals were removed very rapidly, and, in the absence of reinnervation vacated thickenings persisted for at least 6 months. If the preganglionic chain

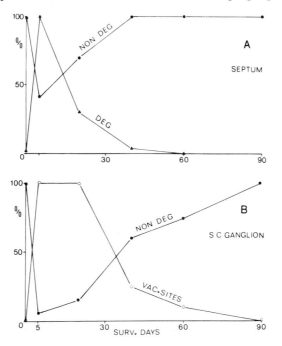

Figure 73. A schematic representation to compare the rate of reinnervation of denervated sites. A. Collateral reinnervation by adjacent, intact axon terminals in the septal neuropil (Septum) selectively denervated by cutting the ipsilateral fimbria. B. Reinnervation of the superior cervical sympathetic ganglion (S.C.Ganglion) by regeneration of the cut preganglionic axons. NON DEG = nondegenerating axon terminals; DEG = axon terminals showing the reaction of electron-dense orthograde degeneration 2 days after section of the parent fibers; VAC. SITES = vacated postsynaptic sites identified by the presence of synaptic thickenings unapposed by axon terminals. [Raisman]

was allowed to regenerate back to the ganglion (e.g., after a freeze-lesion of the chain), synapses began to reappear in the ganglion 1 month after the operation. At the same time, the vacated synaptic thickenings disappeared. Two months after the operation, the number of synapses reached normal levels and there was no further change. The new synapses could be shown to be of preganglionic origin, since they disappeared after surgical section of the regenerated preganglionic chain. Furthermore, measurement of two neurotransmitter enzymes revealed that the biochemical properties of the newly formed synapses were comparable to those of synapses in normal ganglia. Reinnervation caused a reappearance of choline acetyltransferase and a normal transsynaptic TOH response to reserpine.

Comparison of the reinnervation processes in the septal nuclei and the sympathetic ganglion revealed that the former is the result of collateral sprouting by undamaged axons, whereas the latter represents a true regeneration of the severed axons. The septal nuclei, however, were only partially deafferented, whereas the sympathetic ganglia underwent an almost complete interruption of the afferent supply. The absence of appreciable collateral sprouting in the ganglion, therefore, may not be due to any intrinsic inability of the preganglionic axons to show such a reaction, but simply that there were not enough surviving axons to produce a detectable amount of collateral reinnervation. The longer time course for the appearance of new synaptic connections in the ganglion reflected the longer distance the regenerating axons had to travel, as compared with the collateral reinnervation of denervated septal sites, which was carried out by adjacent intact axon terminals and which seemed to follow immediately upon the removal of the degenerating presynaptic elements. However, the difference in time course was partially obscured by the much longer time taken for the removal of the degenerating presynaptic elements in the septal neuropil as opposed to that in the ganglion. In the septum, where the sites were reinnervated almost immediately upon removal of the degeneration, the interval before reinnervation was characterized by the presence of degenerating endings (Figure 73). In contrast, in the ganglion, the degeneration was removed very rapidly, and there was a long interval before the preganglionic axons grew back into the ganglion; this interval was characterized, therefore, by the presence of vacated synaptic thickenings (Figure 73).

From a morphological point of view, the two processes are similar in that, in both areas, postsynaptic sites persisted after deafferentation and these sites were fully reoccupied. As far as can be determined, new postsynaptic sites were not formed, and, in any case, the total number of synapses was unchanged. Such data are consistent with the hypothesis* of Diamond and co-workers and also support the application of a peripheral model to central regeneration. The type of injury produced and the method of study of the regenerative process are important to the conclusions drawn.

The finding that the postsynaptic specialization persists in the absence of the presynaptic terminal brings into question the relative roles played by factors in the presynaptic, as opposed to the postsynaptic, elements in the control of synaptogenesis. At least for regenerative processes in the septal nuclei, the postsynaptic element controls not only the site but also the total number of synapses. However, this does not answer the question as to the determination of the number of synaptic sites during development. A number of models have been proposed for the process of synaptogenesis and these are discussed more fully in Chapter VII. From the work of Olson and Malmfors (1970), Björklund and co-workers (1974), and Raisman and Field (1973a), the target organ would appear to be the controlling factor. Hyperinnervation, however, can also be produced by blocking neuronal transport in some axons supplying an innervation field with colchicine (see Diamond above), suggesting that neurons may also play a role in regulating synaptogenesis. Furthermore, Emmelin and Perec (1968) showed that decentralization can reduce the ability of SCG neurons to sprout. In the following section, Black examines the role of transsynaptic factors in the regulation of the ontogeny of target organ innervation.

Transsynaptic Regulation of the Development of Target Organ Innervation: I. B. Black

To examine the regulation of development of end organ innervation, Black and Mytilineou (1976), using biochemical and histofluorescent approaches, studied the superior cervical ganglion and two of its target organs, the iris and pineal gland (see Chapter II).

---

*Raisman hypothesizes that the maximum number of nerve endings that make synapses is fixed, whereas in the sensory system investigated by Diamond sprouting continues until the balance between sprouting and antisprouting factors is restored. It is possible that in different systems various limitations set an upper level to the number of branches or synapses achieved by a single neuron; in some instances this number may be more dependent on the target tissues; in others, more on the neuron's capacity.

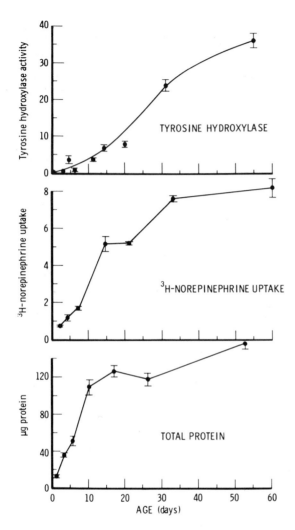

Figure 74. Development of iris innervation and total protein. Groups of rats were taken from litters of different ages, irides were removed, and TOH activity, [3H] norepinephrine uptake, or total protein was determined. Each point represents the mean of determinations performed on irides from 6 to 8 animals and vertical bars indicate S.E.M. TOH activity is expressed as pmoles/iris/hour, [3H] norepinephrine uptake as cpm/iris, and total protein as μg/iris. [Black and Mytilineou, 1976]

During postnatal ontogeny the activity of TOH, which is localized to adrenergic neurons, increased 50-fold in the iris and 34-fold in the pineal nerve terminals of the rat. These increases paralleled the in vitro rise in iris ^{3}H-norepinephrine (^{3}H-NE) uptake, a measure of the presence of functional nerve terminal membrane (Figure 74). These biochemical indices of end organ innervation correlated well with developmental increases in density of innervation, adrenergic plexus ramification, and nerve fiber fluorescence intensity as determined by fluorescence microscopy.

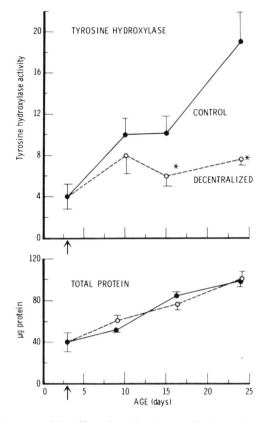

Figure 75. Time course of the effect of ganglion decentralization on the development of TOH activity and total protein in the iris. Ganglia were unilaterally decentralized in 3-day-old rats (arrow) and the animals were killed at the indicated times. Parallel determinations of TOH activity and total protein were performed on aliquots taken from the same iris homogenates. Results for TOH activity are expressed as pmoles/iris/hour, and total protein is expressed as μg/iris for contralateral control irides (solid line) and ipsilateral decentralized irides. Each point represents the mean of determinations on 6 to 8 irides. For total protein, none of the pairs of points differs significantly. *differs from respective control at P<0.01. [Black and Mytilineou, 1976]

Unilateral transection of the presynaptic cholinergic nerves innervating the SCG in 2- to 3-day-old rats prevented the normal development of end organ innervation; TOH activity (Figure 75), ^{3}H-NE uptake, innervation density, plexus ramification, and fluorescence intensity failed to develop normally in irides innervated by decentralized ganglia. These findings led Black and Mytilineou to conclude that transsynaptic factors regulate the maturation of adrenergic nerve terminals and the development of end organ innervation by SCG.

Summary

The study of the relationships between neurons and their innervation fields highlights the complex neuron-target cell inter-relationships that, as a system, result in the specific connectivity patterns and functional characteristics of neural circuits. The concept of a delicate balance of molecular and temporal factors of a continuously responsive nature, whether in the central or peripheral nervous system, is brought out clearly in the studies on sprouting-antisprouting factors in innervation fields and the hypothesis of Diamond and collaborators (see above). The vital role of the target organ in these relationships, either in supplying sprouting factors or in providing a determined number of postsynaptic sites and, hence, synaptic and/or receptor density, should not be underemphasized as the search for neural factors is continued. When the experiments of Diamond, Raisman, and Lynch are considered together, they clearly indicate that neither the neuron nor the target cell acts in isolation. Although the neuron may specify the number of synaptic sites very early in development, from that point on this number becomes a rather stable feature of the target cell and/or organ. The neuronal functions responsible for the biochemical and biophysical maturation of newly formed synaptic connections, as well as of the entire target cell, then become *relatively* more important.

VII. PATHOLOGY OF NEURON-TARGET CELL INTERACTIONS

Whereas the preceding chapters dealt with the importance of neuron-target cell molecular exchange for the normal functions of not only target cells but also of neurons themselves, this chapter will consider the pathology of such interactions. While the concept of an ongoing neuron-target cell and neuron-neuron molecular exchange as a prerequisite to normal function provides a useful perspective on various diseases, our major goal is to identify the pathologic states that may provide useful models for the further elucidation of neuron-target cell and neuron-neuron interactions.

It would seem that three general propositions are possible: (1) the neuron supplies the wrong molecular signal to the target cell or vice versa, or (2) the neuron fails to supply either enough, or any, molecular signal. It is also possible that the neuron supplies too much of a given signal. (3) The ability of the target cell or neuron to respond to the signal is lost or reduced. Although the bulk of the present evidence relates to a failure in the supply of the signal, it is still very difficult to distinguish between the alternatives in many cases. Despite the difficulties of classification, the fact that the neuron plays an active role in causing pathology has been known for some time.

Muscle Diseases

Realistically, of course, we cannot regard the problem in too simple a way. The conflict over the neurogenic versus myogenic hypotheses of muscular dystrophy is particularly instructive. Whether the primary problem is neurogenic or myogenic, the resulting disturbed relationship is likely to mean that abnormalities will result in both elements; i.e., the final pathology will be the result of this complex interaction. Indeed, this is likely to be the case in most of the disease states that are examined closely and is the reason why Rathbone's and Peterson's approaches to the problem, as described in Chapter II, are particularly important. In Rathbone's experiments, an early inductive effect of the neural tube is shown to specify the subsequent development of the muscle. At a later stage in development, it might appear that the muscle is the prime cause. That conclusion, of course, would be erroneous. So, in looking at disease, it is important to sort out such factors and to take them into account in formulating experimental designs.

At present, the central theme in all investigations on muscle disease concerns neural influence on muscle (see Chapter II, "The Proof of Trophism," for a detailed discussion of this influence). The theory of McComas and collaborators (1974a,b), that muscular dystrophies in humans are neurogenic disorders, is a matter of current debate. McComas and co-workers (see McComas and Mrozek, 1967; McComas et al., 1974a,b) were originally led to this suggestion by the finding that muscle fibers tend to drop out as motor units. However, there are a number of studies that challenge the concept of a neurogenic factor in human muscular disease. These include the experiments of Bradley and co-workers (1974; Bradley and Jenkison, 1975), Engel and co-workers (1974), and Gilliatt and colleagues (1974). For example, according to Engel, morphometric analysis of the ultrastructure of neuromuscular junctions from patients with Duchenne's dystrophy showed no evidence of partial denervation. Clearly, analytical techniques, such as those of Rathbone and Peterson, will be required to solve some of these questions.

Another important experimental issue concerns the use of animal models. At the Work Session, Arnason argued that present animal models are not applicable to human disease. For example, in animals murine muscular dystrophy consists of multiple abnormalities that include not only the end-plate and extrajunctional receptor spread but also the peripheral nerves and neurons of the anterior horn. Although the CNS of humans with Duchenne's muscular dystrophy is not normal, there is no receptor spread. Duchenne's dystrophy has long been considered a myogenic disease, but the crucial analytical work has not yet been done.

When Albuquerque* applied the technique that he developed for the study of the neuromuscular junction and neurotrophic effects in animals to humans with muscular dystrophy, he found that the ACh sensitivity of the junctional region was normal. Confirming previous work, he did not observe extrajunctional ACh receptors or a TTX-resistant action potential (Lebeda et al., 1974). However, he did find that the presynaptic nerve terminal underwent degenerative changes. Furthermore, the postjunctional action potential underwent a decremental suppression with a widening that resembles that seen in myasthenia gravis. Also, disruption and fragmentation of the sarcoplasmic reticulum occurred (observed in two patients), coupled with an abnormality in transmitter release or in postsynaptic potential.

*E. X. Albuquerque, unpublished observations.

An early inductive effect of an abnormal human tube may, as in the chick, set the muscle on its dystrophic course with resultant further abnormalities in central neurons. Again, great care must be exercised in drawing any conclusions from present animal studies. Future models, if they are to be applicable to the human problem, will have to take into account time (developmental) parameters, extrajunctional receptor spread, and abnormalities in axoplasmic flow and transport, as well as in central motoneurons and synapses. Analyses of human disease must become increasingly sophisticated with regard to biochemical techniques, such as membrane phosphorylation, ribosomal aggregation, and alteration of genetic expression in muscles and neurons. By using such approaches, it may be possible to gain more knowledge from necessarily limited human material.

Neuron-Neuron Interaction Pathology

Transneuronal Degeneration

Perhaps the best starting point in considering the pathology of neuron-neuron interactions is the phenomenon of transneuronal degeneration, which has been known since the nineteenth century. A basic aspect of this phenomenon is that an injury to one neuron is reflected in the metabolism and morphology of other neurons in the same circuit but one, two, or even more synapses removed from the injured neuron. Examples from human pathology include (1) the degeneration of the lateral geniculate neurons after syphilitic destruction of the retina, (2) hypertrophy of the inferior olive after ipsilateral central tegmental tract lesions or contralateral dentate nucleus lesions, as well as inferior olive atrophy after focal cerebellar lesions, and (3) an unrepeated observation that after amputation of a limb there is degeneration of the corresponding area of the motor cortex (Shorey, 1909). It has also been suggested that Friedreich's ataxia involves transneuronal degeneration as well.

Transneuronal degeneration has been studied much more extensively in animals and can be shown to be anterograde or retrograde (Figure 76). In the case of anterograde transneuronal degeneration, retinal lesions result in characteristic shrinkage and atrophy, and even in the death of neurons of the dorsal nucleus of the lateral geniculate. Furthermore, there can be a statistically significant loss of dendritic spines of the apical dendrites of certain Purkinje cells

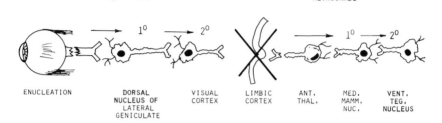

Figure 76. Anterograde and retrograde transneuronal degeneration. In the example given for anterograde transneuronal degeneration, eye enucleation results in structural changes across at least two synapses. Following limbic cortex lesions, retrograde transsynaptic degeneration can be shown in both the medial mammillary nucleus and ventral tegmental nucleus. Whereas transmitter and/or activity can be implicated in anterograde degeneration, the nature of the retrograde signal is unknown. ANT. THAL. = anterior thalamus. [Smith]

in the visual cortex, suggesting an effect across the second-order synapse. A third-order effect has been described for the peristriate cortex.

Other examples of anterograde transneuronal degeneration may be found in the superior colliculus, ventral cochlear nucleus, vestibular nuclei, superior olive, spinal nucleus of the trigeminal nerve, pontine nuclei, reticular nucleus of the thalamus, and olfactory bulb. An excellent review of these phenomena was provided by Cowan in 1971, and since that time further progress has been made. The work of Pinching and Powell (1971) on transneuronal cell degeneration in the olfactory system of the rabbit and rat is important for its application of ultrastructural analysis to the problem. In both the rat and rabbit, the onset of a change in the transneuronal cell is marked by a distinct decrease in the number of postsynaptic thickenings without presynaptic terminals and by a decrease in the fine terminal parts of dendrites.

Role of Activity

There is the question of whether it is the loss of activity or the specific molecular neurotrophic influences that are responsible for the effects of transneuronal degeneration. As noted in Chapter II, this is a complex issue, and its resolution, particularly in the CNS, is difficult. Wiesel's and Hubel's (1963a,b; see also Valverde, 1971) demonstration of physiological and anatomical changes in the lateral geniculate neurons and visual cortex consequent to light deprivation in the kitten would seem to support the role of activity, particularly since Grafstein and Laureno (1973) reported no relationship of transneuronal transfer to activity. However, other investigations have shown the functional responsiveness of retrograde transport systems (see Chapter IV). It may be that the synthesis and delivery of a neurotrophic substance (other than transmitter) are altered by a lack of functional input.

It has been frequently stated in the literature that transneuronal degeneration is most severe in closed sensory systems where there is only one input to the affected cell. This might suggest a quantitative requirement for a nonspecific neurotrophic substance that could be supplied by other inputs, irrespective of whether they are excitatory or inhibitory, in systems with multiple afferents. The much quoted statement about increased severity of changes in closed sensory systems, however, is not quite true. Marked degenerative changes can be produced by partial deafferentation in some systems. If such deafferentation removes only the excitatory input and leaves inhibitory afferents, then the activity and/or transmitter role is strengthened. Several recent works that shed some further light on this question are discussed below.

Ghetti and collaborators (1975) have reexamined transneuronal degeneration in the simian lateral geniculate nucleus after eye enucleation with special attention to the acute and long-term responses of dendrites. Transneuronal degeneration, which readily appeared following enucleation, led steadily to atrophy and numerical loss of neurons. Dendritic changes first appeared 7 days following enucleation. Some dendritic profiles became electron-lucent and revealed floccular material and a few cytoplasmic organelles, while others became vacuolar and filled with tubulovesicular material. These changes were concurrent with the degeneration of the optic nerve terminals but persisted for months after their disappearance. One hundred and seventy days after enucleation, there was a remarkable reduction in dendrites. This decrease occurred before the significant loss of neurons took place (6 to 12 months after enucleation); thus, dendritic loss preceded cell death by a significant time interval. The soma, then, is not nearly as sensitive to loss of activity as the dendrite. The long course of this degeneration and the soma-dendritic differential suggest that something other than activity is important.

More support for this idea comes from the work of Gelfan (1975), who has examined the dendritic trees of canine spinal neurons surviving temporary lumbosacral ischemia. Neurophysiologically increased excitability is characteristic of the α-motoneurons; hence, activity is, if anything, excessive in these neurons. Despite this, the size of surviving dendritic trees was reduced to one-third of normal. There was also some neuronal loss, which reduced the synaptic density on surviving proximal dendrites to about 35% of normal. Again, it is the dendritic component of the neuron that seems to be most dependent on synaptic connections with other neurons. Since there is bioelectric activity, the loss, particularly of the most sensitive fine-terminal dendrites, must be dependent on other factors. Gelfan hypothesizes that a neuron's morphological integrity and local biochemical homeostasis are dependent upon various "neurotrophic factors* continuously supplied transneuronally by the neurons with which it is in contact."

In their study of the acoustic system, Morest and Jean-Baptiste (1975) described long-lasting transneuronal structural changes in highly specific synaptic endings, the calyces of Held, and in the principal cells contacted by these calyces in the medial trapezoid nucleus following acoustic deafferentation of adult cats. Cochlear ablation resulted in an abrupt and complete cessation of spontaneous electrical activity in most cells of the ipsilateral ventral cochlear nucleus. The rapid onset of such electrophysiological changes contrasted with the slow development of morphological changes; e.g., neurofilamentous hyperplasia in the calyx of Held began at 15 days and was maximal at 30 days, and cellular atrophy appeared at 30 days and was maximal at 60 days. However, these structural effects appeared only after complete degeneration and disappearance of the primary nerve endings; hence, one cannot be sure whether synaptic failure or terminal degeneration (or both) was responsible. The long delay before the appearance of morphological changes could, as the authors point out, be consistent with a slow depletion of a hypothetical neurotrophic substance.

Additional evidence was obtained from studies of the principal neuron of the contralateral medial trapezoid nucleus. Signs of morphological alteration, including perikaryal shrinkage and chromatinic condensation, appeared 30 days after ablation. Even though the time course and intensity of cellular atrophy of these neurons were similar to those of the ventral cochlear nucleus,† there was an important difference in that the calyces of Held persisted for several months and eventually recovered their normal appearance. In other words, the

---

*Gelfan seems to mean metabolic factors such as adenosine, as well as potentially neurotrophic proteins or peptides.

†Morest and Jean-Baptiste (1975) pointed out that it is surprising that the time course of cellular atrophy should be the same for neurons in the ipsilateral ventral cochlear and superior olivary nuclei and in the contralateral medial nucleus of the trapezoid body, because the primary auditory nerve fibers synapse only in the ventral and dorsal cochlear nuclei (Cohen et al., 1972). Thus, a very rapid message traverses the interposed calyceal neuron to cause changes matching those of more directly affected cells.

principal neuron atrophied while still in contact with a major part of its afferent endings. However, these endings were electrically silent. Morest and Jean-Baptiste (1975) concluded that synaptic activity is important for neurotrophic influences, although they seemed to feel that it may be the amino acids or proteins released by or with a transmitter that are the actual trophic agents. It will be of some importance to determine whether the morphological return to normal (resolution of neurofilamentous hyperplasia in particular) is accompanied by a return of spontaneous calyceal electrical activity. If it is so accompanied, if the damage once instituted is not irreversible, and if the transneuronal changes in the principal neurons persist despite resumption of such synaptic activity, then it may be necessary to reexamine their conclusion.

Clearly, activity has an important role in neuron-target cell and neuron-neuron interactions. Just as in the case of the nerve-muscle preparation, it is not activity and/or transmitter alone that accounts for the neurotrophic phenomena. As for the transmitter, its crucial action may be via receptors and ionic coupling to cyclic nucleotide or other intracellular mechanisms (see Chapter VIII). On the other hand, as Hornykiewicz and co-workers (1976) have pointed out (see below), dopamine exerts its metabolic effects on the postsynaptic cell by a route that is independent of receptor blockers. In other words, dopamine appears to have separate transmitter and trophic roles. Also, the work of Kreutzberg and co-workers (Kreutzberg and Schubert, 1975; Kreutzberg et al., 1975a) indicates that materials other than transmitters (such as nucleotides, amino acids, NGF, etc.) are exchanged (see Chapter III) between neurons; hence, these, too, must be considered. The issue is further complicated by considerations of glia-neuronal relations (see the section on the control of sprouting in Chapter V) and the control of the extracellular space by dendritic secretion (Kreutzberg and Schubert, 1975). Again, we return to the notion of a complex array of interacting factors integrated by time as the basis of neuron-neuron interactions; the elucidation of the biochemistry of such interactions is vital to making further progress in unravelling these issues.

Biochemistry of Transneuronal Degeneration

In their discussion of the observed chromatinic condensation and temporary neurofilamentous hyperplasia, Morest and Jean-Baptiste (1975) reviewed the current data on biochemical changes in transneuronal degeneration in an attempt to sort out the mechanisms involved. Unfortunately, relatively little information beyond the morphological data has been obtained over the years. Kupfer and Palmer (1964) found histochemical evidence of decreased levels of oxidative enzymes in the atrophic cells of the lateral geniculate bodies of kittens following eye enucleation. In the monkey, Kupfer and Downer (1967) demonstrated a transitory increase in the level of RNA and a concomitant increase in the incorporation of leucine into proteins in the lateral geniculate body 1 to 2 days after enucleation. Of importance is their finding that the changes began as early as 24 hours after denervation, indicating a rather rapid transmission of an injury signal or, on the other hand, perhaps a lack of a normal signal. It is obvious that in order to sort out the various factors involved, adequate biochemical markers, such as the cholinesterase used in nerve-muscle studies (see Chapter II), must be found.

Retrograde Transneuronal Degeneration

If the available morphological and, particularly, biochemical information is less than satisfactory with regard to anterograde transneuronal degeneration, it is even more unsatisfactory in the case of retrograde phenomena.* A well-documented example is the primary and secondary retrograde degeneration observed in medial mammilary and ventral tegmental nuclei, respectively, after a lesion in the limbic cortex. Similarly, retrograde transneuronal degeneration has been demonstrated in ganglion cells of the retina after ablation of the visual cortex. It is difficult to conclude that retrograde effects result from a loss of transmitter. Although unlikely, it is possible that released transmitter acts on presynaptic receptors to control presynaptic metabolism. After loss of the postsynaptic cell, all of the transmitter released may be bound by the presynaptic terminals, resulting in abnormal metabolism and, ultimately, degenerative changes.

Other Pathology Likely to Involve Abnormalities of Neuron-Neuron Interactions: B. H. Smith and B. Arnason

Transneuronal degeneration, a well-established, if somewhat old, phenomenon, serves to underline the importance of the types of molecular interactions discussed in the above sections. It is, in fact, one

*For a full discussion of retrograde transneuronal degeneration, see Cowan (1971).

of the best lines of evidence for the proposition that the exchange of materials described (transmitter or nontransmitter) is, indeed, of functional significance. The study of disease has shown that the failure or absence of these exchanges has rather devasting consequences. However, lest we view the problem too narrowly, we ought to consider a number of other areas (see Figure 77) where the pathology may be, at least in part, that of abnormal neuron-neuron interactions. It should be noted that, although abnormal interactions of neurons with other neurons, target cells, and glia must surely take place, what has been demonstrated of these phenomena in disease states is very limited. The goal at present is to increase our awareness of these phenomena, to determine where abnormal neuron-neuron interactions are most likely to occur, to suggest where to look for others, and to identify possible model systems. Perhaps the best place to start is with developmental problems.

Developmental Disorders

As Arnason pointed out, it is obvious that an intact CNS is important for development; a lesion a considerable distance from a target organ can affect development. A classic example of an abnormal neuron-target cell interaction is congenital hemiatrophy — a phenom-

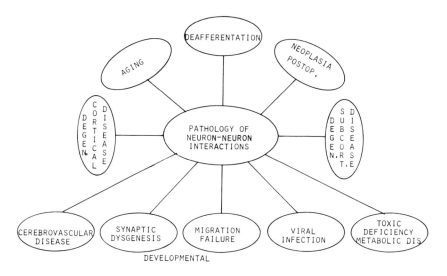

Figure 77. Summary diagram of some neuropathological processes that may involve abnormal neuron-neuron interactions. [Smith]

enon in which the defect is one or more synapses away from the target peripheral tissues (muscle, bone, etc.). The converse of this disease is hemihypertrophy. Patients with Sturge-Weber syndrome, which is a phacomatosis characterized by angiomata of the face and brain, occasionally have abnormal hypertrophy of the affected parts. It is of interest that NGF levels are higher than normal in these patients.

Lissencephaly is an example of a developmental disorder that may have resulted from abnormal or absent neuron-neuron interactions. This disorder, which is also known as agyria, is characterized by the absence of fissures and convolutions and a selective loss of cells of layers 2 and 4 (see Richman et al., 1975). It seems that cells of layer 4 degenerate after a period of cell migration. The sequence of outward cortical neuronal migration is as follows: layers 5, 4, 3, and 2. In lissencephaly the cells of layer 3 are in a normal position and could hardly be expected to have achieved this position unless the cells of layer 4 were normally positioned at the time of migration of cells of layer 3. Since there is a failure of thalamic input into layer 4 in lissencephaly, a reasonable formulation would be that it is input failure that leads to degeneration of the cells of layer 4 after the period of migration.* In other words, this developmental disorder represents a transsynaptic degeneration. Arnason proposed the hypothesis that transneuronal degeneration is a factor in a large number of congenital abnormalities and that the sequencing of neuronal development is a crucial issue. This degeneration is being studied by a number of investigators using animal models (see below).

Adult Diseases

The degenerative diseases of adulthood also merit attention. As Arnason pointed out, such degenerations are initially taken to be idiopathic, but, as the pathophysiology is worked out, a cause for cell death is usually found. The best example of this type of disease is that caused by a slow virus. Although its etiology is unknown, amyotrophic lateral sclerosis (ALS) may provide the prototype of this category of disease. In ALS, anterior horn cells die selectively along with the pyramidal cells with which they synapse. One possibility is that trophic substance X, which is no longer present in anterior horn neurons, results in the death of these neurons and of the pyramidal cells. However, Arnason does not now believe this is the case for ALS,

---

*It was pointed out at the meeting that layers 3 and 5 may or may not be requisite for the development of layers 2 and 4. The evidence is not adequate to resolve this issue at present.

because reverse transcriptase has been identified in anterior horn cells and certain histocompatability types are presented in ALS with unusual frequency, thus suggesting a viral or immunological basis. Nonetheless, it may be useful to apply a similar reasoning to other degenerative diseases.

At the higher levels of degenerative subcortical diseases, and specifically Parkinson's disease, it is known that the primary lesion involves the large nigrostriatal dopaminergic pathway. However, as Hornykiewicz (1972) has pointed out, there are concomitant, although generally more subtle, changes in other putative brain neurotransmitter systems as well. Among these is the decrease in glutamic acid decarboxylase (GAD) of the γ-aminobutyric acid-containing dopaminergic neurons of the nigrostriatal pathway. Hornykiewicz and co-workers (1976) have proposed a model in which GAD-containing neurons are dependent on a continuous trophic influence of the dopaminergic system; thus, a depression of the latter would lead to a lower GAD. If such a postulate is true, then L-dopa might reverse the effect. This, in fact, does happen. However, this action of dopamine is distinct from its effect on postsynaptic dopaminergic receptors (note that the evidence includes the failure of a haloperidol block and the long latency of L-dopa's induction of a GAD increase). It is not clear what role such changes have in the clinical picture of parkinsonism, but the time course of L-dopa's effectiveness on tremor correlates with its effect in increasing GAD activity. The important point is that the relatively gross morphological changes and effects of transneuronal degeneration may not be what should be studied. Rather, it is at the level of the biochemistry of the deafferented neuron that investigations should be made. Such studies should open up enormous possibilities in a field that is relatively untapped at present.

Effects of Aging

The "normal" phenomena of aging are also of interest. The Scheibels and co-workers (1975) have recently shown a correlation between dendritic loss in aging and behavioral changes. Senile changes that take place intracellularly consist of an abnormal aggregation of tubular materials, probably both microtubles and neurofilaments. Such an aggregation of material, thought to be important in dendritic and axonal transport mechanisms, could lead to speculation that the basis of this disorder lies in a failure of neuron-neuron and, especially, dendrodendritic interactions secondary to disrupted axonal and dendritic transport. Although the failure of neuronal molecular interactions is not the primary cause of the problem, dendrites and their neurons die in ever-increasing numbers because of that failure. It is worth emphasizing that, although this failure of molecular exchange need not be primary in any disease, such as ALS, it is certain to be a factor in many diseases of the central and peripheral nervous systems. Studies of neuroaxonal dystrophies (Jellinger and Jirásek, 1971; Berard-Badier et al., 1971; Seitelberger, 1971) and, in fact, of any disease with primary axonal or synaptic lesions (see Sandbank and Bubis, 1974, for a review) should profit from an incorporation of neuron-target cell interaction principles into experimental design.

Deafferentation Phenomena

Another example of abnormal neuron-neuron interactions is the deafferentation phenomena. Deafferentation of the spinal trigeminal nucleus by section of the incoming nerve results in spontaneous hyperactivity (in fact, epileptiform bursting), as if control of this inherent property of the neuron was maintained by the afferent system (Loeser et al., 1968; Westrum, 1974). If the axonal transport systems are functionally responsive, the messages received will be different in the deafferented case, and the metabolism of the whole circuit, including thalamic and, perhaps, cortical neurons, will be altered. Just as in the case of the nerve-muscle preparation, transmitters may have a role in this phenomenon. However, other substances, ranging from nucleosides to proteins, which are transported bidirectionally by both axons and dendrites and then transneuronally delivered to pre- or postsynaptic cells, need to be investigated.

Mirror Focus

The development of the mirror focus in epilepsy may be another example of a transneuronal effect that results in a respecification of the properties of the postsynaptic neuron. Although this is the converse of the deafferentation problem, the principle involved is the same. The mechanism by which the primary epileptogenic focus gives rise to the secondary or mirror focus is unknown. Morrell's (1961) original theory, that it was the continuous neuronal bombardment of the secondary by the primary site, raises again the question of the sufficiency of activity per se. This theory was modified by Goddard's

(1967, 1972) discovery that intermittent stimulation (e.g., in the cat amygdala a daily 2-sec train of biphasic 1-msec pulses at 62.5 Hz and with an amplitude of $200\,\mu V$ peak to peak) rapidly resulted in the establishment of a seizure focus representing a permanent change not requiring further electrode stimulation.

That the establishment of the mirror focus must be dependent on neuronal connections can be shown by sectioning the interhemispheric commissures. When they are sectioned, no mirror focus develops. In the presence of intact pathways, there is rather widespread dissemination of epileptogenic abnormality from a chronic focus. The rate of dissemination (Morrell and Tsuru, 1974, 1976) seems to be a function not of distance but rather of the number of intervening synapses. The slow time course of secondary epileptogenesis and the striking requirement of intermittency required to achieve "kindling" suggested to Morrell and co-workers (1975) that a substance having a slower transit time than an action potential has to pass, perhaps by axonal transport, from the primary to the secondary region. They hypothesized that if such a substance were, for example, a protein in limited supply and requiring synthesis, then only brief periods of stimulation would be effective and that relatively long intervals (minutes) would have to intervene before the system could be reactivated.

To test the postulate that protein synthesis is involved, Morrell and co-workers (1975) induced an epileptogenic focus in the hippocampal cortex of a paralyzed bullfrog. Intraperitoneal administration of cycloheximide (50 mg per gm) resulted in an 88 to 99% reduction in ^{14}C-leucine incorporation into brain protein. Under these conditions spontaneous epileptiform potentials could be induced in the primary hemisphere, but no mirror focus would develop. Cycloheximide did not appear to disturb normal electrogenesis or disrupt the primary after-discharges (clarification in respect to the controls used in the experiment is needed). These investigators are also utilizing local anesthetic application (silastic sheet) to block impulse conduction in the interhemispheric connections and colchicine to block axoplasmic transport in the same system.

Whether the development of the mirror focus can be shown to be dependent on the transsynaptic delivery of a specific protein(s) is perhaps not so important as the attempt to sort out the activity. Furthermore, this is one disease whose underlying principles (if not specific anatomy) can be attacked particularly well by using an animal model.

Synaptogenesis in the Cerebellum: Are Transsynaptic Molecular Interactions Really Necessary? A. Hirano

At this point in the report, we need to put the broad implications of neuron-neuron and neuron-target cell interactions into perspective. The interdependence of neurons and their target cells, whether other neurons, glia, muscle or other cell types, has been strongly emphasized in the preceding chapters. Are there situations in which a given neuron can function independently of such interactions? It is to this issue that Hirano addressed himself in light of his studies on cerebellar synaptogenesis and synaptic maintenance.

The general consensus seems to be that both the pre- and postsynaptic elements are required for synapse formation. In other words, both of these elements form and actively seek out each other in the formation process. As alternatives to this concept, Hirano discussed two other hypotheses: According to the first, synaptic vesicles accumulate at the contact region of the presynaptic element, and this specialization somehow induces the formation of a postsynaptic differentiation in the associated postsynaptic element. The second hypothesis is that characteristic postsynaptic specialization precedes and presumably influences the formation or accumulation of synaptic vesicles in the presynaptic ending. At this point, it is not clear which of these concepts is correct.

Cerebellum as a Model System

Cerebellar synaptic architecture is well understood from both the morphological and functional points of view; moreover, a large body of work has now accumulated regarding the normal development of the cerebellum. Thus, it is possible to study experimentally altered or aberrant developmental processes with some measure of confidence that there is a solid base line for a comparison of the findings. Also, several experimental models are available, and cerebellar development can be altered in a fairly clear-cut manner. Most of these model studies involve the loss or marked diminution of granule cells, a condition that mimics some human conditions (see Hirano and Zimmerman, 1973).

In the study of Margolis and Kilham (1968; Margolis et al., 1971), newborn ferrets were inoculated with feline panleukopenia virus. This led to a severe diminution of granule cells and a profound disruption of normal cerebellar architecture, in which morphologically normal Purkinje cells became abnormally arrayed. There have also been studies in which several toxins have been employed: cytarabine, a chemotherapeutic agent sometimes used in the treatment of malignant neoplasms; cycasin or methylazoxymethanol glucoside, an agent derived from the cycad seed; mercury; and X-irradiation of young animals to destroy granule cells. Finally, a number of spontaneous murine mutations have been discovered in which the granule cells of the cerebellum are mostly missing (Sidman et al., 1965; Sidman, 1968).

In Hirano's laboratory, cycasin-treated mice (Hirano and Jones, 1972; Hirano et al., 1972), as well as the murine mutants "weaver," "staggerer," and "reeler," have been studied. Cycasin administered to mice and hamsters within 1 day after birth produced severe neurologic symptoms and, indeed, necrosis of the external granule cell layer of the cerebellum (this does not happen in adults). These changes could be observed within 1 day after treatment. After a week, almost all the granule cells were absent, and the histoarchitecture of the cerebellar cortex was severely distorted. Despite the destruction of granule cells, the Purkinje cells, while not necessarily in their normal arrangement, were apparently intact, and no degenerative alterations in their fine structure could be detected. The startling and relevant observation was the presence of numerous dendritic spines projecting into a matrix of astrocytic cytoplasm (Figure 78). Such structures occupied the bulk of the cortical mantle and appeared identical to those observed in the untreated control. As in the normal animal, they contained no spine apparatus or mitochondria, and they frequently had the characteristic postsynaptic specialization (a membranous thickening), even though, in the majority of cases, no presynaptic elements were present (Figure 79, A and B). Instead, as already stated, the unattached dendritic spines were buried in the matrix of astrocytic cytoplasm. Furthermore, the space between the unattached spines in the cycasin-treated mice and the apposing astrocytic cytoplasm membrane was about 200 A, i.e., identical to that in the normal case, and contained morphologically identical dense material.

Another model of granule cell loss, the weaver mutant mouse, has been studied by Sidman and associates (Sidman et al., 1965; Rakic and Sidman, 1973a,b,c), as well as by Yoon and Frouhar (1973), Hirano and Dembitzer (1973), and Sotelo (1973). These workers also found unattached dendritic spines identical to those seen after cycasin treatment or virus infection (Herndon et al., 1971; Llinás et al., 1973). Histochemical tests to determine the similarity of the unattached dendritic spines in weaver mice to the attached spines of intact synapses in normal mice included impregnation with phosphotungstic acid,

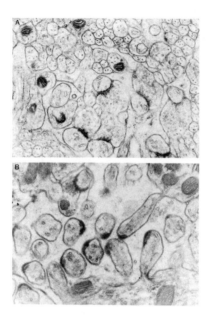

Figure 78. The molecular layer of a normal (A) and cycasin-treated (B) mouse. In the latter, the postsynaptic spines are free of presynaptic endings. ×30,000. [Hirano et al., 1972]

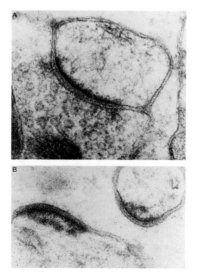

Figure 79. Higher magnification of an intact synapse (A) in a normal mouse and unattached spines (B) in a cycasin-treated mouse. ×120,000, [Hirano et al., 1972]

bismuth iodide, and uranyl acetate. In all cases, the staining properties of the unattached spines were indistinguishable from those seen in either normal mice or even those rarely found in the weaver cerebellum (Hirano, 1972; Hirano and Dembitzer, 1973; Hirano and Zimmerman, 1973). Recent freeze-fracture studies (Hanna et al., 1976) have confirmed the similarity between the attached and the unattached spines.

According to Hirano, the most obvious explanation is that the synapse between the parallel fiber and the Purkinje cell dendritic spine is, in all three cases, formed before the action of the toxic agent or genetic death occurs and that the unattached dendritic spines are simply the remains of synapses once intact. Troubling, however, is the finding of Sidman and co-workers (1965) that destruction of granule cells occurs in the weaver mouse prior to their migration to form the granule layer (which occurs in the second week) and that weaver symptoms occur as early as 8 days, which is before the formation of Purkinje spine-granule cell synapses (Larramendi, 1969). Hirano and Dembitzer (1974) were unable to find any degenerating parallel fibers attached to dendritic spines in the youngest weaver mice they could reliably pick out (11- to 14-days old). In other words, it is unlikely that many (if any) Purkinje cell-granule cell synapses were ever formed in the weaver mouse. The apparently obvious explanation that synaptic connections form and then dissolve simply does not hold up. Can it be that apparently intact postsynaptic terminals develop and survive without the influence of a presynaptic process? Perhaps there is a genetic program for the number and location of postsynaptic specializations.

On the basis of work with virus-infected animals, Hámori (1973a,b) has proposed that it is not the parallel fiber but rather the climbing fiber that acts as a signal for the production of spines over the entire dendritic tree. This suggestion differs from that of a localized one-to-one pre- to postsynaptic element interaction and differentiation by postulating that a remote signal causes widespread dendritic specializations to form. It may be that the postsynaptic specialization is crucial. In any case, climbing fibers are present in the weaver mouse, which does support this theory.

As an experimental test, Hámori (1973a) undercut the cerebellar cortex of untreated animals to sever the climbing fiber input and found no dendritic spines despite the presence of abundant parallel fibers. Refining the procedure to rule out injury of the Purkinje cell axon as a factor, Hámori (1973b) severed the climbing fiber input at the level of the restiform body, which is believed to be the source of the climbing fibers from the inferior olive (Eccles, 1974). As his theory predicted, this resulted in a severe reduction in the number of dendritic spines. Hámori thus concluded that the climbing fiber is necessary not only for the induction of the spines but also for their maintenance.

On the other hand, Seil and Herndon (1970) and Kim (1975) cultured Purkinje cells and demonstrated unattached dendritic spines as well as some spines in synaptic contact with parallel fibers in preparations uninfluenced by the inferior olive. Furthermore, there is other evidence that postsynaptic elements in the olfactory bulb of the chiropter *Desmodus rotundus* form without neuronal presynaptic influences (Palacios Prü and Briceño, 1972). Instead, these postsynaptic specializations form "synaptic-like" relationships with neighboring glia.* Could it be, asks Hirano, that some intrinsic nucleus gives rise to some of the climbing fibers?† To try to answer this question, Hirano and Dembitzer (1975b) turned to staggerer mice, which were reported to be free of dendritic spines but have climbing fibers (Landis, 1971; Sidman, 1972; Landis and Sidman, 1974; Sotelo and Changeux, 1974). Unfortunately, a few dendritic spines were found, thus ruling out the use of staggerer mice as a test of Hámori's theory.

In an attempt to correlate all the data, Hirano and Dembitzer (1974) have suggested a simple variation of Hámori's idea. Since synapses between parallel fibers and dendritic spines occasionally occur in young weaver mouse, it is possible that these ephemeral contacts, though few in number, are sufficient to trigger the differentiation of dendritic spines throughout the dendritic tree. This could explain the presence of spines not only in weaver but also in the cycasin-treated animals (where a few such synapses were found) and, perhaps, in the virus-treated animals. It would also explain the presence of spines in cerebellar cultures. However, Hámori's experiment, in which he was able to reduce the number of dendritic spines in the presence of parallel fibers by cutting the inferior olive, is inconsistent with this explanation.

In summing up this complex discussion, we can only conclude that dendritic spines do not require a one-to-one induction of a presynaptic element. This is not to say, as Hirano and Dembitzer caution, that parallel fibers are totally without influence on the development of dendritic spines. As one might suspect, on closer

---

*The possible maintenance of postsynaptic specializations by glia was discussed in Chapter V, but it seems unlikely that glia have a role in the development of postsynaptic specializations.
†Some authors (see Riviera-Domingues et al., 1974) maintain that not all climbing fibers originate in the inferior olive.

inspection there are minor differences between the spines in the weaver or cycasin-treated mouse. Although the enzyme histochemistry of these structures is normal, there are some structural differences. First, the spines are more common on the larger dendritic branches in the pathological than in the normal animals. Whereas some spines are elongated and have narrow necks and bulbous endings, others show branching at their origin and more than one postsynaptic membranous thickening. Thus, Hirano and Dembitzer (1975a) state: "It seems as though the formation of the spine may be induced by some generalized stimulus but that the resulting structures, in the absence of their normal presynaptic mates, remain unfulfilled and aberrant." As far as the question originally posed concerning the need for transsynaptic interactions, the above answer seems appropriate. Even if such interactions are not required at each developmental step, they appear, at the very least, to be involved in the modulation and functional fulfillment of a single neuron's intrinsic genetic programming.*

New Approaches to Two Major Experimental Problems

Although it seems self-evident that abnormal neuron-neuron and neuron-target cell interactions lead to disease, hard proof of this postulate is rather limited. It seems clear that the neuropathology and, particularly, biochemistry and electrophysiology of transneuronal degeneration have not been exploited fully with regard to their potential for elucidating not only normal mechanisms of neuron-target and neuron-neuron interactions but also those of disease. With the techniques presently available, it is reasonable to expect that at least some of the disease issues can be attacked rather directly. Two major problems exist: The first concerns the need for improvement in the collection and analysis of human neuropathological data. The second problem, which is related to the first, involves defining guidelines for the development of suitable animal models. In other words, we can pose the question: "Are there any suitable models of animal trans-neuronal disease that illuminate human disease problems?"

---

*Important issues in these studies, i.e., how does a localized stimulus influence an entire cell and the more difficult problem of how does a generalized stimulus or influence result in only a very localized metabolic or structural response, are dealt with in more detail in Chapter IX, "Research Issues and Strategies."

Much of the work described in this chapter has involved experimental animals. Yet, as Arnason pointed out with regard to attempts to relate murine to human muscular dystrophy, the animal data may not bear immediately or directly on the human problem. In fact, such data may even be misleading. However, a counterargument is that, even if animal models are not directly relevant, they may provide us with sufficient insight to accelerate our study, understanding, and treatment of human transneuronal disease. In the following section, fairly direct comparisons of the animal and human data in some situations are discussed.

Formalin-Fixed Human Material and Mutant Mice

A particulary good example of using a relevant experimental model is the study by Hirano and co-workers (1973) of a human case of granule-cell type of cerebellar degeneration. By applying both conventional pathological processing procedures and phosphotungstic acid staining to formalin-fixed human brain tissue, they were able to determine that the alterations were morphologically similar in both the human disease and the murine mutant weaver. Both showed an almost complete absence of granule cells and an abundance of unattached Purkinje cell dendritic spines, which seemed, at least at the levels of resolution achieved, identical to those found in the respective normal tissues. Furthermore, the unattached spines retained their postmembranous specialization and were embedded in a matrix of astrocytic cytoplasm. So, at least in this case, the weaver mouse seems to be a suitable model for studying human disease. Although the actual pathophysiological mechanisms have not been determined, the opportunity is now available for their study.

The demonstration that the phosphotungstic acid technique can be applied to human materials stored in formalin is important. By using this and other techniques yet to be developed, some of the vast neuropathological material, traditionally stored in formalin, can be made accessible to fine structural and, perhaps, histochemical evaluation of synaptic sites and, hence, to transneuronal interaction analysis. One would like to be able to study human brain tissue from the point of view of dynamic biochemistry without the constraints of formalin or other fixation. Ideally, the techniques used in the study of animal models should be applicable to the study of human material.

Enzyme Biochemistry in Disorders of the
Autonomic Nervous System

Black, in collaboration with Petito,* has examined discrete brain areas and sympathetic ganglia obtained at autopsy from seven controls and three patients with the rare degenerative neurological disease, idiopathic orthostatic hypotension (IOH). In this disease widespread degeneration of cranial nerve nuclei, striatum, substantia nigra, pontine nuclei, inferior olives, cerebellar cortex, spinal cord, and autonomic ganglia leads to postural hypotension, incontinence, sexual impotence, and disorders of movement. The specimens were examined anatomically and were assayed for TOH, the rate-limiting enzyme, and dopamine-β-hydroxylase (DBH), the final enzyme in NE biosynthesis. Both central and peripheral noradrenergic neurons were abnormal in the IOH patients: DBH activity was decreased by 7.5-fold in sympathetic ganglia, while TOH activity was reduced more than 50-fold in the pontine nucleus locus coeruleus. The differences were not attributable to such variables as postmortem delay, age, sex, race, and medications, suggesting that the enzyme deficits reflect the disease process itself. These observations indicate that both brain and ganglion noradrenergic neurons are affected, but suggest that the central and peripheral biochemical deficits differ. Moreover, the findings imply that, in diseased human neurons, either TOH or DBH activity may be decreased selectively, without an apparent change in the other enzyme. Although it is too early in the course of this research to discuss the dynamics of metabolic deregulation or any transneuronal effects, Black and Petito have shown that techniques developed for animal systems can be usefully applied to the study of human material.

Another disorder of the autonomic nervous system, which has been cited as a dystrophic disease (Smith and Hui, 1973) and seems amenable to Black's analysis, is familial dysautonomia or Riley-Day syndrome. This degenerative disorder appears genetically transmitted as an autosomal recessive trait and is limited primarily to Ashkenazic Jews. Clinically, it is characterized by defective lacrimation, hyperhidrosis, episodic hypertension, hyperpyrexia, vomiting, and attacks of epilepsy. Most patients also show dysphagia, ageusia, areflexia, and a relative insensitivity to pain. Several pathological features have been described and include (1) a marked reduction in sympathetic post-

*I. B. Black and C. K. Petito, manuscript in press.

ganglionic neurons in the peripheral axons, (2) marked reduction in sensory dorsal root ganglia neurons, (3) small myelinated and non-myelinated axons in the peripheral nerves, (4) variable reduction in submucosal sensory axons of neurons thought to be parasympathetic in nature in the submucosa of the tongue, and (5) variable reduction in mucosal papillae and taste buds (see Pearson et al., 1974).

The coexistence of abnormal taste buds and a diminution of tongue submucosal neurons in children with familial dysautonomia suggests a dystrophic relationship. The primary deficit is not clear and may possibly reflect that of an abnormal neural crest. The combined sensory and sympathetic nervous systems lesions resemble defects caused by an antibody to NGF at certain critical stages of development. The fact that sensory neurons continue to transport NGF throughout their existence despite a change in their response to it (see Thoenen, Chapter II) may indicate that these neurons have a life-long sensitivity to such a factor. It may be that the sympathetic degeneration results from a loss of the trophic influence of the preganglionic neurons on the sympathetic ganglia.

At present, there is no completely suitable in vivo or in vitro model for the study of familial dysautonomia. The logic and techniques described in the preceding chapters and particularly those of Black, Thoenen, and Diamond, offer real opportunities for progress in research. Another example of a useful approach is that of Coughlin (1975), who is attempting to use target organ stimulation of para-sympathetic nerve growth in the developing mouse submandibular gland as a model system for this disease.* Rogers and co-workers (1975) are trying to exploit the anatomical and physiological similari-ties between familial dysautonomia and mammals immunosym-pathectomized by treatment with antibodies to mouse NGF. Using immunological techniques, they have already shown elevated levels of β-NGF in familial dysautonomia. However, it is not clear whether there is only one pathogenic defect, and, until the variables can be sorted out with respect to time and what is primary and secondary, this issue cannot be resolved. Riley (1974) believes that the condition arises from an abnormality in a single gene and, perhaps, a single enzyme. If this is so, then the Riley-Day syndrome as an "experiment of nature" may be a very fruitful avenue for the study of neuron-target cell interaction.

*Also M. Coughlin, personal communication.

Conclusions

As a final reprise, it is fair to say that human dystrophic disease represents an untapped resource in the study of the pathology of neuron-target cell interactions. Much more useful data can be collected from patients, and fresh or fixed autopsy material offers some valuable opportunities. Albuquerque has shown the practicality of applying analytical muscle receptor techniques to Duchenne's dystrophy. The use of α-bungarotoxin in the study of receptors in biopsy material was suggested at the Work Session by both Greene and Lentz. The new technique of Lentz and co-workers (1975), utilizing HRP-labeled α-bungarotoxin, appears to be particularly useful. The studies of Peterson, Rathbone, Diamond, and their collaborators are important for the insights they offer into the primary and secondary factors in muscular dystrophy, as well as experimental model design. Black and Petito have started to look at the biochemical correlates of degenerative autonomic disease. In regard to NGF, Arnason has shown its abnormalities in various situations, including limb hypertrophy in Sturge-Weber disease.

The interface between basic and clinical science with regard to neuron-target cell interactions seems to be a particularly fruitful one. To the clinician, of course, the major goal is improved patient care, and, it does not seem unreasonable to expect advances from collaborative efforts at this time. We can now perceive the dim outlines of a day when a trophic factor, such as has been isolated by Lentz, Rathbone, and Oh, a nerve growth factor, or factors that may be identified from systems, such as Lynch's hippocampal slice, may be able to be used clinically to prevent or arrest degenerative neurological processes. With sprouting factors we may even be able to promote and/or direct central nervous system regeneration.

VIII. MECHANISMS OF NEURON-TARGET
CELL INTERACTIONS

Having discussed in the preceding chapters a number of
neuron-target cell interaction phenomena, as well as the candidates for
the molecular signals involved, we can now consider the mechanisms by
which the signals act. For example, when such interactions result in
changes in enzymes levels, as in the case of cholinesterase at the nerve
muscle junction, how does the molecular signal involved achieve its
effect? Stated another way, how does the signal regulate the synthesis
and assembly of polypeptides that result in normal cholinesterase
levels? At what levels are the controls exerted? Are synthesis, release,
and/or activity affected? The same questions could be asked for virtually
all of the phenomena we have described, from the signalling of
secretory export in the chick ciliary ganglion to the control of neuron
transmitter synthesis, regenerative sprouting, and innervation field, as
well as the control of alterations in dendritic membrane length
constants and synaptic efficiency that may be involved in information
processing. What are the available answers?

The Role of Cyclic Nucleotides

Nerve-Muscle Preparation

In conducting in vitro studies on neurotrophism at the
nerve-muscle junction, Lentz (1972a,b, 1974b; see also Carlsen, 1975;
Oh, 1975; Rathbone et al., 1975a; Chapter II) found that cyclic
adenosine monophosphate (cAMP) plus theophylline could mimic the
effects of the trophic, neural extract peptide, which he has isolated and
partially characterized. Furthermore, this extract increases cAMP levels
in muscle. These findings suggest that the trophic effects of nerve and
muscle are mediated by cAMP formed in response to trophic influences
of the motoneuron.

To check this possibility, Lentz (1975) studied the changes in
cAMP with (1) denervation, (2) nerve extract replacement, and (3) reinnervation. A few days after denervation, cAMP decreased; however, it
then rose to levels considerably higher than those in normally
innervated muscle. With reinnervation, it fell to normal levels. After
being cultured for a short time, muscle treated with nerve extracts

showed a higher level of cAMP than untreated muscle. When cultured for long periods, the untreated muscles (comparable to denervated muscle in vivo) revealed higher levels of cAMP than treated muscles. In other words, extract-treated muscle in culture behaved as reinnervated muscle.

The initial decrease in cAMP in denervated muscle and the initial increase in cAMP in muscle treated with extracts are consistent with the hypothesis that trophism is mediated by neuronal regulation of cAMP levels. However, the large subsequent increase in cAMP levels in denervated muscle, as well as the lower levels in muscles either reinnervated or treated with extracts in long-term cultures, seems to indicate that innervation normally suppresses cAMP levels. At this point, then, it appears that the nerve supply influences both cAMP and ChE levels* and that cAMP affects muscle cholinesterase. However, the precise relationship is not known.

The Role of Cyclic Nucleotides in Central Synaptic Function and Neuron-Target Cell Interactions: F. E. Bloom

As for the nerve-muscle junction, cyclic nucleotides have also been suspected of being involved in central synaptic transmitter function. Despite great interest and effort, the role of cyclic nucleotides in synaptic function and other long-term (trophic) neurobiological phenomena is only beginning to be outlined (see Bloom, 1975, for a review). In terms of satisfying the criteria for the involvement of cyclic nucleotide mechanisms in a given transmitter's effects, three lines of evidence — the biochemical, electrophysiological, and histochemical — can be utilized. Brain slices, microiontophoresis, and immunocyto-chemical localization have all been used to advantage.

The evidence obtained from such studies suggests that cyclic nucleotides can mediate the effects of norepinephrine synapses on the following target cells: cerebellar Purkinje cells, hippocampal pyramidal cells, cerebral cortical pyramidal tract neurons, and caudate nucleus neurons postsynaptic to dopamine projections. Microiontophoretic studies showed that cAMP can simulate intracellularly or extra-cellularly the effects elicited by stimulation of the NE pathway originating in the locus coeruleus (Siggins et al., 1969, 1971a-d, 1974; Hoffer et al., 1971a,b,c, 1972, 1973; Lake et al., 1972, 1973; Anderson et al., 1973; Lake and Jordan, 1974; Segal and Bloom, 1974a,b; Bloom,

---

*Diisopropyl fluorophosphate studies indicate that this is an effect on synthesis and not on activity.

1975). Moreover, the effects of catecholamines, cAMP, and NE pathway stimulation can be potentiated by phosphodiesterase inhibitors and antagonized by substances that, at least in the peripheral nervous system, antagonize the effects of catecholamine on cAMP synthesis. The number of cerebellar Purkinje cells showing a positive reaction for cAMP immunocytochemically increased after stimulation of the NE pathway from the locus coeruleus (Siggins et al., 1973). Cyclic guanosine monophosphate may also be involved in some central transmitter systems since, at least in sympathetic ganglia, dopamine can regulate cAMP synthesis and ACh can regulate cGMP. Furthermore, each nucleotide produced a specific biophysical response – a slow inhibitory synaptic potential for cyclic AMP and an excitatory potential for cGMP (Greengard and Kebabian, 1974).

Taking evidence from his own, as well as Greengard's (1975; Greengard and Kebabian, 1974) and Rodbell's (Rodbell et al., 1971, 1975) studies, Bloom proposed that the following processes occur at the target cell in cyclic nucleotide-mediated events (Figure 80): Hormones and neurotransmitters activate the formation of cAMP in the presence of appropriate amounts of calcium and adenyl nucleotides. This cAMP then becomes involved in the following reactions in the target cell: (1) it is catabolized by phosphodiesterase to 5^1-adenosine monophosphate with a resultant increase in intracellular adenosine; (2) it is bound to cAMP regulatory protein to activate protein kinases that, in turn, may alter enzyme activity, ionic pumps, microtubule assembly, gene activity, and membrane permeability by phosphorylation. Bloom and co-workers have tested twenty-one cAMP derivatives for their ability (1) to be substrates for phosphodiesterase, (2) to activate protein kinase, or (3) to penetrate the cell membrane. The efficiency of these derivatives in producing a biophysical response could be directly correlated with the degree to which they activated brain protein kinases. Moreover, it could be shown that intracellular iontophoresis in hippocampal neurons was more effective than extracellular application.

It is not clear that the effects of transmitters in this central catecholaminergic system are, indeed, trophic. The role of transmitters in electrical transmission is not neurotrophic because of the brief duration of the effect; but it is possible that long-term changes may be induced by receptor-mediated responses to a transmitter. As Bloom pointed out at the Work Session, there is evidence for a specific trophic effect of locus coeruleus neurons on the cerebral cortical pyramidal cells.

As shown by thymidine autoradiography, locus coeruleus neurons appear 3.5 to 4 days before the hippocampal pyramidal cells, cerebral cortex pyramidal cells, and the cerebellar Purkinje cells begin to differentiate. This may be coincidental; but, as Maeda and co-workers (1974) have shown, the cortical pyramidal cells fail to mature on the side of the rat brain in which the locus coeruleus has been lesioned. These findings seem to indicate that the pyramidal cells require interaction with the locus coeruleus neurons for their final development. The nature of this relationship and whether catecholaminergic cells are sufficient for the maturation process to occur are issues that require clarification. Part of this maturation process may, of course, be transmitter-mediated as well.

An interesting experiment would be to determine whether stimulation of the axonal collaterals of locus coeruleus pathways might accelerate or otherwise change the maturation of cortical pyramidal cells. It is known that locus coeruleus neurons will form axon collaterals with minimal provocation; i.e., they will not only reinnervate areas that have lost some of their NE fibers but will even hyperinnervate them. According to Bloom, this ability of the central catecholaminergic system to form functionally conducting axon collaterals and thus trigger the differentiation of specific target cells in the developing brain, as well as the repair of the mature organ, is an important trophic function. It is separate from, although perhaps ultimately linked to, the role of the locus coeruleus in biasing target systems in such a way as to potentiate their response to other inputs. Utilization of the cAMP system can provide tremendous amplification (as demonstrated in nonneuronal tissue to date); thus, a relatively small group of neurons can achieve widespread and powerful effects.

Bloom was careful to point out that cAMP cannot explain all the effects of catecholamines. Furthermore, not all trophic effects can be explained by cyclic nucleotide mechanisms (see the section on NGF in this chapter). Nonetheless, cyclic nucleotides are ubiquitous, and both cAMP and cGMP influence functions such as neurite formation, axonal elongation, glial nucleic acid synthesis, and the maintenance of the neuromuscular junction in culture. They have been postulated to be involved in cell division, secretion, microtubule assembly, enzyme induction, and even in long-term behavioral events, such as opiate dependence, human affective disorders, neuroendocrine functions, and learned feeding behavior (see Bloom, 1975).

It is well known that cyclic nucleotides not only interact with other modulatory molecules (such as Ca^{2+} and ATP) present in the cell but are also regulated by these molecules (Figure 80).   Bloom (1975) suggested that these complex   interrelationships   require   a   three-dimensional matrix for their analysis; however, this is also true for all neuron-target cell interactions, because none of them operates in isolation. The complexity of these interrelationships in the aggregate yields a system with great responsiveness and coding potential. Finally, it is worth considering, as Bloom does, that the electrical events, traditionally regarded as the end-product of all neuronal processes, may not be the primary objective of every synaptic transmission.

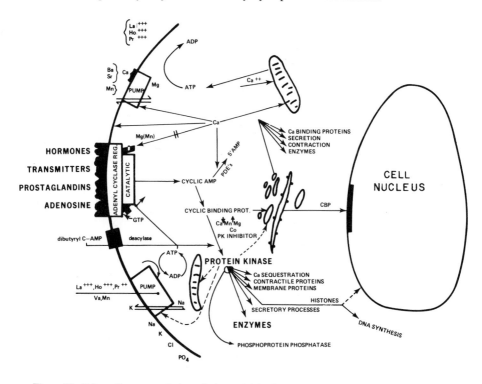

Figure 80. Schematic representation of the multiple lines of interreactive systems by which cyclic nucleotides, ATP, and metallic cations can influence the functional status of biochemical and bioelectrical properties of neurons. The multivalent cations used experimentally to interfere with Ca^{2+} fluxes and Ca^{2+}-dependent monovalent pumps are indicated for future references, although such data for central neurons are still lacking. Dibutyryl cAMP is shown entering the cell after partial deacylation, but this deacylase is relatively inactive in brain. Ca^{2+}-related events (storage, binding, and translocation) are emphasized in the upper half of the hypothetical cell, while cAMP-related events are emphasized in the lower half. The interreactions on adenylate cyclase substrates, cofactors, and protein kinases are indicated at the interface between the two systems. PDE's = phosphodiesterase. [Bloom, 1975]

cAMP-Mediated Phosphorylation of Membrane
Proteins: S. A. Rudolph

One of the cAMP-mediated intracellular processes described by Bloom is that of membrane protein phosphorylation. If such phosphorylation were related to synaptic activity, it would be relatively short-lived (i.e., the duration of the postsynaptic potential), being terminated by phosphatase activity. Phosphorylation of neuropil protein in *Aplysia* abdominal ganglia has a 4-hour half-life, suggesting that it can be involved in more sustained processes than neurotransmission (Levitan and Barondes, 1974; Levitan et al., 1974). Phosphorylation of structural membrane protein implies a functional change, and, if it persists, then a relatively permanent change in a functional neuronal parameter, such as membrane permeability, might be induced. This would be an important neuron-target cell interaction.

Basing their studies on the hypothesis that synaptic transmission and, specifically, the generation of certain postsynaptic membrane potentials are dependent on cAMP-mediated membrane protein phosphorylation, Rudolph, Greengard, and their collaborators have attempted to identify the proteins phosphorylated in some nonnervous tissues and directly correlate protein phosphorylation with membrane permeability (see Ueda et al., 1973, 1975; Greengard and Kebabian, 1974; Maeno et al., 1974, 1975; Rudolph and Greengard, 1974; Greengard, 1975; Sloboda et al., 1975).

The endogenous phosphorylation of synaptic membrane proteins shows a high degree of specificity (Johnson et al., 1972; Ueda et al., 1973). Solubilized synaptic membrane proteins, subjected to SDS-polyacrylamide gel electrophoresis, protein staining, and autoradiography in order to determine the amount of radioactivity incorporated into individual protein bands, showed six bands with a measurable level of phosphate incorporation. Of these six, the phosphorylation of only two (designated Proteins I and II) was markedly affected by the presence of cAMP (Figure 81).

The time course (see Figure 82) of phosphorylation and dephosphorylation of these two membrane proteins was of particular interest because of their hypothesized role in synaptic transmission. Ueda and co-workers (1973) found that the phosphorylation of Proteins I and II was maximal within 5 sec, which was the shortest incubation time that could be accurately studied. The kinetics are consistent with the hypothesis that phosphorylation is involved in

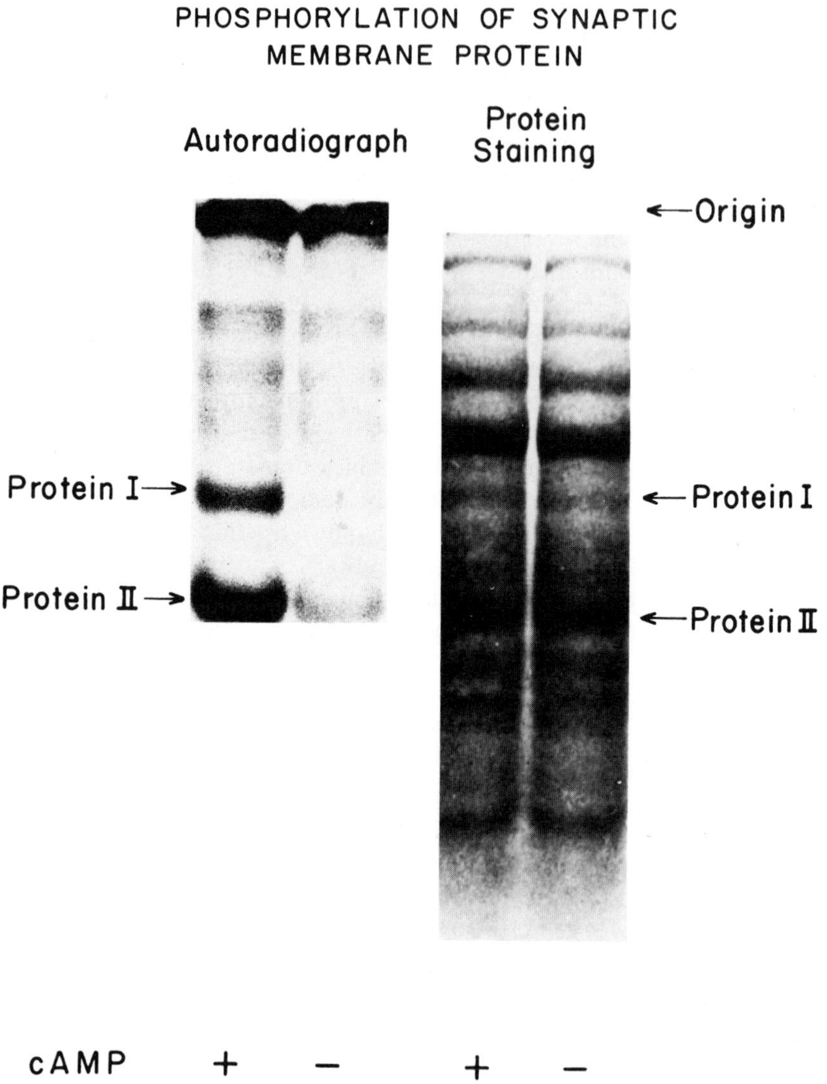

PHOSPHORYLATION OF SYNAPTIC
MEMBRANE PROTEIN

Figure 81. Effect of cAMP on the endogenous phosphorylation of synaptic membrane preparation from rat cerebrum. The synaptic membrane preparation was incubated with $\gamma[^{32}P]$ ATP in the presence or absence of cAMP. The reaction was stopped by the addition of sodium dodecyl sulfate, and the solubilized protein was subjected to slab gel electrophoresis, protein staining, and autoradiography. The resulting autoradiograph is shown on the left side, and a photograph of the protein staining pattern of the dried gel is shown on the right side. The plus and minus signs at the bottom of the gel indicate the presence and absence, respectively, of 5×10^{-6} M cAMP in the incubation mixture. The arrows identify the positions of the gel of Proteins I and II, the phosphorylation of which was markedly increased in the presence of cAMP. [Ueda et al., 1973]

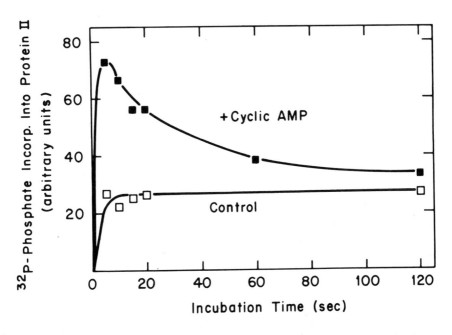

Figure 82. Endogenous phosphorylation of Protein II in synaptic membrane preparation from rat cerebrum as a function of incubation time in the absence or presence of 5×10^{-6} M cAMP. The amount of [^{32}P]phosphate incorporated from γ[^{32}P]ATP into Protein II was calculated from the intensity of the darkness of the band corresponding to Protein II on the X-ray film and is expressed in arbitrary units [Ueda et al., 1973]

synaptic transmission. However, direct correlation is technically very difficult in this system, because the duration of the postsynaptic potential is so short.

Because of such difficulties, Rudolph and Greengard (1974) have examined the turkey erythrocyte membrane. They found that the β-adrenergic agonist, ℓ-isoproterenol, stimulated the incorporation of ^{32}P into a single membrane-bound protein of the intact turkey erythrocyte with a concomitant increase of membrane permeability. The incorporation of ^{32}P reached half its maximal value within 6 min after the addition of ℓ-isoproterenol at 1×10^{-8} M. The β-adrenergic blocking agent, propanolol, abolished this effect, whereas exogenous cAMP and N^6-monobutyrl cAMP mimicked the effect of isoproterenol (Figure 83).* The phosphoprotein, identified on SDS-polyacrylamide

---

*Greengard's laboratory (DeLorenzo et al., 1973) has also reported that the mechanism by which the polypeptide hormone, vasopressin, increases the sodium permeability of the toad bladder may involve cAMP-dependent regulation of the state of phosphorylation of a membrane protein.

gels, was estimated to have an apparent molecular weight of 240,000 and appeared to be coincident with the protein band characteristic of human erythrocyte plasma membranes known as Band II (Figure 83). Increased phosphorylation of this protein correlated with increased cAMP levels and increased sodium uptake in response to various agents.

Rudolph also presented data (Sloboda et al., 1975) on the cAMP-dependent endogenous phosphorylation of microtubule-associated proteins. Microtubules prepared from chick brain homogenates by successive cycles of assembly-disassembly were found to contain two high-molecular weight ($\sim$300,000) proteins designated

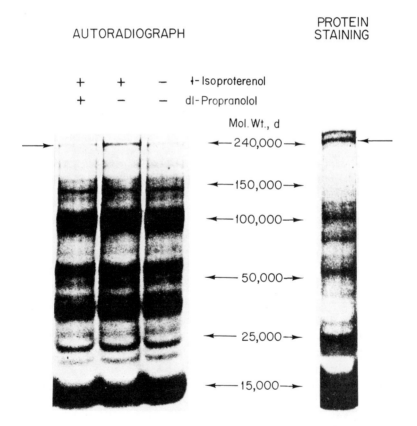

Figure 83. Effect of l-isoproterenol (3×10^{-7} M) and dl-propranolol (2×10^{16} M) on the net incorporation of ^{32}P into proteins of the intact turkey erythrocyte. Erythrocytes were incubated in the presence of the test agents for 10 min. Incorporation of ^{32}P into the 240,000-molecular-weight protein band in the experiment illustrated was 1,200 and 2,500 cpm in the absence and presence of l-isoproterenol, respectively. [Rudolph and Greengard, 1974]

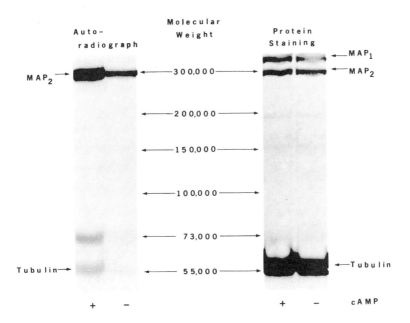

Figure 84. Effect of cAMP on the endogenous phosphorylation of microtubule proteins. Fifty μg of microtubule protein, polymerized three times, were phosphorylated for 30 sec, in the standard reaction mixture, in the presence or absence of 10^{-5} M cAMP. An aliquot containing 25 μg of the protein, solubilized in sodium dodecyl sulfate, was then subjected to polyacrylamide gel electrophoresis. The autoradiograph showing ^{32}P incorporation is at the left, and the protein staining pattern is at the right. MAP = microtubule-associated protein. [Sloboda et al., 1975]

microtubule-associated proteins, MAP_1 and MAP_2 (Figure 84). MAP_2 was the preferred substrate for an endogenous cAMP-dependent protein kinase that appeared to be an integral component of microtubles. cAMP enhanced the initial rate of phosphorylation of MAP_2 4- to 6-fold and, under optimal conditions, almost doubled the incorporation of labeled phosphate (Figure 85, A and B). cAMP also stimulated the phosphorylation of tubulin, but at a rate only 0.15% that of MAP_2. Thus, protein phosphorylation mediated by cAMP-dependent protein kinase is involved in membrane permeability and may also play a role in microtubule assembly or function. It is conceivable that this phosphorylation is involved in regenerative neural sprouting as described by Lynch (see Chapter V).*

*As discussed in a later section of this chapter, NGF appears to stimulate neurite outgrowth by increasing cellular microtubule levels. cAMP can also stimulate neurite outgrowth, but this appears to be on the basis of a different mechanism (Hier et al., 1972, 1973).

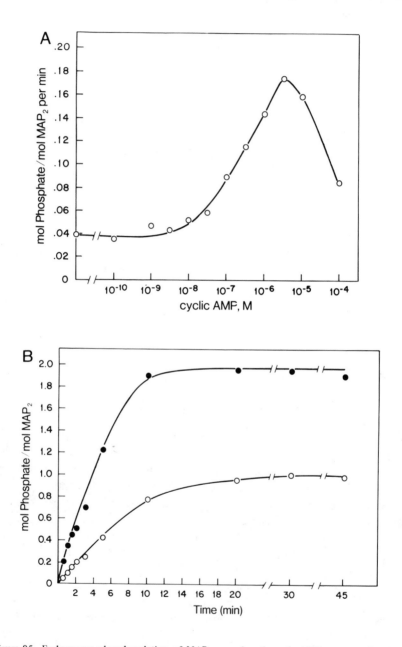

Figure 85. Endogenous phosphorylation of MAP$_2$ as a function of cAMP concentration (A) and incubation time in the absence (O) or presence (●) of 10^{-5} M cAMP (B). Standard reaction conditions were used, except for the changes indicated. [Sloboda et al., 1975]

Adenosine Derivatives from Neurons and Possible Functional Implications: P. Schubert

The discovery of cAMP-mediated membrane phosphorylation and permeability changes and their implications for neuronal membrane electrical characteristics prompted Schubert and his collaborators (Kreutzberg and Schubert, 1975; Schubert and Kreutzberg, 1975a,b) to look at the CNS release, uptake, and transcellular transfer of adenosine, which is recognized as a potent stimulator of cAMP synthesis (Sattin and Rall, 1970). Using the visual corticothalamic system of rabbits (Figure 86), Schubert and Kreutzberg (1974, 1975a) injected ^{3}H-adenosine into areas 17 and 18 of the striate cortex and found that adenosine and/or its trichloroacetic acid-soluble derivatives were transported to and released from axon terminals and were preferentially taken up by the neurons of the target area (see Figure 87, A and B).

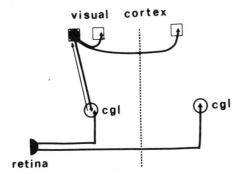

Figure 86. Visual pathways used for studying nucleoside transfer. Solid symbols = injection sites; open symbols = target areas. [Schubert]

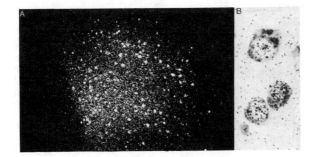

Figure 87. Transport of ^{3}H-adenosine derivatives to the lateral geniculate nucleus target area. Silver grains are scattered over the neuropil (axon terminals) and are highly accumulated over the nerve cells (indicating transfer of the adenosine derivatives). Autoradiography: left, dark-field illumination, ×80; right, ×800. [Schubert and Kreutzberg, 1975a]

Since the blood-brain barrier is relatively impermeable to adenosine (Berne et al., 1974), the local extracellular concentration of this biologically active substance in the CNS seems to be largely determined by its intracerebral distribution and by the processes controlling its release from neurons. It has been already shown by McIlwain (1973) that the release of adenosine derivatives from brain slices can be considerably enhanced by electrical stimulation in vitro. Recent experiments, performed by Schubert in collaboration with Lynch and co-workers (1976), produced direct evidence for a release of adenosine derivatives from entorhinal axon terminals to the postsynaptic granule cells; this release could be considerably enhanced by electrical stimulation of the entorhinal cortex.

Speculating on the functional meaning of an activity-related interneuronal nucleoside transfer, Schubert proposed the following system for altering information processing in the postsynaptic neuron: If the repetitive activation of afferent fibers terminating on the dendritic tree of their target neuron causes a prolonged release of adenosine derivatives, the concentration of these derivatives will rise at the postsynaptic membrane sites and may reach a level that is sufficient to trigger the formation of cAMP.* This may, in turn, lead to local phosphorylation of membrane protein and altered membrane permeability and electrical characteristics. A change in the ion conductivity, which would imply a change in the apparent membrane resistance, may, for example, alter the length constant and, thus, the cable properties and signal transmission of that dendrite (Lux and Schubert, 1975). The information processing within the neurons of a defined network can thus be altered by previous repetitive activation of that network.

As Bloom (1975) pointed out, the central catecholamine pathways provide a useful system for the analysis of "where and how" cyclic nucleotides might participate in synaptic transmission since the catecholamines are known to influence adenylate cyclase or cAMP levels in various regions of the nervous system and since the source and target neurons are known and accessible to experimental manipulation. For the projection of locus coeruleus neurons onto cerebellar Purkinje cells or hippocampal pyramidal cells, the following mechanism (see review by Bloom, 1975) seems to be operative:

Locus coeruleus activity → release of NE → formation of cAMP in
target neuron (hippocampal, pyramidal cell, or cerebellar Purkinje

*The release of nucleoside derivatives may also serve to increase a restricted pool of RNA precursors in the postsynaptic neuron.

cell) → cAMP activation of cAMP-dependent protein kinase → increased membrane resistance and hyperpolarization of long duration.

There is evidence that other cells have similar mechanisms. Almost all pyramidal tract neurons, for example, respond to NE by slowing their spontaneous discharge rates. More than 75% of the cells responding to NE were also depressed by cAMP. Whether there is a direct anatomical or physiological influence of the locus coeruleus on these neurons remains unknown.

In addition to the directed transfer of nucleoside derivatives from axon terminals to target neurons, Schubert and Kreutzberg (1975b,c) have noted a nonspecific release from dendrites following intraneuronal iontophoresis of ^{3}H-adenosine (Figure 88). This activity-related release of adenosine may have implications for the control of the local environment by the neuron. It is known from the experiments of Berne and co-workers (1974) that adenosine causes a vasodilation in cerebral vessels, just as it does in the coronary arteries. The experimental finding of Kato and co-workers (1974) that a photic stimulation

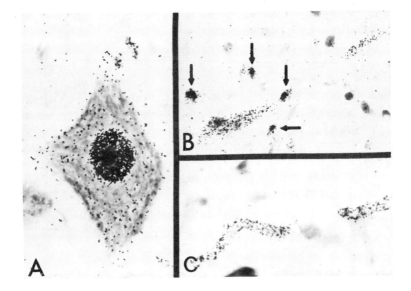

Figure 88. Incorporation of ^{3}H-adenosine derivatives in soma and nucleus (A) and transport of same in dendrites (B) and in axons (C). ^{3}H-Adenosine is released from soma and dendrites, as indicated by the heavy labeling of glial cells (arrows). A, ×600; B, ×400; C, ×400. [Schubert and Kreutzberg, 1975b]

of the retina causes a localized increase of blood flow in the visual cortex and Ingvar's (1973, 1974) clinical observation of an increased blood flow in active brain areas point to a neural regulation of regional blood flow that may operate via the adenosine mechanism.

Evidence for Noncyclic Nucleotide-Mediated Mechanisms of Neuron-Target Cell Interactions

As has already been pointed out, cyclic nucleotides can act at several levels of gene expression. On the other hand, there are data to indicate that they are not involved in all neuron-target cell interactions. Furthermore, there is some question about their true role at the nerve-muscle junction. For example, Rathbone and co-workers (1973,1974) have found that the cholinesterase-maintaining effect of the nerve can be mimicked by the addition of cAMP and theophylline or N^6,O^2-dibutyryl cAMP alone or with theophylline in organ cultures of denervated newt muscles. Because ChE in muscles and organ cultures is also maintained by adrenergic agonists (Lentz, 1974a,b), Rathbone investigated the relationship between the ChE-maintaining ability of adrenergic agonists and their ability to increase cAMP levels or to stimulate the muscle adenylate cyclase of cultured muscles.

Cholinesterase is maintained best by NE, which has predominantly α adrenergic effects, slightly by epinephrine, which has both α and β effects, and not at all by isoproterenol, which has predominantly β effects. However, NE does not increase the intracellular cAMP in these muscles, whereas epinephrine and isoproterenol do. Therefore, in this case, maintenance of ChE in cultured muscles is not associated with a rise in intracellular cAMP. Furthermore, following denervation in vivo, newt muscles lose up to 60% of their ChE activity after 1 week, during which time no significant fall in muscle cAMP levels occurs. Rathbone concluded that changes in intracellular cAMP levels and the stimulation of adenylate cyclase are not the sole mediators of trophic effects of nerves despite the ChE-maintaining effect of cAMP analogues on cultured muscle.

There is also debate in the literature over the involvement of cAMP in neural enzyme induction in the adrenal medulla (Costa and Guidotti, 1973; Guidotti et al., 1973a; Otten et al., 1974b). Although the evidence required to resolve these issues is not yet available, it is important to consider other possibile mechanisms so that experimental designs can take them into account.

Transsynaptic Enzyme Induction in the Peripheral Sympathetic Nervous System: Regulation of Transcription vs. Cyclic Nucleotide Mechanisms

An increased activity of the cholinergic fibers supplying the adrenal medulla elicits an induction of tyrosine hydroxylase. This increased synthesis of new enzyme protein is often preceded by an increase in cAMP in the adrenal medulla. Costa, Guidotti, and their collaborators (Costa and Guidotti, 1973; Guidotti and Costa, 1973, 1974; Guidotti et al., 1973a,b,1975) have proposed that the transsynaptic induction of TOH, which results from appropriate environmental or pharmacological stimuli, is causally related to and, in fact, triggered by the increased cAMP. Other investigators (Otten et al., 1973a; Mueller et al., 1974; Otten et al., 1974a,b; Thoenen and Otten, 1976) have found that TOH induction can take place in the absence of a stimulus-coupled increase in cAMP content. In reserpine-initiated TOH induction in the adrenal medulla, the data (Mueller et al., 1974) indicated that the turnover of cAMP actually decreases during the critical interval of splanchnic nerve stimulation, and that there are marked differences between the changes in cAMP and subsequent induction of the enzyme. Prior treatment of the rats with propanolol reduced the medullary reserpine-induced cAMP increase (40% vs. 410% in controls), while the TOH activity was not affected (Otten et al., 1974a,b).

In studies to determine the presence of an isoproterenol-responsive cAMP pool in adrenergic nerve cell bodies, Otten and co-workers (1974a) treated newborn rats with NGF antiserum or 6-hydroxydopamine, which caused destruction of 61 to 85% of the adrenergic nerve cell bodies in the superior cervical ganglion. This treatment, however, led to only a 16 to 28% decrease in cAMP, indicating that a relatively small portion of cAMP is localized in the adrenergic neurons. Isoproterenol produced a 12-fold increase in cAMP only in this neuronal pool, but neither single nor repeated injections of isoproterenol led to induction of TOH. In the rat adrenal medulla, treatment with reserpine led to both a brief increase in cAMP and a subsequent induction of TOH. Propanolol almost completely prevented the increase of cAMP (40% vs. 320%), but, again, the enzyme induction was not diminished.

In another study, Otten and co-workers (1975) examined the effect of hypophysectomy on cAMP changes in rat adrenal medulla evoked by catecholamines and carbamylcholine. Carbamylcholine, adrenocorticotropic hormone, histamine, norepinephrine, and dopamine all produced marked (500 to 900%) increases in both adrenal cortical and medullary cAMP. Interestingly enough, neither isoproterenol nor epinephrine influenced cAMP levels, even at excessively high doses. In all cases studied, transection of the splanchnic fibers supplying the adrenals reduced the increase in medullary cAMP by no more than 25 to 30%, suggesting that cAMP levels in the adrenal medulla are predominantly under the control of nonneuronal mechanisms. Additional evidence for this was obtained with the observation that hypophysectomy completely abolished the 500 to 600% increase in cAMP produced by dopamine and reduced the 700% increase resulting from carbamylcholine to 70%. In spite of the marked increase in cAMP produced by single and repeated doses of dopamine, there was no induction of TOH. Moreover, single high doses of carbamylcholine evoked TOH induction only in innervated animals.

On compiling the evidence, Otten and co-workers concluded that direct cholinergic mechanisms, which are responsible for TOH induction, play, at the most, only a small part in the regulation of adrenal medullary cAMP. On the other hand, Costa and collaborators (see Costa et al., 1974, for review) feel that their studies on the cyclic nucleotide concentrations in the adrenal medulla during increased stimulation support the view that TOH induction is preceded by a stimulus-coupled increase of cAMP. In their experiments carbamylcholine increased cAMP and TOH in decentralized and intact adrenal medulla. When medullary adenyl cyclase decreased 2 weeks after denervation, carbamylcholine no longer increased TOH.

An increase in the cAMP/cGMP concentration of a stimulus-coupled biochemical change can be measured in the adrenal medulla during the transsynaptic induction of TOH. Nonetheless, as Guidotti and co-workers (1975) pointed out, a crucial role for cAMP and/or cGMP in the transsynaptic induction of TOH cannot be proved definitively by merely confirming or denying that the medullary content of these nucleotides changes coincidentally with the induction of the enzyme by the stimulus. These investigators have gone on to study protein kinase activation in rat adrenal medulla. When reserpine (16 μmoles per kg injected intraperitoneally) alone or reserpine and propanolol (40 μmoles per kg administered intraperitoneally 30 min before reserpine) were administered to rats exposed to 4°C for 4 hours, the extent and duration of the increase of the cAMP/cGMP concentration ratio were sufficient to activate the protein kinases. This activation, which outlasted the cAMP/cGMP change, appeared in their system to be an obligatory event, perhaps preceding changes in ribosome function in the transsynaptic induction of TOH (see below).

If cAMP is not involved in this process, as Thoenen suggests above, then what is the mechanism for the transsynaptic induction of TOH? On finding that reserpine induction of TOH can be blocked by both cycloheximide and actinomycin D, Mueller and co-workers (1969) concluded that the primary site of regulation of this induction process was at the transcription level.

Otten and co-workers (1973b) followed up these earlier studies with an examination of the time requirement for each of the steps involved in TOH induction in the adrenal medulla and superior cervical and stellate ganglia. They found that an intermittent swimming stress of 1 hour was sufficient to lead to a statistically significant increase in TOH activity 48 hours later in the adrenal medulla, whereas a 2-hour stress was necessary to produce the same effect in the superior cervical and stellate ganglia. Administration of the ganglionic blocking agent chlorisondamine (5 mg per kg injected intraperitoneally) immediately and 1 hour after termination of the swimming stress reduced the increase in TOH activity. However, if chlorisondamine was administered 2 hours after the stress, it had no effect, indicating that either enhanced preganglionic activity outlasts the stress or ganglionic transmission is only necessary in the initiation of the process. Administration of actinomycin D (a single dose of 0.8 mg per kg subcutaneously) immediately before or after the swimming stress completely abolished the TOH induction. By 6 or 12 hours after the stress, the increase in TOH was reduced but not abolished, and by 24 hours actinomycin D administration had no effect, indicating that the transcription phase of transsynaptic induction was completed 24 hours after the stress. The fact that increased synthesis of TOH continued up to 48 hours after the stress suggests that the turnover of the RNA is relatively slow. As the investigators pointed out, it is not possible to determine from their data whether the changes at the transcription step involve an increased synthesis of messenger RNA or a regulatory factor acting at the translation step. Additionally, if the TOH increase is roughly proportional to the duration of the increased activity (as was found), and if increased activity of periods as short as 1 hour are sufficient, then every nerve impulse may affect protein synthesis. Such effects on protein synthesis in a region of a single dendrite may have important functional consequences.

Control of Ribosomal Aggregation:
R. J. Wurtman

At the Work Session, Wurtman emphasized the potential importance of control of the state of ribosomal aggregation as a mechanism for influencing gene expression and, thus, neuron-target cell interactions. In support of this, he discussed data showing that both serotonin (Weiss et al., 1973) and dopamine (Weiss et al., 1971, 1974, 1975; Munro et al., 1973; Roel et al., 1974; Moskowitz et al., 1975) cause the disaggregation of brain polysomes and thereby act at a translational level to inhibit rat brain protein synthesis. The L-dopa-induced disaggregation of brain polysomes is suppressed in animals pretreated with drugs blocking the conversion of L-dopa to dopamine or with drugs blocking dopamine receptors (Weiss et al., 1972, 1974); hence, the disaggregation of polysomes would seem to result from a direct action of dopamine on a "receptor" controlling the machinery of cellular protein synthesis.

Weiss and collaborators (1975) have demonstrated that the change in state of polysome aggregation is caused by the interactions of dopamine and serotonin with specific receptor sites. Thus, L-dopa-induced disaggregation is blocked if rats are pretreated with haloperidol or pimozide, while 5-hydroxytryptophan (5HTP)-induced disaggregation is blocked by methysergide or cyproheptadine. Pretreatment of rats with MK-486, a drug that inhibits dopa decarboxylase in blood vessels and peripheral tissues but not in brain, does not block the effect, indicating that the critical dopamine receptors are in the brain parenchyma. Since neither intraperitoneal apomorphine nor intracisternal dopamine caused polysome disaggregation, as would be expected if the responsible receptors were in the postsynaptic membrane, the possibility must be entertained that the brain monoamines formed from exogenous dopa or 5HTP act directly on intracellular receptors associated with perikaryal organelles and not on postsynaptic receptors.

The magnitude of polysomal disaggregation (see Figure 89) observed in these studies is also better explained on the basis of intracellular "receptors," since dopa would have to be acting on many more neurons[*] than are presently known to receive monoaminergic synaptic inputs. Studies are now in progress to determine whether

---

[*]Most likely on glial cells as well, as Weiss and co-workers (1974) have shown.

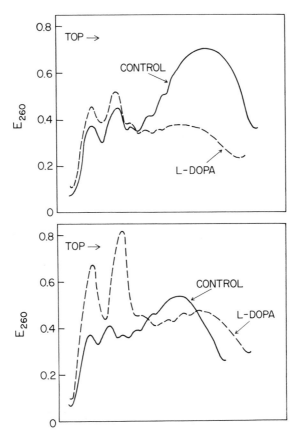

Figure 89. Effects of L-dopa on brain polysome profiles in 20- and 100-gm rats. Brains were taken 60 min after the administration of either L-dopa dissolved in 0.05 M HC1 or the diluent alone. Twenty-gm rats (upper graph, 7- to 9-days old) received 200 mg of the amino acid per kg; 100-gm rats (lower graph) received 500 mg/kg. Polysomes were isolated with discontinuous sucrose gradients, and samples were spun on continuous 10 to 40% sucrose density gradients for 70 min at 38,000 rpm to obtain polysome profiles. Solid line indicates controls; dash line, L-dopa. The arrows indicate top of gradient. [Weiss et al., 1971]

serotonin, dopamine, or drugs active in these transmitter systems can affect the synthesis of proteins in cell-free brain systems. d-Amphetamine, which was shown to cause disaggregation of brain polysomes via a dopaminergic mechanism in vivo, also appears effective in vitro.*

As Weiss and co-workers (1973) have emphasized, the mechanism by which dopamine and serotonin disaggregate brain polysomes and

*R. J. Wurtman, unpublished data.

suppress brain protein synthesis is still an open question. cAMP may be involved and, in fact, a cAMP-dependent protein kinase has been identified in adrenocortical ribosomes (Walton and Gill, 1973). Costa and co-workers (1974), while believing that cAMP has a role here and knowing that phosphorylation of ribosomal proteins decreases their binding to intraperikaryal organelles, have stated that present know-ledge does not allow for a determination of the functional significance of ribosomal phosphorylation. It is interesting, however, to note that in peripherally deprived and normal neurons undergoing cell death the state of polysome aggregation was different, suggesting a functional correlation with a lack of a molecular signal from the periphery (see Landmesser, Chapter IV). It has also been shown that some neurons in monkey occipital cortex lack polysomes (Palay et al., 1974), and, in a recent study, LeVay (1975) reported that deprivation of visual input results in polysomal disaggregation.

Mechanism of Action of NGF

Perhaps the clearest example of a noncyclic nucleotide-mediated process is that of the neurite outgrowth produced by NGF. In studies by Hier and collaborators (1972,1973), explanted chick embryo sensory ganglia were treated with NGF, and the cellular concentration of microtubule protein (as a measure of neurite outgrowth) was measured chemically by a colchicine-binding assay. The data demon-strated that NGF markedly increases the microtubule content of sensory ganglia by de novo synthesis of subunit protein and that this effect precedes neurite extension.

Both cAMP and dibutyryl cAMP stimulate extension of cytoplasmic processes from neoplastic fibroblast lines (Hsie and Puck, 1971; Johnson et al., 1971), from neuroblastoma cells (Prasad and Hsie, 1971), and from embryonic sensory ganglia (Haas et al., 1972, Hier et al., 1972, 1973; Roisen et al., 1972). However, while it stimulates neurite extension, dibutyryl cAMP does not increase cellular microtubule levels (Hier et al., 1973). Conversely, NGF does not act in the sensory ganglia system to increase amounts of adenosine 3',5'-monophosphate in intact glia or to stimulate adenylate cyclase activity in broken ganglia cells. Thus, although both cAMP and NGF achieve the same end result, they do so by different mechanisms. It has been suggested that cAMP stimulates neurite extension by enhancing the assembly of microtubule subunits into polymers (Kirkland and Burton, 1972; Roisen et al., 1972; see also Rudolph above). On the other hand, NGF acts through stimulation of synthesis of microtubule subunit protein and cAMP is not the "second messenger." The detailed mechanism of NGF action in producing neurite outgrowth remains to be determined.

The results of Hier and co-workers (1972) differ from those of Yamada and Wessells (1971), who observed that NGF-treated ganglia displayed no increase in microtubule protein when compared with controls during 16 hours of culture. The reasons for this discrepancy are not clear. Yamada and Wessells routinely incorporated chick embryo extract into their culture media. Hier and co-workers have observed that these extracts promote not only neurite extension but also microtubule synthesis, when compared to cultures incubated without embryo extract. They pointed out that perhaps the stimulation of neurite outgrowth and microtubule synthesis by chick embryo extracts masked the effect of NGF.

Conclusions

Much remains to be determined as to the mechanisms by which the molecular signals involved in neuron-target cell interactions act. Several facts have emerged, however, which deserve emphasis.

Cyclic nucleotides seem to be involved in some but not all such interactions, and they may, or may not, act as "second messengers." The changes in membrane permeability that result from cAMP-mediated phosphorylation of membrane proteins have important implications for the electrical properties and, hence, information-processing activities of neurons. On the other hand, the mechanism of action of NGF in promoting neurite extension is not cAMP-dependent, and the neurotrophic induction of TOH synthesis in the adrenal medulla can be shown to occur independently of cyclic nucleotide pathways. Question has been raised as to cAMP involvement at the neuromuscular junction as well. The cholinergic nicotinic synapse itself does not appear to have cAMP-mediated processes.

At present, we have only suggestions as to what the alternative mechanisms are. TOH induction in the adrenal medulla involves control of gene expression at the level of transcription, and NGF acts to increase the synthesis of microtubule subunits. However, the direct or indirect means by which the effects are achieved are not known.

Control of the state of polysomal aggregation is likely to be important for both cAMP and noncyclic nucleotide neuron-target cell interaction mechanisms whether the molecular signal is specifically neurotrophic or is also involved in neurotransmission.

To develop a balanced view of neuron-target cell interaction mechanisms, it is essential to remember that, while the two cells are interacting, multiple processes, set in motion by several molecular signals reaching the target cell, interact within the cell to produce unique patterns of metabolic and electrical activity. The potential of such interactions for the production of complex and highly sensitive cellular behavior is great.

IX. RESEARCH ISSUES AND STRATEGIES

At the 1968 NRP Work Session (Guth, 1969), the participants, after deliberating whether neurotrophism could be so defined as to provide a useful basis for experimental investigations, decided that trophic effects are "interactions between nerves and other cells which initiate or control molecular modification* in the other cell." Increasingly clear is the fact that both neuron-to-target-cell and target-cell-to-neuron trophisms exist in a dynamic, interdependent system. Whereas the term "neurotrophic" has been retained through the years to emphasize the importance of neural trophism directed at target cells, it is now better to use the term "neuron-target cell interactions," in recognition of bidirectional trophic balance. The complexity of the phenomena involved makes clear identification of issues and the proper choice of research strategies critical to further progress in understanding neuron-target cell interactions. Drachman (1974b), at a New York Academy of Sciences conference on "Trophic Functions of the Neuron," made the point that "one cannot assume a priori that the rules that govern neurotrophic control in one system should also apply in another system." Merely organizing the available data into a useful format is a considerable task. One approach is to sort the data along a single dimension such as time. In this chapter we will (1) look at the data from the perspective of time, (2) review the experimental issues and research strategies on a chapter-by-chapter basis, and, finally, (3) make a general concluding statement.

Time and Neuron-Target Cell Interactions

Time is a useful, if ultimately limited, parameter around which to organize the data on neuron-target cell interactions. It can be used in several different ways, and "time" measurements, i.e., milliseconds, seconds, minutes, hours, and days, represent only one facet. Other "times" that may be useful to consider include developmental time, aging time, circadian time, chemical time, and, possibly, "coincident" and intraneuronal time. Measurement "time," as such, needs no explanation. In one dimension it provides a useful device to categorize the numerous molecular signals. In Kreutzberg's time-based scheme (see

*Implicit in this definition is a *long-term* modification in the target cell. Production of a postsynaptic potential by a neurotransmitter is of short duration and thus not "trophic."

Figure 1 in Chapter I), adenosine is in a different category of structural and functional significance than is nerve growth factor. There is, of course, some risk in making restrictive temporal categories, because boundaries between categories may be blurred or one substance may appear in more than one category of function or mechanism. This seems particularly true for neurotransmitters.

Developmental Time

Developmental time, which includes both embryonic and postnatal maturational time, is generally divided into blocks, such as gestational days, stages, or periods. Although its existence is well known, it is too often neglected in experimental design.

A particularly cogent example of the importance of developmental time is the controversy over whether the nerve or the muscle is primary in dystrophic disease of muscle. As discussed in Chapter II, when muscle from 12-day-old dystrophic chick embryos was transplanted to normal chicks, it did not undergo phenotypic alteration. Therefore, it seemed reasonable to conclude that there were no extramuscular, or especially neural, influences that made the muscle dystrophic, and that the muscle, itself, was genetically dystrophic. However, by transplanting the neural tube from dystrophic to normal chicks before the first-known inductive neural influences on somites occurred, Rathbone and collaborators (see Chapter II) showed that an early inductive effect of the neural tube on presumptive myoblasts set their subsequent normal or dystrophic developmental course. Thus, the neuron becomes the villain in chick muscular dystrophy, which is precisely the opposite conclusion to that reached in the previous experiment. Similarly, Peterson, using mouse chimeras, has been able to establish a role for an extramuscular factor(s) in murine muscular dystrophy.

Another example of the importance of developmental time is the response of sensory ganglion neurons to NGF. For a brief period during development, these cells emit neurites in response to NGF; however, the mature sensory neurons cease responding in this way (see Thoenen; Chapter III). If one were to test NGF only on adult sensory neurons, one might erroneously conclude that this is without effect.

One interesting point brought out by these experiments is that one trophic signal may have different roles at different developmental times. Curiously, although mature sensory neurons lose their ability to sprout in response to NGF, they continue to transport it rapidly from their terminals to their somata. This finding suggests that NGF plays a different role in adult sensory neurons than in developing ones, similar, perhaps, to its maintenance of normal tyrosine hydroxylase in adult sympathetic ganglia. Other molecular signals involved in neuron-target cell interactions may also have similar dual or multiple, developmental, time-dependent roles. That the "different times-different roles" principle is of general relevance in development is worth emphasizing (see McMahon, 1974).

Aging Time

Aging time is in the same continuum as developmental and maturational time, and much the same case can be made for it. The point in time in adult life when a particular neurotrophic phenomenon is examined may be critical. During maturity, the adult organism undergoes continuous subtle changes that may be irreversible or cyclical. In advanced aging, the changes may be extreme. The age-related intraneuronal aggregation of tubular materials, probably both microtubules and neurofilaments (see section on "Effects of Aging" in Chapter VII), may disrupt normal transport mechanisms, and failure to find a response to a given target-cell-to-neuron signal in an adult may reflect that disruption. A different example is that of adult salamander neurons, which show seasonal changes in their ability to sprout. Similar changes in higher organisms, including man, are likely to be found and to have their basis in cyclical hormonal changes of daily, monthly, or longer duration.

Cyclical Time

In considering circadian and cyclical times, peripherally produced hormones, as well as their releasing factors, acting back on the nervous system deserve examination (see discussion in Chapter IV). In these cases both metabolism and electrical activity of neurons are influenced. The postnatal presence or absence of estrogen determines whether a genetic female will support a normal estrus cycle, which is, in turn, coupled to cyclic behavioral changes. The daily rhythm of glucocorticoid production by the adrenal medulla correlates with the inducibility of TOH; in the sympathetic ganglia, induction occurs when glucocorticoid levels are high, while in the adrenal medulla, induction is only possible when glucocorticoid levels are low. Conclusions about a neurotrophic effect, then, are only valid if they have a basis in cyclical or "endocrine" time.

Chemical Time

Still another facet is "chemical" time. This refers to the kinetics of the biochemical reactions underlying neuron-target cell interactions (see Chapter VIII). In this way kinetic parameters form a useful standard for determining the likelihood of any given mechanism in a neurotrophic effect. Where there is a time discrepancy, another mechanism should be considered. For example, phosphorylation of membrane protein, secondary to activation of cyclic nucleotide mechanisms, has been postulated to have a role not only in the production of postsynaptic potentials but also in processes lasting up to several hours. An important key to the different requirements of these two situations may lie in differential local phosphatase activity. A neurotrophic effect of several hours duration will require different chemical mechanisms than one lasting days, weeks, or even the organism's lifetime. Lifetime effects may require constant renewal to maintain permanence.

Intraneuronal Time

Is there an intraneuronal clock genetically programming a self-destructive mechanism for cells that fail to make appropriate connections by a given stage? This does not seem to be the case for chick ciliary ganglia in Landmesser's studies (see Chapter IV). However, if dendritic spine formation in cerebellar Purkinje cells does not require a postsynaptic trigger, then timed intraneuronal programming may exist in this system. Herrup* thinks that the change in responsiveness of sensory ganglion cells to NGF is related to receptor loss, and the timing of this event may well prove to be intrinsic to the cell itself. However, more evidence is required to prove the existence of such a neuronal clock.

"Coincident" Time

"Coincident" time, a composite of all time elements, serves to emphasize that a neurotrophic effect does not occur in isolation. For example, in addition to intact innervation, testosterone must be present for the effective neurotrophic regulation of taste bud formation. As noted above, the neural induction of TOH depends on high levels of

---

*K. Herrup, personal communication.

glucocorticoid in sympathetic ganglia and low levels in the adrenal medulla. The coincidence of multiple factors, such as thyroid hormone, corticosteroids estrogen and androgen, and perhaps glial and other sprouting factors, as well as specifically neurotrophic factors, is crucial to normal central nervous system development. In fact, coincident time is too restrictive a term, because the sequence of events ("sequential" time) is also important (e.g., plowing a field is required before planting). If one or more extraneuronal factors are abnormal or absent, then a neurotrophic effect may not occur. Furthermore, as was pointed out by Grafstein, development may be sequential without the necessity of a *causal* relationship in the sequence itself. In designating a "neurotrophic effect" perhaps the "permissive" nonneural factors should be specified.

While useful as a heuristic device and important in research strategy, time must still be viewed in the perspective of still other factors. In cases where an inappropriate neuron forms a connection with a target cell but is later displaced by the correct neuron, time is clearly overridden.

The Proof of Trophism

Having explored time as an approach to the organization of neuron-target cell interaction data, we may find it useful to outline the major issues of the preceding chapters. "The Proof of Trophism" (Chapter II), perhaps the most basic issue, serves as a good starting point.

At the 1968 NRP Work Session (Guth, 1969), where experimental approaches to the problem of the trophic functions of the neuron were discussed, the participants concluded that the strategy of denervation was unlikely to further the analysis of the trophic influence, since the major problems, the roles of disuse and transmitter, could not be sorted out. More recently, colchicine has been used in an elimination strategy to block delivery of a hypothetical trophic substance to the nerve terminal and, hence, to the target muscle cell. It has been argued that this blockade of delivery takes place without changes in electrical activity and usage and so avoids the problems of denervation. However, colchicine has other effects on the muscle membrane that are not mediated by the nerve.* Albuquerque's use of

*These objections to the use of colchicine do not appear to apply to studies of sensory systems and innervation fields in salamander skin (see Diamond, Chapter VI).

batrachotoxin (see Chapter II) to block both slow and fast transport, as well as to produce an irreversible depolarization, seems to offer a way around objections to colchicine usage in nerve-muscle systems. The strategy of replacement, whose employment was suggested at the 1969 Work Session, has been demonstrated to be useful by Lentz, Rathbone, and Oh. On the basis of the available data, which now represent much more than that obtained from nerve-muscle studies, we can conclude that there are neurotrophic effects independent of transmitter action and activity per se. At the same time, molecules with synaptic transmission as one function *are* involved in anterograde neurotrophism both through metabolic processes linked to postsynaptic receptors and through other actions that are independent of transmission-related receptors or even receptors at all.

The identification of the molecular signals in neuron-target cell interactions has only begun. As the number of suspected and proven molecular signals grows, the ability to sort out the multiple factors involved will be increasingly important. Some factors will be primary; others will be secondary, tertiary, or, perhaps, coincidental. Systems that provide for such sorting are much to be desired. These include the nerve-muscle culture of Lentz (presented in Chapter II) and the chimera approaches of Peterson (1974) and LaVail and Mullen (1976; Mullen and LaVail, 1976). Greene suggested that α-bungarotoxin could be profitably used to monitor such trophic influences in nerve-nerve interactions, as well as in nerve-muscle interactions. Several recent studies have shown that the toxin binds to what appear to be cholinergic receptors in peripheral and central nervous tissue (Greene et al., 1973; Salvaterra and Moore, 1973; Eterović and Bennett, 1974; Freeman, 1976). In several instances, it has been possible by autoradiographic means to localize the binding of toxin to particular groups of neurons or to the dendritic processes of a particular group of neurons (Polz-Tejera et al., 1975; Freeman, 1976).* Such findings suggest that the toxin could be used to assay the effects of denervation, cross innervation, blockade of synaptic transmission, or deprivation of first synaptic contacts on the number and distribution of neuronal acetylcholine receptors. Furthermore, in a suitable test system, such as cell cultures, the toxin could be of great aid in assaying for the effects of putative trophic substances.

*See also E. Kouvelas, L. Greene, and J. H. LaVail, unpublished data.

Pathways of Intraneuronal Transport and
Transneuronal Exchange

Much has been learned about anterograde and retrograde axonal and dendritic transport – the intracellular pathways in transneuronal exchange. Although the phenomenological lore has increased greatly, the molecular mechanism(s) of these intracellular pathways remains obscure. The extracellular and transcellular pathways remain unknown, and it is uncertain how specificity of transfer is achieved. At present, the study of transcellular molecular interchange pathways (anterograde or retrograde) in in vivo nerve-muscle preparations is not useful owing to inadequate spatial resolution. The pursuit of the study of the gap junction and of target cell uptake mechanisms as devices for specific transfer seems promising. Incidentally, functional neuroanatomical mapping, such as that provided by the "Sokoloff method" (see Kennedy et al., 1975; Plum et al., 1976), may yield further information as to which central nervous system structures are functionally connected, as well as to the time sequence in which they are activated. This information should aid in determining the "when and where" of neuron-target cell interactions.

Target Cell-Neuron Relationships

The importance of the target cell for the development, health, and even viability of its innervating neuron has been established. Of the signals involved in direct target-cell-to-neuron interactions, only NGF has been identified. Identification of another such signal (e.g., the signal for the peripheral control of neuronal death in the chick ciliary ganglion or for the induction of the synthesis of choline acetyltransferase in muscle) is a necessary next step. The "indirect" target-cell-to-neuron signals, such as hormones and hormone-releasing factors, must also be determined. Not only which agents are active but also the mechanisms by which they exert their effects need to be elucidated.

The functional responsiveness of the retrograde uptake and transport systems to changed physiological demands remains to be defined. Both the identification of the signals and the evaluation of the functional responsiveness demand the right system. The chick retinoisthmooptic nucleus model used by Halperin and LaVail seems to be a useful strategy. The sympathetic nervous system, particularly the superior cervical ganglion, as used by Black, Thoenen, and others, provides ease of manipulation as well as quantitation. Bisby's motor neuron-sensory neuron system represents still another approach.

Glia-Neuron Interactions

The complex structural and functional interdependency of neurons and glia is a subject of increasing interest. Elucidation of the role of glia in neuron-target cell interactions requires high resolution methodology, but the analytical techniques that have been used lack adequate biochemical markers for clearly distinguishing the two cell types in a mixed population. The culture of clonal lines of neurons and glia and the methods for selectively growing neurons or glia in a mixed culture, such as those of Patterson, seem to offer the necessary resolution. These in vitro methods have already shown that glia (at least cloned tumor lines, such as the C6 glioma) produce NGF, a neuroblastoma sprouting factor, and another, as yet uncharacterized, agent(s) with implications for neuronal development and differentiation. A more complex system, the hippocampal slice method of Lynch and co-workers, looks promising. It may be useful not only for the isolation of a potential glial sprouting factor but also for the assay of its effects. Perhaps this model could be used to study the neuron-to-glia signal for glial mitosis after neuronal injury. The further elucidation of these and other neuron-glia interactions involved in circuit formation, modulation of neuronal electrical activity, maintenance of neuronal health, and repair and regeneration of neurons will make for significant conceptual advance in neuroscience.

Target Cell Innervation

Several issues regarding the development and control of innervation fields remain unsettled: (1) To what degree can peripheral models be applied to regeneration in the central nervous system? (2) Can the respective roles of the neuron and target cell in determining an innervation pattern be clarified? It is not likely to be an either-or situation. Time may be a crucial factor. (3) Are competition models and, particularly, the sprouting-antisprouting hypothesis of Diamond and collaborators valid? If NGF or a like substance is the sprouting factor, can the postulated antisprouting factor be identified? (4) Is there a "concept of body space" in neurons? (5) Is the specificity of neuron-target cell interactions related to the specificity of the formation of neuronal connections?

Each of the three experimental systems presented in Chapter VI (see above) offers opportunities to get at Issues 1 to 3, while Diamond's system is particularly suited to Issues 4 and 5. The sympathetic nervous system, particularly as used by Black, is remarkably adaptable to a wide variety of experimental conditions.

In regard to Issue 5, our present knowledge about neuron-target cell interactions is such that we cannot directly answer the question of how specificity of neuronal connections, let alone how their subsequent stability or modifiability, is achieved. These interactions, however, do point to mechanisms that may be involved in the production of this specificity. The fact that one salamander spinal nerve will not invade the territory of another despite massive denervation, or, similarly, that entorhinal fiber input to the hippocampal pyramidal cell dendrites will not expand into the commissural associational zone with denervation, indicates strong specificity or unusual stability. Forcing the salamander nerve to grow down the stump of the nerve to the foreign territory, however, overcomes the territorial restrictions. Denervating the entorhinal zone of the hippocampal pyramidal cells results in expansion of the remaining undamaged afferents — a sort of unidirectional specificity. The rotated skin experiments in the salamander would seem to indicate that the neuron, in fact, has some inherent "concept" of space.

The demonstrated compression and expansion of retinotectal fields (Edds et al., 1976) raise the alternative possibilities of respecification vs. systems matching on a spatial basis. For retinotectal system specificity, two general hypotheses have been put forward: The first, stemming from Sperry's concepts of neuronal specificity, is that each retinal cell acquires position-related properties (expressed at the level of the cell membrane molecules) that are matched with those of corresponding tectal cells. In other words, each retinal and tectal cell has a unique address, perhaps molecularly specified. The alternative model is based on the properties of populations of cells. In this theory the relative position of a cell along a gradient axis is crucial; hence, specificity is achieved not by virtue of the properties of a single cell but rather by complex interactions between the population units. The final explanation may have elements of both. The evidence presented in this

Bulletin suggests that there is cellular specificity in the sense that a parasympathetic nerve cannot maintain muscle cholinesterase at normal levels whereas a motor nerve can. Whereas only gustatory neurons can produce taste bud differentiation, they are unable to do so in the absence of testosterone. The coincidence of several factors in time and space may result in a highly specified pattern of connection. Absence of any one factor may reduce such specificity or actually produce a failure of connections in any pattern. Whatever the detailed explanation, the elucidation of the basis of population properties seems to be a crucial task.

Pathology of Neuron-Target Cell Interactions

The pathology of neuron-target cell interactions represents an as yet untapped resource. Areas of interest include anterograde and retrograde transneuronal degeneration; deafferentation phenomena; aging; cortical, subcortical, and spinal degenerative or dystrophic diseases; synaptic dysgenesis; migration failure; viral infection, toxic and deficiency diseases; and surgical trauma. Animal models are valuable for study, but, as Black and Hirano have shown, basic science strategies and techniques can be applied to human material (in some cases even after formalin fixation). Much more effort in this direction seems worthwhile, not only for the further elucidation of neuron-target cell interactions but also for improved understanding and treatment of human disease.

Molecular Mechanisms of Neuron-Target Cell Interactions

While the phenomenology of neuron-target cell interactions has burgeoned in the last few years, the molecular mechanisms by which the trophic signals exert their effects are only beginning to be appreciated. This area is at a catalytic stage and can be expected to grow rapidly. Present candidates for the multiple mechanisms likely to be involved include cyclic nucleotides, control of the RNA at the transcriptional level, and control of the state of polysome aggregation. Although we know that cAMP is not involved in the action of NGF, no other mechanism has emerged. Their studies on the adrenal medulla in vivo and in vitro have led Thoenen and co-workers to question the involvement of cyclic nucleotides in the neural induction of medullary TOH; these investigators favor control at the level of RNA transcription. Control of the state of polysome aggregation, which apparently can be exerted by a transmitter like dopamine and which may also involve cyclic nucleotide or other mechanisms, merits further investigation.

How should we regard the molecular interactions we have been describing? On the one hand, they may represent mechanisms for the recycling or reutilization of valuable nutrients such as adenosine, which cannot cross the blood-brain barrier. On the other hand, the observed transcellular molecular flux may represent a true signalling device. Although the signals may, like hormones, not be metabolized themselves, they, nonetheless, can profoundly affect the metabolism of the target cell. They may include small peptides or macromolecules carrying sequentially coded information to alter not only metabolism but also membrane structure and, hence, neuronal function.

Another fundamental question is whether there can be restriction of the response to a given signal, e.g., to one region of a dendritic membrane. Alternatively, is the whole cell affected? Does the induction of one dendritic spine cause other spines to form on the same dendrite or, perhaps, on other dendrites to form spines? If there is collateral sprouting in one axonal branch on the same cell, is there sprouting in all the others?* The answer seems to be that there can be both restricted and general responses. One might argue that a restricted response may occur simply because the delivery of the signal is restricted. However, the soma, as the synthetic center of the cell, must certainly be involved. It may be that the restricted delivery zone is in some way prepared (e.g., by increased membrane fluidity) by the same or another molecular signal to express the somal activity in a manner that "unprepared" regions of the dendrite are not.†‡ This could explain a restricted response in one dendrite to a circulating hormone arriving at the soma.

---

*Diamond and co-workers are actively investigating this phenomenon in the salamander.

†Structural mosaicism of dendritic membranes could accomplish this without invoking a second signal.

‡E. X. Albuquerque cited the work of Jacobson and Papahadjopoulos (1975) showing that there are differences in the phase transition behavior of normal and denervated muscle membrane. This is at least consistent with a "preparedness" hypothesis. How the nerve accomplishes regulation of membrane lipids is not known.

As Black pointed out, there is virtually no evidence at the biochemical level to indicate that only one molecule or species, e.g., a transmitter system enzyme, increases in response to a given signal. Generally, other proteins accumulate as well, suggesting a more general "switching on" of protein synthesis. What may restrict the response are one or more modulating factors that, when acting in concert, might result in cell death, but, when occurring in lesser aggregates, might yield "local growth."

Strategies for Analyzing Molecular Interactions

The diversity and ubiquity of the molecular interactions between neurons and their target cells "speak" for their importance in the formation, function, maintenance, and reparative capability of the nervous system. The evidence presented challenges us to view neuronal and brain function from new perspectives in which active, bidirectional molecular transfer may be just as important as the transmission of electrical impulses. One wonders, in fact, whether the production of a postsynaptic potential represents the primary message of every synaptic event or whether metabolic changes are the real objective. Bloom (1975, p. 77), writing about the role of cyclic nucleotides in central synaptic function, stated it particularly well when he wrote:

> The range of functions which could be controlled through cyclic nucleotide-sensitive protein kinases may currently be said to know no limits, since so few studies have as yet been reported in which substrate proteins of known function have been evaluated . . . . In the face of such a powerful biochemical lever for the regulation of neuronal and possibly glial metabolism, it might be wondered whether the electrophysiological effects of postsynaptic inhibition represent the primary message of such synaptic events or whether these electrophysiological effects might not be epi-phenomena of a more pervasive, but covert, shift in cellular metabolism which is evoked by these cyclic nucleotide-mediated synaptic stimuli.
>   . . . Thus, even though the electrical activity of neurons has long been their most striking functionally-related property, electrical changes which accompany synaptic events may not be the primary objective of every synaptic transmission.

It is not unreasonable to think of chemical as well as electrical circuits, fields, and information processing. Connectivity in chemical circuits need not be defined solely by synaptic specializations; such circuits might well add not only considerable complexity but also new dimensions of functional capability to the nervous system.

As has been pointed out many times in this *Bulletin*, the molecular signals involved in phenomena ranging from the maintenance of muscle cholinesterase to the development of complex innervation patterns do not act singly or in isolation. The aggregate effects of multiple interacting factors or systems are not likely to be predictable on a simple one- or two-factor basis. Not only the number of molecular signals but also their interaction with, and modulation by, other intracellular and extracellular signals require new modes of analysis if we are to understand the emergent system properties. In fact, the development of adequate concepts and techniques for the required interactional or systems analysis may be one of the greatest challenges in neurobiology today.

ABBREVIATIONS

ACh	acetylcholine
AChE	acetylcholinesterase
ALS	amylotrophic lateral sclerosis
ATP	adenosine triphosphate
ATPase	adenosine triphosphatase
BTX	batrachotoxin
cAMP	cyclic adenosine monophosphate
cGMP	cyclic guanosine monophosphate
ChAc	choline acetyltransferase
ChE	cholinesterase
CNS	central nervous system
DBH	dopamine β-hydroxylase
EDL	extensor digitorum longus
ER	endoplasmic reticulum
FSH	follicle-stimulating hormone
GABA	γ-aminobutyric acid
GAD	glutamic acid decarboxylase
^{3}H-NE	^{3}H-norepinephrine
HRP	horseradish peroxidase
5HTP	5-hydroxytryptophan
IOH	idiopathic orthostatic hypotension
LGA	lateral giant axon
LGB	lateral geniculate body
LGN	lateral geniculate nucleus
LH	luteinizing hormone
LH-RH	luteinizing hormone-releasing hormone
MEPP's	miniature end-plate potentials
NE	norepinephrine
NGF	nerve growth factor
6-OHDA	6-hydroxydopamine
POA	preoptic area
Rc	Retzius cell
RNA	ribonucleic acid
SCG	superior cervical ganglion
SDS	sodium dodecyl sulfate
TCA	trichloroacetic acid
TOH	tyrosine hydroxylase
TRH	thyrotropin-releasing hormone
TTX	tetrodotoxin
VMH	ventromedial hypothalamic nucleus
VMN	ventromedial nucleus

BIBLIOGRAPHY

This bibliography contains two types of entries: (1) citations given or work alluded to in the report, and (2) additional references to pertinent literature by conference participants and others. Citations in group (1) may be found in the text on the pages listed in the right-hand column.   Page

Abe, T., Haga, T.T., and Kurokawa, M. (1974): Retrograde axoplasmic transport: 274
its continuation as anterograde transport. *FEBS Lett.* 47:272-275.

Aguayo, A.J., Terry, L.C., and Bray, G.M. (1973): Spontaneous loss of axons in sympathetic unmyelinated nerve fibers of the rat during development. *Brain Res.* 54:360-364.

Aguilar, C.E., Bisby, M.A., Cooper, E., and Diamond, J. (1973): Evidence that   260,261,
axoplasmic transport of trophic factors is involved in the regulation of peripheral   337
nerve fields in salamanders. *J. Physiol.* 234:449-464.

Aguilar, C.E., Bisby, M.A., and Diamond, J. (1972): Impulses and the transfer of trophic factors in nerves. *J. Physiol.* 226:60P-61P.

Aiken, J. and Reit, E. (1969): A comparison of the sensitivity to chemical stimuli   326
of adrenergic and cholinergic neurons in the cat stellate ganglion. *J. Pharmacol. Exp. Ther.* 169:211-223.

Albuquerque, E.X., Barnard, E.A., Porter, C.W., and Warnick, J.E. (1974a): The density of acetylcholine receptors and their sensitivity in the postsynaptic membrane of muscle endplates. *Proc. Nat. Acad. Sci.* 71:2818-2822.

Albuquerque, E.X., Daly, J.W., and Witkop, B. (1971a): Batrachotoxin: Chemistry   220,229,
and pharmacology. *Science* 172:995-1002.   231

Albuquerque, E.X., Deshpande, S.S., Kauffman, F.C., Garcia, J., and Warnick, J.E.   232,233,
(1975): Neurotrophic control of the fast and slow skeletal muscle. *In:*   234
Neurotransmission, Vol. 2. (Proceedings of the Sixth International Congress of Pharmacology, Helsinki, Finland.) Forssa: Forssan Kirjapaino Oy, pp. 185-194.

Albuquerque, E.X. and McIsaac, R.J. (1969): Early development of acetylcholine   227
receptors in fast and slow mammalian muscle. *Life Sci.* 8:409-416.

Albuquerque, E.X. and McIsaac, R.J. (1970): Fast and slow mammalian muscles   220
after denervation. *Exp. Neurol.* 26:183-202.

Albuquerque, E.X., Schuh, F.T., and Kauffman, F.C. (1971b): Early membrane   227
depolarization of the fast mammalian muscle after denervation. *Pfluegers Arch.* 328:36-50.

Albuquerque, E.X. and Warnick, J.E. (1971): Electrophysiological observations in   227
normal and dystrophic chicken muscles. *Science* 172:1260-1263.

Albuquerque, E.X. and Warnick, J.E. (1972): The pharmacology of batrachotoxin.   231
IV. Interaction with tetrodotoxin on innervated and chronically denervated rat skeletal muscle. *J. Pharmacol. Exp. Ther.* 180:683-697.

Albuquerque, E.X., Warnick, J.E., and Sansone, F.M. (1971c): The pharmacology   231
of batrachotoxin. II. Effect on electrical properties of the mammalian nerve and skeletal muscle membranes. *J. Pharmacol. Exp. Ther.* 176:511-528.

Page

Albuquerque, E.X., Warnick, J.E., Sansone, F.M., and Daly, J. (1973): The   229
pharmacology of batrachotoxin. V. A comparative study of membrane properties and the effect of batrachotoxin on sartorius muscles of the frogs *Phyllobates
aurotaenia* and *Rana pipiens. J. Pharmacol. Exp. Ther.* 184:315-329.

Albuquerque, E.X., Warnick, J.E., Sansone, F.M., and Onur, R. (1974b): The   227,261
effects of vinblastine and colchicine on neural regulation of muscle. *Ann. N.Y.
Acad. Sci.* 228:224-243.

Albuquerque, E.X., Warnick, J.E., Tasse, J.R., and Sansone, F.M. (1972): Effects of   220,227,
vinblastine and colchicine on neural regulation of the fast and slow skeletal   261
muscles of the rat. *Exp. Neurol.* 37:607-634.

Altman, J. (1973): Experimental reorganization of the cerebellar cortex. III. Regeneration of the external germinal layer and granule cell ectopia. *J. Comp. Neurol.*
149:153-180.

Alvarez, J. and Püschel, M. (1972): Transfer of material from efferent axons to   276
sensory epithelium in the goldfish vestibular system. *Brain Res.* 37:265-278.

Anderson, E.G., Haas, H., and Hösli, L. (1973): Comparison of effects of   377
noradrenaline and histamine with cyclic AMP on brain stem neurones. *Brain Res.*
49:471-475.

Anderson, L.E. and McClure, W.O. (1973): Differential transport of protein in   274
axons: Comparison between the sciatic nerve and dorsal columns of cats. *Proc.
Nat. Acad. Sci.* 70:1521-1525.

Appeltauer, G.S.L. and Korr, I.M. (1975): Axonal delivery of soluble, insoluble and   276
electrophoretic fractions of neuronal proteins to muscle. *Exp. Neurol.*
46:132-146.

Appenzeller, O. and Ogin, G. (1975): Pathogenesis of muscular dystrophies.
Sympathetic neurovascular components. *Arch. Neurol.* 32:2-4.

Autilio-Gambetti, L., Gambetti, P., and Shafer, B. (1975): Glial and neuronal
contribution to proteins and glycoproteins recovered in myelin fractions. *Brain
Res.* 84:336-340.

Bárány, M. and Close, R.I. (1971): The transformation of myosin in cross-   236
innervated rat muscles. *J. Physiol.* 213:455-474.

Barber, P.C. and Raisman, G. (1974): An autoradiographic investigation of the
projection of the vomeronasal organ to the accessory olfactory bulb in the
mouse. *Brain Res.* 81:21-30.

Bargmann, W. (1949a): Uber die neurosekretorische Verknüpfung von Hypothal-   217
amus und Hypophyse. *Klin. Wochenschr.* 27:617-622.

Bargmann, W. (1949b): Uber die neurosekretorische Verknüpfung von Hypothal-   217
amus und Neurohypophyse. *Z. Zellforsch. Mikrosk. Anat.* 34:610-634.

Barker, D. and Ip, M.C. (1966): Sprouting and degeneration of mammalian motor   237
axons in normal and de-afferented skeletal muscle. *Proc. R. Soc. B* 163:538-554.

Barondes, S.H. (1967): Axoplasmic transport. *Neurosciences Res. Prog. Bull.*   270
5:307-419. Also *In: Neurosciences Research Symposium Summaries, Vol. 3.*
Schmitt, F.O. et al., eds. Cambridge, Mass.: M.I.T. Press, 1969, pp. 191-299.

Neurosciences Res. Prog. Bull., Vol. 14, No. 3   415

Page

Barron, D.H. (1946): Observations on the early differentiation of the motor   294
neuroblasts in the spinal cord of the chick. *J. Comp. Neurol.* 85:149-169.

Bennett, M.R., McLachlan, E.M., and Taylor, R.S. (1973): The formation of
synapses in mammalian striated muscle reinnervated with autonomic preganglionic nerves. *J. Physiol.* 233:501-517.

Bennett, M.V.L. and Dunham, P.B. (1970): Sucrose permeability of junctional   290
membrane at an electrotonic synapse. *Biophys. J.* 10:117. (Abstr.)

Bennett, M.V.L. and Goodenough, D.A. (1976): Electrotonic junctions. *Neuro-*   290
sciences Res. Prog. Bull. (In press)

Berard-Badier, M., Gambarelli, D., Pinsard, N., Hassoun, J., and Toga, M. (1971):   364
Infantile neuroaxonal dystrophy or Seitelberger's disease. II. Peripheral nerve
involvement: electron microscopic study in one case. *Acta Neuropathol.*
5(Suppl. 5):30-39.

Berg, D.K. and Hall, Z.W. (1974): Fate of α-bungarotoxin bound to acetylcholine
receptors of normal and denervated muscle. *Science* 184:473-475.

Berne, R.M., Rubio, R., and Curnish, R.R. (1974): Release of adenosine from   388,389
ischemic brain. *Circ. Res.* 35:262-272.

Binaglia, L., Goracci, G., Porcellati, G., Roberti, R., and Woelk, H. (1973): The
synthesis of choline and ethanolamine phosphoglycerides in neuronal and glial
cells of rabbit *in vitro. J. Neurochem.* 21:1067-1082.

Binaglia, L., Roberti, R., Goracci, G., Francescangeli, E., and Porcellati, G. (1974):
Enzymic synthesis of ethanolamine plasmogens through ethanolaminephospho-
transferase activity in neurons and glial cells of rabbit in vitro. *Lipids* 9:738-747.

Bisby, M.A. (1975a): Inhibition of axonal transport in nerves chronically treated   307
with local anesthetics. *Exp. Neurol.* 47:481-489.

Bisby, M.A. (1975b): Retrograde axonal transport of protein: differences between   273,308
motor and sensory axons. *Proc. Can. Fed. Biol. Sci.* 18:8. (Abstr.)

Bisby, M.A. (1976): Orthograde and retrograde axonal transport of labelled protein   270
in motoneurons. *Exp. Neurol.* 50:628-640.

Bisby, M.A., Fillenz, M., and Smith, A.D. (1973): Evidence for the presence of   276
dopamine-β-hydroxylase in both populations of noradrenaline storage vesicles in
sympathetic nerve terminals of the rat vas deferens. *J. Neurochem.* 20:245-248.

Bjerre, B., Björklund, A., Mobley, W., and Rosengren, E. (1975): Short- and
long-term effects of nerve growth factor on the sympathetic nervous system in
the adult mouse. *Brain Res.* 94:263-277.

Bjerre, B., Björklund, A., and Stenevi, U. (1974): Inhibition of the regenerative
growth of central noradrenergic neurons by intracerebrally administered
anti-NGF serum. *Brain Res.* 74:1-18.

Björklund, A., Bjerre, B., and Stenevi, U. (1974): Has nerve growth factor a role in   336,349
the regeneration of central and peripheral catecholamine neurons? *In: Dynamics*
of Degeneration and Growth in Neurons, Vol. 22. (Proceedings of the
International Symposium held in Wenner-Gren Center, Stockholm, May, 1973.)
Fuxe, K., Olson, L., and Zotterman, Y., eds. New York: Pergamon Press,
pp. 389-409.

  Page

Björklund, A., Johansson, B., Stenevi, U., and Svendgaard, N.-A. (1975):   336
Re-establishment of functional connections by regenerating central adrenergic
and cholinergic axons. *Nature* 253:446-448.

Björklund, A. and Lindvall, O. (1975): Dopamine in dendrites of substantia nigra
neurons: Suggestions for a role in dendritic terminals. *Brain Res.* 83:531-537.

Black, I.B. (1974): Growth and development of cholinergic and adrenergic neurons
in a sympathetic ganglion: Reciprocal regulation at the synapse. *In: Dynamics of
Degeneration and Growth in Neurons, Vol. 22.* (Proceedings of the International
Symposium held in Wenner-Gren Center, Stockholm, May, 1973.) Fuxe, K.,
Olson, L., and Zotterman, Y., eds. New York: Pergamon Press, pp. 455-467.

Black, I.B., Bloom, F.E., Hendry, I.A., and Iversen, L.L. (1971a): Growth and   250
development of a sympathetic ganglion: maturation of transmitter enzymes and
synapse formation in the mouse superior cervical ganglion. *J. Physiol.*
215:24P-25P.

Black, I.B. and Geen, S.C. (1973): Trans-synaptic regulation of adrenergic neuron   250,255
development: inhibition by ganglionic blockade. *Brain Res.* 63:291-302.

Black, I.B. and Geen, S.C. (1974): Inhibition of the biochemical and morphological   250
maturation of adrenergic neurons by nicotinic receptor blockade. *J. Neurochem.*
22:301-306.

Black, I.B., Hendry, I., and Iversen, L.L. (1971b): Differences in the regulation of   250
tyrosine hydroxylase and DOPA decarboxylase in sympathetic ganglia and
adrenals. *Nature New Biol.* 231:27-29.

Black, I.B., Hendry, I.A., and Iversen, L.L. (1971c): Regulation of the development   250
of choline acetyl transferase in presynaptic nerves by post-synaptic neurones in
mouse sympathetic ganglion. *J. Physiol.* 216:41P-42P.

Black, I.B., Hendry, I.A., and Iversen, L.L. (1971d): Trans-synaptic regulation of   250,252,
growth and development of adrenergic neurones in a mouse sympathetic   253
ganglion. *Brain Res.* 34:229-240.

Black, I.B., Hendry, I.A., and Iversen, L.L. (1972a): Effects of surgical decentrali-   250,254
zation and nerve growth factor on the maturation of adrenergic neurons in a
mouse sympathetic ganglion. *J. Neurochem.* 19:1367-1377.

Black, I.B., Hendry, I.A., and Iversen, L.L. (1972b): The role of post-synaptic   250,253,
neurones in the biochemical maturation of presynaptic cholinergic nerve   256,257,
terminals in a mouse sympathetic ganglion. *J. Physiol.* 221:149-159.   294

Black, I.B., Joh, T.H., and Reis, D.J. (1974): Accumulation of tyrosine hydroxylase   250,251,
molecules during growth and development of the superior cervical ganglion.   254
Brain Res. 75:133-144.

Black, I.B. and Mytilineou, C. (1976): Trans-synaptic regulation of the develop-   250,349,
ment of end organ innervation by sympathetic neurons. *Brain Res.*   350,351
101:503-521.

Black, I.B. and Reis, D.J. (1975): Ontogeny of the induction of tyrosine
hydroxylase by reserpine in the superior cervical ganglion, nucleus locus
coeruleus and adrenal gland. *Brain Res.* 84:269-278.

Blinzinger, K. and Kreutzberg, G. (1968): Displacement of synaptic terminals from   322
regenerating motoneurons by microglial cells. *Z. Zellforsch. Mikrosk. Anat.*
85:145-157.

Neurosciences Res. Prog. Bull., Vol. 14, No. 3   417

Page

Bloom, F.E. (1972): Amino acids and polypeptides in neuronal function.   318,320
Neurosciences Res. Prog. Bull. 10:122-251. Also *In: Neurosciences Research
Symposium Summaries, Vol. 7.* Schmitt, F.O. et al., eds. Cambridge, Mass.,
M.I.T. Press, 1974, pp. 122-251.

Bloom, F.E. (1973): Dynamic synaptic communication: Finding the vocabulary.
Brain Res. 62:299-305.

Bloom, F.E. (1975): The role of cyclic nucleotides in central synaptic function.   377,378,
Rev. Physiol. Biochem. Pharmacol. 74:1-103.   379,380,
          388,410

Boegman, R.J. and Wood, P.L. (1975): Drug-induced alterations in the rate of   306
rapid axoplasmic flow. *Proc. Can. Fed. Biol. Sci.* 18:64. (Abstr.)

Boegman, R.J., Wood, P.L., and Pinaud, L. (1975): Increased axoplasmic flow   306,308
associated with pargyline under conditions which induce a myopathy. *Nature*
253:51-52.

Bradley, W.G. and Jaros, E. (1973): Axoplasmic flow in axonal neuropathies.
II. Axoplasmic flow in mice with motor neuron disease and muscular dystrophy.
Brain 96:247-258.

Bradley, W.G. and Jenkison, M. (1973): Abnormalities of peripheral nerves in
murine muscular dystrophy. *J. Neurol. Sci.* 18:227-247.

Bradley, W.G. and Jenkison, M. (1975): Neural abnormalities in the dystrophic   354
mouse. *J. Neurol. Sci.* 25:249-255.

Bradley, W.G., Jenkison, M., and Montgomery, A. (1974): The significance of   354
neural abnormalities in muscular dystrophy. *Excerpta Med. Int. Congr. Series*
334:82. (Abstr.)

Bradley, W.G. and Williams, M.H. (1973): Axoplasmic flow in axonal neuropathies.
I. Axoplasmic flow in cats with toxic neuropathies. *Brain* 96:235-246.

Brazeau, P. and Guillemin, R. (1974): Somatostatin: newcomer from the   318
hypothalamus (editorial). *N. Engl. J. Med.* 290:963-964.

Brightman, M.W. and Reese, T.S. (1969): Junctions between intimately apposed   322
cell membranes in the vertebrate brain. *J. Cell Biol.* 40:648-677.

Brown, M. and Vale, W. (1975): Central nervous system effects of hypothalamic   318
peptides. *Endocrinology* 96:1333-1336.

Brown-Grant, K. (1972): Recent studies on the sexual differentiation of the brain.   310
In: Foetal and Neonatal Physiology. Comline, R.S., Cross, K.W., Dawes, G.S.,
and Nathanielsz, P.W., eds. Cambridge: Cambridge University Press, pp. 527-545.

Bueker, E.D. (1943): Intracentral and peripheral factors in the differentiation of   294
motor neurons in transplanted lumbo-sacral spinal cords of chick embryos. *J.
Exp. Zool.* 93:99-129.

Buller, A.J., Eccles, J.C., and Eccles, R.M. (1960a): Differentiation of fast and slow   236
muscles in the cat hind limb. *J. Physiol.* 150:399-416.

Buller, A.J., Eccles, J.C., and Eccles, R.M. (1960b): Interactions between   236
motoneurones and muscles in respect of the characteristic speeds of their
responses. *J. Physiol.* 150:417-439.

Page

Burnham, P., Raiborn, C., and Varon, S. (1972): Replacement of nerve-growth   323
factor by ganglionic non-neuronal cells for the survival in vitro of dissociated
ganglionic neurons. *Proc. Nat. Acad. Sci.* 69:3556-3560.

Burnstock, G. (1972): Purinergic nerves. *Pharmacol. Rev.* 24:509-581.

Burt, D.R. and Snyder, S.H. (1975): Thyrotropin releasing hormone (TRH):   318
apparent receptor binding in rat brain membranes. *Brain Res.* 93:309-328.

Byers, M.R., Fink, B.R., Kennedy, R.D., Middaugh, M.E., and Hendrickson, A.E.   307
(1973): Effects of lidocaine on axonal morphology, microtubules, and rapid
transport in rabbit vagus nerve in vitro. *J. Neurobiol.* 4:125-143.

Cangiano, A. (1973): Acetylcholine supersensitivity: the role of neurotrophic   228
factors. *Brain Res.* 58:255-259.

Cangiano, A. and Fried, J.A. (1974): Neurotrophic control of skeletal muscle of the   228
rat. *J. Physiol.* 239:31P-33P.

Cangiano, A. and Fried, J.A. (1976): The production of denervation-like changes in 228,261
rat muscle by colchicine, without interference with axonal transport or muscle
activity. *J. Physiol.* (In press)

Cannon, W.B. and Rosenbleuth, A. (1949): *The Supersensitivity of Denervated
Structures. A Law of Denervation.* New York: The MacMillan Co.

Carlsen, R.C. (1975): The possible role of cyclic AMP in the neurotrophic control   376
of skeletal muscle. *J. Physiol.* 247:343-361.

Carlsson, A. and Lindqvist, M. (1974): Studies on the neurogenic short-term
control of adrenomedullary hormone synthesis. *J. Neural Trans.* 35:181-196.

Casey, E.G., Jellife, A.M., Le Quesne, P.M., and Millett, Y.L. (1973): Vincristine
neuropathy. Clinical and electrophysiological observations. *Brain* 96:69-86.

Chalazonitis, A., Greene, L.A., and Nirenberg, M. (1974): Electrophysiological
characteristics of chick embryo sympathetic neurons in dissociated cell culture.
Brain Res. 68:235-252.

Charcot, J.M. (1881): *Lectures on the Diseases of the Nervous System. Delivered at*   218
La Salpetrière. (Translated by George Sigerson.) London: The New Sydenham
Society, 1877-1889. Published under the same title as above by the Library of
the New York Academy of Medicine, Hafner Publishing Co., New York, 1962.

Clement-Cormier, Y.C., Parrish, R.G., Petzold, G.L., Kebabian, J.W., and Greengard, P. (1975): Characterization of a dopamine-sensitive adenylate cyclase in
the rat caudate nucleus. *J. Neurochem.* 25:143-149.

Close, R.I. (1972): Dynamic properties of mammalian skeletal muscles. *Physiol.*   236
Rev. 52:129-197.

Cockett, S.A. and Kiernan, J.A. (1973): Acceleration of peripheral nervous   317
regeneration in the rat by exogenous triiodothyronine. *Exp. Neurol.*
39:389-394.

Coggeshall, R.E. and Fawcett, D.W. (1964): The fine structure of the central
nervous system of the leech, *Hirudo medicinalis. J. Neurophysiol.* 27:229-289.

Neurosciences Res. Prog. Bull., Vol. 14, No. 3   419

Page

Cohen, A.M. (1972): Factors directing the expression of sympathetic nerve traits in   326
cells of neural crest origin. *J. Exp. Zool.* 179:167-182.

Cohen, E.S., Brawer, J.R., and Morest, D.K. (1972): Projections of the cochlea to   358
the dorsal cochlear nucleus in the cat. *Exp. Neurol.* 35:470-479.

Cook, R.D. and Wiśniewski, H.M. (1973): The role of oligodendroglia and astroglia
in Wallerian degeneration of the optic nerve. *Brain Res.* 61:191-206.

Cooper, E. and Diamond, J. (1976): A quantitative study of the mechanosensory
innervation of the salamander skin. *J. Physiol.* (In press)

Cooper, E., Diamond, J., Leslie, R., Parducz, A., and Turner, C. (1976a): Touch
receptors of the salamander skin. *J. Physiol.* (In press)

Cooper, E., Diamond, J., MacIntyre, L., and Turner, C. (1975): Control of
collateral sprouting in mechanosensory nerves of salamander skin. *J. Physiol.*
252:20P-21P.

Cooper, E., Diamond, J., and Turner, C. (1976b): The effects of nerve section and   338
of colchicine treatment on the density of mechanosensory nerve endings in
salamander skin. *J. Physiol.* (In press)

Costa, E. and Guidotti, A. (1973): The role of 3',5'-cyclic adenosine monophos-   390,391
phate in the regulation of adrenal medullary function. *In: New Concepts in
Neurotransmitter Regulation.* Mandell, A.J., ed. New York: Plenum Press,
pp. 135-152.

Costa, E., Guidotti, A., and Hanbauer, I. (1974): Do cyclic nucleotides promote the   392,396
trans-synaptic induction of tyrosine hydroxylase. *Life Sci.* 14:1169-1188. Also
In: Minireviews of the Neurosciences. Brodie, B.B. and Bressler, R., eds.
New York: Pergamon Press, pp. 195-214.

Cotman, C.W. and Banker, G.A. (1974): The making of a synapse. *In: Reviews of
Neuroscience, Vol. I.* Ehrenpreis, S. and Kopin, I.J., eds. New York: Raven Press,
pp. 1-62.

Coughlin, M. (1975): Target organ stimulation of parasympathetic nerve growth in   374
the developing mouse submandibular gland. *Dev. Biol.* 43:140-158.

Cowan, W.M. (1970): Anterograde and retrograde transneuronal degeneration in
the central and peripheral nervous system. *In: Contemporary Research Methods
in Neuroanatomy.* Nauta, W.J.H. and Ebbesson, S.O.E., eds. New York:
Springer-Verlag, pp. 217-251.

Cowan, W.M. (1971): The maintenance of neurons in the developing visual system   356,360
of the chick. *In: Cellular Aspects of Neural Growth and Differentiation.* Pease,
D.C., ed. Berkeley: University of California Press, pp. 177-222.

Cowan, W.M. and Wenger, E. (1968): Degeneration in the nucleus of origin of the   294
preganglionic fibers to the chick ciliary ganglion following early removal of the
optic vesicle. *J. Exp. Zool.* 168:105-124.

Cragg, B.G. (1970): What is the signal for chromatolysis? *Brain Res.* 23:1-21.

Cragg, B.G. (1975): The development of synapses in kitten visual cortex during
visual deprivation. *Exp. Neurol.* 46:445-451.

Cragg, B.G. (1975): The development of synapses in the visual system of the cat. *J. Comp. Neurol.* 160:147-166.

Crain, S.M. and Peterson, E.R. (1974): Development of neural connections in culture. *Ann. N.Y. Acad. Sci.* 228:6-34.

Curran, M. and Parry, D.J. (1975): Neuromuscular function in fast and slow muscles of genetically dystrophic mice. *Exp. Neurol.* 47:150-161.

Dahlström, A. (1967): The transport of noradrenaline between two simultaneously performed ligations of the sciatic nerves of the rat and cat. *Acta Physiol. Scand.* 69:158-166.

Dahlström, A. and Häggendal, J. (1967): Studies on the transport and life-span of   307
amine storage granules in the adrenergic neuron system of the rabbit sciatic nerve. *Acta Physiol. Scand.* 69:153-157.

Das, G.D. and Hine, R.J. (1972): Nature and significance of spontaneous degeneration of axons in the pyramidal tract. *Z. Anat. Entwicklungsgesch.* 136:98-114.

DeLorenzo, R.J., Walton, K.G., Curran, P.F., and Greengard, P. (1973): Regulation   383
of phosphorylation of a specific protein in toad-bladder membrane by antidiuretic hormone and cyclic AMP, and its possible relationship to membrane permeability changes. *Proc. Nat. Acad. Sci.* 70:880-884.

De Vito, J.L., Clausing, K.W., and Smith, O.A. (1974): Uptake and transport of horseradish peroxidase by cut ends of the vagus nerve. *Brain Res.* 82:269-271.

Diamond, J., Cooper, E., Turner, C., and MacIntyre, L. (1976): Trophic regulation   337
of nerve sprouting: neuron-target interactions and spatial relations control mechanosensory nerve fields in salamander skin. *Science* (In press)

Dolan, L., Chew, L., Morgan, G., and Kidman, A.D. (1975): Enzyme studies of skeletal muscle in mice with different types of neural impairment and muscular dystrophy. *Exp. Neurol.* 47:105-117.

Drachman, D.B. (1974a): The role of acetylcholine as a neurotrophic transmitter.   226
Ann. N.Y. Acad. Sci. 228:160-176.

Drachman, D.B., ed. (1974b): Trophic functions of the neuron. *Ann. N.Y. Acad.*   226,399
Sci. 228:1-423.

Drachman, D.B., Murphy, S.R., Nigam, M.P., and Hills, J.R. (1967): "Myopathic" changes in chronically denervated muscle. *Arch. Neurol.* 16:14-24.

Dräger, U.C. (1974): Autoradiography of tritiated proline and fucose transported   280
transneuronally from the eye to the visual cortex in pigmented and albino mice. *Brain Res.* 82:284-292.

Droz, B., Koenig, H.L., and Di Giamberardino, L. (1973): Axonal migration of   280
protein and glycoprotein to nerve endings. I. Radioautographic analysis of the renewal of protein in nerve endings of chicken ciliary ganglion after intracerebral injection of [^{3}H]lysine. *Brain Res.* 60:93-127.

Droz, B., Rambourg, A., and Koenig, H.L. (1975): The smooth endoplasmic   261
reticulum: structure and role in the renewal of axonal membrane and synaptic vesicles by fast axonal transport. *Brain Res.* 93:1-13.

Page

Frizell, M. and Sjöstrand, J. (1974): Transport of proteins, glycoproteins and   308
cholinergic enzymes in regenerating hypoglossal neurons. *J. Neurochem.*
22:845-850.

Furstman, L., Saporta, S., and Druger, L. (1975): Retrograde axonal transport of   274
horseradish peroxidase in sensory nerves and ganglion cells of the rat. *Brain Res.*
84:320-324.

Gainer, H. and Barker, J.L. (1974): Synaptic regulation of specific protein synthesis
in an identified neuron. *Brain Res.* 78:314-319.

Galambos, R. (1961): A glia-neural theory of brain function. *Proc. Nat. Acad. Sci.*   322
47:129-136.

Galambos, R. (1967): Brain correlates of learning. *In: The Neurosciences: A Study*   322
Program. Quarton, G.C., Melnechuk, T., and Schmitt, F.O., eds. New York:
Rockefeller University Press, pp. 637-643.

Galindo, A., Krnjević, K., and Schwartz, S. (1967): Micro-iontophoretic studies on
neurones in the cuneate nucleus. *J. Physiol.* 192:359-377.

Gallup, B. and Dubowitz, V. (1973): Failure of "dystrophic" neurones to support
functional regeneration of normal or dystrophic muscle in culture. *Nature*
243:287-289.

Garcia, J., Pierce, R.S., Albuquerque, E.X., Deshpande, S.S., and Warnick, J.E.   231
(1975): Axonal changes in rat spinal cord induced by batrachotoxin. *In:*
Symposium on Nerve Growth Factor. (Sixth International Congress of
Pharmacology, Helsinki, Finland, July 20-25.) New York: Pergamon Press,
p. 36. (Abstr.)

Gaze, R.M. (1970): *The Formation of Nerve Connections.* New York: Academic
Press.

Geffen, L.B., Livett, B.G., and Rush, R.A. (1970): Immunohistochemical locali-   276
zation of chromogranins in sheep sympathetic neurones and their release by
nerve impulses. *In: New Aspects of Storage and Release Mechanisms of*
Catecholamines. (Bayer Symposium II.) Schümann, H.J. and Kroneberg, G.,
eds. Berlin: Springer-Verlag, pp. 58-72.

Geffen, L.B. and Rush, R.A. (1968): Transport of noradrenaline in sympathetic   307
nerves and the effect of nerve impulses on its contribution to transmitter stores.
J. Neurochem. 15:925-930.

Gelfan, S. (1975): Denervation and neuronal interdependence. *In: Advances in*   357
Neurology, Vol. 12. Physiology and Pathology of Dendrites. Kreutzberg, G.W.,
ed. New York: Raven Press, pp. 425-438.

Gewirtz, G.P. and Kopin, I.J. (1970): Release of dopamine-beta-hydroxylase with   276
norepinephrine during cat splenic nerve stimulation. *Nature* 227:406-407.

Ghetti, B., Horoupian, D.S., and Wiśniewski, H.M. (1975): Acute and long-term   357
transneuronal response of dendrites of lateral geniculate neurons following
transection of the primary visual afferent pathway. *In: Advances in Neurology,*
Vol. 12. Physiology and Pathology of Dendrites. Kreutzberg, G.W., ed. New
York: Raven Press, pp. 401-424.

Giller, E.L., Jr., Schrier, B.K., Shainberg, A., Fisk, H.R., and Nelson, P.G. (1973): Choline acetyltransferase activity is increased in combined cultures of spinal cord and muscle cells from mice. *Science* 182:588-589.   294,322, 325

Gilliatt, R.W., Hopf, H.C., Rudge, P., and Baraitser, M. (1974): The range of conduction velocity in motor fibres to a single muscle. *Excerpta Med. Int. Congr. Series* 334:133. (Abstr.)   354

Gilman, A.G. and Nirenberg, M. (1971a): Effect of catecholamines on the adenosine 3′:5′-cyclic monophosphate concentrations of clonal satellite cells of neurons. *Proc. Nat. Acad. Sci.* 68:2165-2168.   322

Gilman, A.G. and Nirenberg, M. (1971b): Regulation of adenosine 3′,5′-cyclic monophosphate metabolism in cultured neuroblastoma cells. *Nature* 234: 356-358.   322

Gilman, A.G. and Schrier, B.K. (1972): Adenosine cyclic 3′,5′-monophosphate in fetal rat brain cell cultures. I. Effect of catecholamines. *Mol. Pharmacol.* 8:410-416.   322

Globus, A., Lux, H.D., and Schubert, P. (1968): Somatodendritic spread of intracellularly injected glycine in cat spinal motoneurons. *Brain Res.* 11:440-445.   282,283

Globus, A., Lux, H.D., and Schubert, P. (1973): Transfer of amino acids between neuroglia cells and neurons in the leech ganglion. *Exp. Neurol.* 40:104:113.   287,323

Goddard, G.V. (1967): Development of epileptic seizures through brain stimulation at low intensity. *Nature* 214:1020-1021.   365

Goddard, G.V. (1972): Long term alteration following amygdaloid stimulation. *In: The Neurobiology of the Amygdala.* Eleftheriou, B.E., ed. New York: Plenum Press, pp. 581-596.   365

Goodman, R., Otten, U., and Thoenen, H. (1975): Organ culture of the rat adrenal medulla: A model system for the study of trans-synaptic enzyme induction. *J. Neurochem.* 25:423-427.   315,316

Goracci, G., Blomstrand, C., Arienti, G., Hamberger, A., and Porcellati, G. (1973): Base-exchange enzymic system for the synthesis of phospholipids in neuronal and glial cells and their subfractions: A possible marker for neuronal membranes. *J. Neurochem.* 20:1167-1180.

Grafstein, B. (1971): Transneuronal transfer of radioactivity in the central nervous system. *Science* 172:177-179.   276

Grafstein, B. (1975): Principles of anterograde axonal transport in relation to studies of neuronal connectivity. *In: The Use of Axonal Transport for Studies of Neuronal Connectivity.* Cowan, W.M. and Cuénod, M., eds. New York: Elsevier, pp. 47-67.   276

Grafstein, B. and Laureno, R. (1973): Transport of radioactivity from eye to visual cortex in the mouse. *Exp. Neurol.* 39:44-57.   276,279, 280,356

Grafstein, B. and Murray, M. (1969): Transport of protein in goldfish optic nerve during regeneration. *Exp. Neurol.* 25:494-508.   308

Grafstein, B., Murray, M., and Ingoglia, N. (1972): Axonal transport of protein in optic system of mice lacking visual receptors. *Brain Res.* 44:37-48.   307

Page

Greene, L.A., Sytkowski, A.J., Vogel, Z., and Nirenberg, M.W. (1973): α-Bungar-   404
otoxin used as a probe for acetylcholine receptors of cultured neurons. *Nature*
243:163-166.

Greengard, P. (1975): Cyclic nucleotides, protein phosphorylation, and neuronal   378,381
function. *Adv. Cyclic Nucleotide Res.* 5:585-601.

Greengard, P. (1976): Possible role for cyclic nucleotides and phosphorylated
membrane proteins in postsynaptic actions of neurotransmitters. *Nature*
260:101-108.

Greengard, P. and Kebabian, J.W. (1974): Role of cyclic AMP in synaptic   378,381
transmission in the mammalian peripheral nervous system. *Fed. Proc.*
33:1059-1066.

Greengard, P., Nathanson, J.A., and Kebabian, J.W. (1973): Dopamine-, octopa-
mine-, and serotonin-sensitive adenylate cyclases: possible receptors in aminergic
neurotransmission. *In: Frontiers in Catecholamine Research.* Usdin, E. and
Snyder, S.H., eds. New York: Pergamon Press, pp. 377-382.

Guidotti, A. and Costa, E. (1973): Involvement of adenosine 3',5'-monophosphate   391
in the activation of tyrosine hydroxylase elicited by drugs. *Science*
179:902-904.

Guidotti, A. and Costa, E. (1974): A role for nicotinic receptors in the regulation   391
of the adenylate cyclase of adrenal medulla. *J. Pharmacol. Exp. Ther.*
189:665-675.

Guidotti, A., Kurosawa, A., Chuang, D.M., and Costa, E. (1975): Protein kinase   392
activation as an early event in the trans-synaptic induction of tyrosine
3-monooxygenase in adrenal medulla. *Proc. Nat. Acad. Sci.* 72:1152-1156.

Guidotti, A., Mao, C.C., and Costa, E. (1973a): Transsynaptic regulation of   390,391
tyrosine hydroxylase in adrenal medulla: possible role of cyclic nucleotides. *In:*
Frontiers in Catecholamine Research. Usdin, E. and Snyder, S.H., eds. New
York: Pergamon Press, pp. 231-236.

Guidotti, A., Zivkovic, B., Pfeiffer, R., and Costa, E. (1973b): Involvement of   316,391
3',5'-cyclic adenosine monophosphate in the increase of tyrosine hydroxylase
activity elicited by cold exposure. *Naunyn-Schmiedebergs Arch. Pharmakol.*
278:195-206.

Guth, L. (1958): Taste buds on the cat's circumvallate papilla after reinnervation   219
by glossopharyngeal, vagus, and hypoglossal nerves. *Anat. Rec.* 130:25-37.

Guth, L. (1969): "Trophic" effects of vertebrate neurons. *Neurosciences Res. Prog.* 218,220,
Bull. 7:1-73. Also *In: Neurosciences Research Symposium Summaries, Vol. 4.*   225,259,
Schmitt, F.O. et al., eds. Cambridge, Mass.: M.I.T. Press, 1970, pp. 327-396.   399,403

Guth, L. (1971a): Degeneration and regeneration of taste buds. *In: Handbook of*   219
Sensory Physiology, Vol. IV. Chemical Senses. Part 2. Taste. Beidler, L.M., ed.
New York: Springer-Verlag, pp. 63-74.

Guth, L. (1971b): A review of the evidence for the neural regulation of gene
expression in muscle. *In: Contractility of Muscle Cells and Related Processes.*
Podolsky, R.J., ed. Englewood Cliffs, N.J.: Prentice-Hall, Inc., pp. 189-201.

Guth, L. (1972): Regulation of metabolic and functional properties of muscle. *In:*
Regulation of Organ and Tissue Growth. New York: Academic Press, pp. 61-75.

Page

Guth, L. (1974a): Axonal regeneration and functional plasticity in the central   317
nervous system. *Exp. Neurol.* 45:606-654.

Guth, L. (1974b): "Trophic" functions. *In: The Peripheral Nervous System.*   219,225,
Hubbard, J.I., ed. New York: Plenum Press, pp. 329-343.   236

Guth, L. and Bernstein, J.J. (1961): Selectivity in the re-establishment of synapses
in the superior cervical sympathetic ganglion of the cat. *Exp. Neurol.* 4:59-69.

Guth, L. and Wells, J.B. (1972): Physiological and histochemical properties of the   236
soleus muscle after denervation of its antagonists. *Exp. Neurol.* 36:463-471.

Guth, L. and Yellin, H. (1971): The dynamic nature of the so-called "fiber types"
of mammalian skeletal muscle. *Exp. Neurol.* 31:277-300.

Haas, D.C., Hier, D.B., Arnason, B.G.W., and Young, M. (1972): On a possible   396
relationship of cyclic AMP to the mechanism of action of nerve growth factor.
Proc. Soc. Exp. Biol. Med. 140:45-47.

Halperin, J.J. and LaVail, J.H. (1975): A study of the dynamics of retrograde   302,303,
transport and accumulation of horseradish peroxidase in injured neurons. *Brain*   308
Res. 100:253-269.

Hamburger, V. (1934): The effects of wing bud extirpation on the development of   222,294,
the central nervous system in chick embryos. *J. Exp. Zool.* 68:449-494.   336

Hamburger, V. (1948): The mitotic patterns in the spinal cord of the chick embryo   294
and their relation to histogenetic processes. *J. Comp. Neurol.* 88:221-283.

Hamburger, V. (1958): Regression versus peripheral control of differentiation in 294,297
motor hypoplasia. *Am. J. Anat.* 102:365-408.

Hamburger, V. (1975): Cell death in the development of the lateral motor column   297
of the chick embryo. *J. Comp. Neurol.* 160:535-546.

Hámori, J. (1973a): Developmental morphology of dendritic postsynaptic speciali-   369
zations. *In: Recent Developments of Neurobiology in Hungary, Vol. IV. Results*
in Neuroanatomy, Neuroendocrinology, Neurophysiology and Behaviour,
Neuropathology. Lissák, K., ed. Budapest: Akadémiai Kiadó, pp. 9-32.

Hámori, J. (1973b): The inductive role of presynaptic axons in the development of   369
postsynaptic spines. *Brain Res.* 62:337-344.

Hanna, R.B., Hirano, A., and Pappas, G.D. (1976): Membrane specializations of   369
dendritic spines and glia in the weaver mouse cerebellum: A freeze-fracture
study. *J. Cell Biol.* 68:403-410.

Harris, A.J., Kuffler, S.W., and Dennis, M.J. (1971): Differential chemosensitivity
of synaptic and extrasynaptic areas on the neuronal surface membrane in
parasympathetic neurons of the frog, tested by microapplication of acetylcholine. *Proc. R. Soc. B* 177:541-553.

Harris, G.W. (1970): Hormonal differentiation of the developing central nervous   312
system with respect to patterns of endocrine function. *Phil. Trans. R. Soc. B*
259:165-176.

Harris, G.W. and Campbell, H.J. (1966): The regulation of the secretion of   309
luteinizing hormone and ovulation. *In: The Pituitary Gland, Vol. 2.* Harris, G.W.
and Donovan, B.T., eds. Berkeley, Calif.: University of California Press,
pp. 99-165.

Page

Harvey, J.E. and Srebnik, H.H. (1967): Locomotor activity and axon regeneration   317
following spinal cord compression in rats treated with L-thyroxine. *J.
Neuropathol. Exp. Neurol.* 26:661-668.

Hawken, M.J., Bray, J.J., and Hubbard, J.I. (1974): Evidence for a soluble trophic   226
factor affecting muscle fibre resting potential. *Proc. Univ. Otago Med. School*
52:17-18.

Hayes, B.P. and Roberts, A. (1973): Synaptic junction development in the spinal
cord of an amphibian embryo: An electron microscope study. *Z. Zellforsch.
Mikrosk. Anat.* 137:251-269.

Heacock, A.M. and Agranoff, B.W. (1975): Axonal transport of unincorporated   280
³H-proline and its release from labeled protein both contribute to transneuronally labeled protein. *In: Neuroscience Abstracts, Vol. I.* (Fifth Annual Meeting
of the Society for Neuroscience, New York City, Nov. 2-6, 1975.) P. 796.

Hedqvist, P. (1973): Prostaglandin as a tool for local control of transmitter release   320
from sympathetic nerves. *Brain Res.* 62:483-488.

Heidenhain, R.P.H. (1878): Uber secretorische und trophische Drüsen-nerven.   218,219
Pfluegers Arch. Physiol. 17:1-67.

Heimer, L. and Nauta, W.J.H. (1969): The hypothalamic distribution of the stria   310
terminalis in the rat. *Brain Res.* 13:284-297.

Hendry, I.A. (1975a): The effects of axotomy on the development of the rat   268
superior cervical ganglion. *Brain Res.* 90:235-244.

Hendry, I.A. (1975b): The response of adrenergic neurones to axotomy and nerve   268
growth factor. *Brain Res.* 94:87-97.

Hendry, I.A. (1975c): The retrograde trans-synaptic control of the development of
cholinergic terminals in sympathetic ganglia. *Brain Res.* 86:483-487.

Hendry, I.A. and Iversen, L.L. (1973): Reduction in the concentration of nerve   294
growth factor in mice after sialectomy and castration. *Nature* 243:500-504.

Hendry, I.A., Stöckel, K., Thoenen, H., and Iversen, L.L. (1974): The retrograde   262
axonal transport of nerve growth factor. *Brain Res.* 68:103-121.

Henn, F.A., Goldstein, M.N., and Hamberger, A. (1974): Uptake of the   322
neurotransmitter candidate glutamate by glia. *Nature* 249:663-664.

Henrikson, C.K. and Vaughn, J.E. (1974): Fine structural relationships between   322
neurites and radial glial processes in developing mouse spinal cord. *J.
Neurocytol.* 3:659-675.

Hermann, A., Rieske, E., Kreutzberg, G.W., and Lux, H.D. (1975): Transjunctional   290,291
flux of radioactive precursors across electrotonic synapses between lateral giant
axons of the crayfish. *Brain Res.* 95:125-131.

Herndon, R.M., Margolis, G., and Kilham, L. (1971): The synaptic organization of   367
the malformed cerebellum induced by perinatal infection with the feline
panleukopenia virus (PLV). II. The Purkinje cell and its afferents. *J. Neuropathol. Exp. Neurol.* 30:557-580.

Herrup, K. and Shooter, E.M. (1975): Properties of the β-nerve growth factor   270
receptor in development. *J. Cell Biol.* 67:118-125.

Page

Hier, D.B., Arnason, B.G.W., and Young, M. (1972): Studies on the mechanism of   385,396,
action of nerve growth factor. *Proc. Nat. Acad. Sci.* 69:2268-2272.   397

Hier, D.B., Arnason, B.G.W., and Young, M. (1973): Nerve growth factor: 385,396
Relationship to the cyclic AMP system of sensory ganglia. *Science* 182:79-81.

Hines, J.F., Garwood, M.M., and Forsyth, L.A. (1974): In vitro release of protein   276
from axons during rapid axonal transport. *In: Program and Abstracts, Society
for Neuroscience, Fourth Annual Meeting,* St. Louis, Missouri, p. 257.

Hirano, A. (1972): Cytochemical observations of weaver mouse cerebellum. *In:*   369
*Proceedings of the Fourth International Congress of Histochemistry and
Cytochemistry.* Takeuchi, T., Ogawa, K., and Fugita, S., eds. Kyoto, Japan:
Japan Society of Histochemistry and Cytochemistry, pp. 513-514.

Hirano, A. and Dembitzer, H.M. (1973): Cerebellar alterations in the weaver mouse.   367,369
J. Cell Biol. 56:478-486.

Hirano, A. and Dembitzer, H.M. (1974): Observations on the development of the   369,370
weaver mouse cerebellum. *J. Neuropathol. Exp. Neurol.* 33:354-364.

Hirano, A. and Dembitzer, H.M. (1975a): Aberrant development of the Purkinje   371
cell dendritic spine. *In: Advances in Neurology, Vol. 12. Physiology and
Pathology of Dendrites.* Kreutzberg, G.W., ed. New York: Raven Press,
pp. 353-360.

Hirano, A. and Dembitzer, H.M. (1975b): The fine structure of staggerer   370
cerebellum. *J. Neuropathol. Exp. Neurol.* 34:1-11.

Hirano, A., Dembitzer, H.M., Ghatak, N.R., Fan, K.-J., and Zimmerman, H.M.   372
(1973): On the relationship between human and experimental granule cell type
cerebellar degeneration. *J. Neuropathol. Exp. Neurol.* 32:493-502.

Hirano, A., Dembitzer, H.M., and Jones, M. (1972): An electron microscopic study   367,368
of cycasin-induced cerebellar alterations. *J. Neuropathol. Exp. Neurol.*
31:113-125.

Hirano, A. and Jones, M. (1972): Fine structure of cycasin-induced cerebellar   367
alterations. *Fed. Proc.* 31:1517-1519.

Hirano, A. and Zimmerman, H.M. (1973): Aberrant synaptic development.   366,369
A review. *Arch. Neurol.* 28:359-366.

Hironaka, T. and Miyata, Y. (1975): Transplantation of skeletal muscle in normal
and dystrophic mice. *Exp. Neurol.* 47:1-15.

Hoffer, B.J., Siggins, G.R., and Bloom, F.E. (1971a): Studies on norepinephrine-   377
containing afferents to Purkinje cells of rat cerebellum. II. Sensitivity of
Purkinje cells to norepinephrine and related substances administered by
microiontophoresis. *Brain Res.* 25:523-534.

Hoffer, B.J., Siggins, G.R., Oliver, A.P., and Bloom, F.E. (1971b): Cyclic AMP   377
mediation of norepinephrine inhibition in rat cerebellar cortex: A unique class
of synaptic responses. *Ann. N.Y. Acad. Sci.* 185:531-549.

Hoffer, B.J., Siggins, G.R., Oliver, A.P., and Bloom, F.E. (1972): Cyclic adenosine   377
monophosphate mediated adrenergic synapses to cerebellar Purkinje cells. *Adv.
Cyclic Nucleotide Res.* 1:411-423.

Hoffer, B.J., Siggins, G.R., Oliver, A.P., and Bloom, F.E. (1973): Activation of the pathway from locus coeruleus to rat cerebellar Purkinje neurons: pharmacological evidence of noradrenergic central inhibition. *J. Pharmacol. Exp. Ther.* 184:553-569.

Hoffer, B.J., Siggins, G.R., Woodward, D.J., and Bloom, F.E. (1971c): Spontaneous   377
discharge of Purkinje neurons after destruction of catecholamine-containing afferents by 6-hydroxydopamine. *Brain Res.* 30:425-430.

Hofmann, W.W. and Peacock, J.H. (1973): Postjunctional changes induced by partial interruption of axoplasmic flow in motor nerves. *Exp. Neurol.* 41:345-356.

Hofmann, W.W., Peacock, J.H., and Forno, L.S. (1975): Studies on neuromuscular responses to long-term axonal colchicine treatment. *Exp. Neurol.* 46:355-367.

Hoffmann, W.W. and Thesleff, S. (1972): Studies on the trophic influence of nerve on skeletal muscle. *Eur. J. Pharmacol.* 20:256-260.

Hogan, P.M. and Albuquerque, E.X. (1971): The pharmacology of batrachotoxin.   231
III. Effect on the heart Purkinje fibers. *J. Pharmacol. Exp. Ther.* 176:529-537.

Hökfelt, T., Efendic, S., Johansson, O., Luft, R., and Arimura, A. (1974):   318
Immunohistochemical localization of somatostatin (growth hormone release-inhibiting factor) in the guinea pig brain. *Brain Res.* 80:165-169.

Hökfelt, T., Fuxe, K., Johansson, O., Jeffcoate, S., and White, N. (1975): Thyrotropin releasing hormone (TRH)-containing nerve terminals in certain brain stem nuclei and in the spinal cord. *Neurosciences Lett.* 1:133-139.

Hökfelt, T., Meyerson, B., Nilsson, G., Pernow, B., and Sachs, C. (1976):   319
Immunohistochemical evidence for substance P-containing nerve endings in the human cortex. *Brain Res.* 104:181-186.

Holtzman, E., Novikoff, A.B., and Villaverde, H. (1967): Lysosomes and GERL in   305
normal and chromatolytic neurons of the rat ganglion nodosum. *J. Cell Biol.* 33:419-435.

Hooisma, J., Slaaf, D.W., Meeter, E., and Stevens, W.F. (1975): The innervation of chick striated muscle fibers by the chick ciliary ganglion in tissue culture. *Brain Res.* 85:79-85.

Hornykiewicz, O. (1972): Neurochemistry of parkinsonism. *In: Handbook of*   363
Neurochemistry, Vol. 7. Lajtha, A., ed. New York: Plenum Press, pp. 465-501.

Hornykiewicz, O., Lloyd, K.G., and Davidson, L. (1976): The GABA system,   359,363
function of the basal ganglia, and Parkinson's disease. *In: GABA in Nervous System Function.* (Kroc Foundation Series, Vol. 5.) Roberts, E., Chase, T.N., and Tower, D.B., eds. New York: Raven Press, pp. 479-485.

Hsie, A.W. and Puck, T.T. (1971): Morphological transformation of Chinese   396
hamster cells by dibutyryl adenosine cyclic 3':5'-monophosphate and testosterone. *Proc. Nat. Acad. Sci.* 68:358-361.

Hubel, D. (1975): An autoradiographic study of the retino-cortical projections in   280
the tree shrew *(Tupaia glis). Brain Res.* 96:41-50.

Hubel, D.H., LeVay, S., and Wiesel, T.N. (1975): Mode of termination of   346
retinotectal fibers in macaque monkey: an autoradiographic study. *Brain Res.* 96:25-40.

Neurosciences Res. Prog. Bull., Vol. 14, No. 3   429

Page

Hughes, A. (1961): Cell degeneration in the larval ventral horn of *Xenopus laevus*   294,297
(Daudin). *J. Embryol. Exp. Morphol.* 9:269-284.

Hughes, A. and Tschumi, P.A. (1958): The factors controlling the development of   294
the dorsal root ganglia and ventral horn in *Xenopus laevis* (Daudin). *J. Anat.*
92:498-527.

Hughes, J., Smith, T.W., Kosterlitz, H.W., Fothergill, L.A., Morgan, B.A., and   320
Morris, H.R. (1975): Identification of two related pentapeptides from the brain
with potent opiate agonist activity. *Nature* 258:577-579.

Hydén, H. (1967): Biochemical changes accompanying learning. *In: The Neuro-*   322
sciences: A Study Program. Quarton, G.C., Melnechuk, T., and Schmitt, F.O.,
eds. New York: Rockefeller University Press, pp. 765-771.

Illis, L.S. (1973a): Experimental model of regeneration in the central nervous
system. I. Synaptic changes. *Brain* 96:47-60.

Illis, L.S. (1973b): Experimental model of regeneration in the central nervous   322
system. II. The reaction of glia in the synaptic zone. *Brain* 96:61-68.

Ingoglia, N.A., Grafstein, B., and McEwen, B.S. (1974): Effect of actinomycin-D on   282
labelled material in the retina and optic tectum of goldfish after intraocular
injection of tritiated RNA precursors. *J. Neurochem.* 23:681-687.

Ingoglia, N.A., Grafstein, B., McEwen, B.S., and McQuarrie, I.G. (1973): Axonal
transport of radioactivity in the goldfish optic system following intraocular
injection of labelled RNA precursors. *J. Neurochem.* 20:1605-1615.

Ingvar, D.H. (1973): Cerebral blood flow and metabolism in complete apallic   390
syndromes, in states of severe dementia, and in akinetic mutism. *Acta Neurol.*
Scand. 49:233-244.

Ingvar, D.H. (1974): Regional cerebral blood flow in organic dementia and in   390
chronic schizophrenia. *Triangle* 13:17-23.

Iversen, L.L., Stöckel, K., and Thoenen, H. (1975): Autoradiographic studies of the   262
retrograde axonal transport of nerve growth factor in mouse sympathetic
neurones. *Brain Res.* 88:37-43.

Jacobowitz, D.M. and Greene, L.A. (1974): Histofluorescence study of chromaffin
cells in dissociated cell cultures of chick embryo .sympathetic ganglia. *J.*
Neurobiol. 5:65-83.

Jacobson, K. and Papahadjopoulos, D. (1975): Phase transitions and phase   409
separations in phospholipid membranes induced by changes in temperature, pH,
and concentration of bivalent cations. *Biochemistry* 14:152-161.

James, N.T. and Meek, G.A. (1975): Ultrastructure of muscle spindles in dystrophic
mice. *Nature* 254:612-613.

Jankowska, E., Lubińska, L., and Niemierko, S. (1969): Translocation of   307
AChE-containing particles in the axoplasm during nerve activity. *Comp.*
Biochem. Physiol. 28:907-913.

Jansson, S.-E., Albuquerque, E.X., and Daly, J. (1974): The pharmacology of   232
batrachotoxin. VI. Effects on the mammalian motor nerve terminal. *J.*
Pharmacol. Exp. Ther. 189:525-537.

  Page

Jean, D.H., Guth, L., and Albers, R.W. (1973): Neural regulation of the structure of   236
myosin. *Exp. Neurol.* 38:458-471.

Jellinger, K. and Jirásek, A. (1971): Neuroaxonal dystrophy in man: character and   364
natural history. *Acta Neuropathol.* 5(Suppl. 5):3-16.

Johnson, E.M., Ueda, T., Maeno, H., and Greengard, P. (1972): Adenosine   381
3',5'-monophosphate-dependent phosphorylation of a specific protein in synaptic membrane fractions from rat cerebrum. *J. Biol. Chem.* 247:5650-5652.

Johnson, G.S., Friedman, R.M., and Pastan, I. (1971): Restoration of several   396
morphological characteristics of normal fibroblasts in sarcoma cells treated with
adenosine-3':5'-cyclic monophosphate and its derivatives. *Proc. Nat. Acad. Sci.*
68:425-429.

Johnston, B.T., Schramek, J.E., and Mark, R.F. (1975): Re-innervation of axolotl   342
limbs. II. Sensory nerves. *Proc. R. Soc. B* 190:59-75.

Jones, D.P. and Singer, M. (1969): Neurotrophic dependence of the lateral-line   281
sensory organs of the newt, *Triturus viridescens. J. Exp. Zool.* 171:433-442.

Jones, R. and Vrbová, G. (1974): Two factors responsible for the development of
denervation hypersensitivity. *J. Physiol.* 236:517-538.

Kalix, P., McAfee, D.A., Schorderet, M., and Greengard, P. (1974): Pharmacological
analysis of synaptically mediated increase in cyclic adenosine monophosphate in
rabbit superior cervical ganglion. *J. Pharmacol. Exp. Ther.* 188:676-687.

Kato, M., Ueno, H., and Black, P. (1974): Regional cerebral blood flow of the main   389
visual pathways during photic stimulation of the retina in intact and split-brain
monkeys. *Exp. Neurol.* 42:65-77.

Kauffman, F.C., Warnick, J.E., and Albuquerque, E.X. (1974): Uptake of [^{3}H]-   228
colchicine from silastic implants by mammalian nerves and muscles. *Exp.*
Neurol. 44:404-416.

Kebabian, J.W., Steiner, A.L., and Greengard, P. (1975): Muscarinic cholinergic
regulation of cyclic guanosine 3',5'-monophosphate in autonomic ganglia:
possible role in synaptic transmission. *J. Pharmacol. Exp. Ther.* 193:474-488.

Keen, P. and McLean, W.G. (1974): The effect of nerve stimulation on the axonal
transport of noradrenaline and dopamine-β-hydroxylase. *Br. J. Pharmacol.*
52:527-531.

Kelly, J.P. and Van Essen, D.C. (1974): Cell structure and function in the visual   322
cortex of the cat. *J. Physiol.* 238:515-547.

Kennedy, C., Des Rosiers, M.H., Jehle, J.W., Reivich, M., Sharpe, F., and Sokoloff,   405
L. (1975): Mapping of functional neural pathways by autoradiographic survey
of local metabolic rate with [^{14}C] deoxyglucose. *Science* 187:850-853.

Kerkut, G.A., Shapira, A., and Walker, R.J. (1967): The transport of ^{14}C-labelled   307
material from CNS to and from muscle along a nerve trunk. *Comp. Biochem.*
Physiol. 23:729-748.

Kiernan, J.A. and Rawcliffe, P.M. (1971): Effects of triiodothyronine on the   317
cerebellar cortex of the new-born rat in tissue culture. *Experientia* 27:678-679.

Page

Kim, S.V. (1975): Formation of unattached spines of Purkinje cell dendrite in   370
organotypic culture of mouse cerebellum. *Brain Res.* 88:52-58.

Kirkland, W.L. and Burton, P.R. (1972): Cyclic adenosine monophosphate-   397
mediated stabilization of mouse neuroblastoma cell neuritis microtubules
exposed to low temperature. *Nature New Biol.* 240:205-207.

Komiya, Y. and Austin, L. (1974): Axoplasmic flow of protein in the sciatic nerve
of normal and dystrophic mice. *Exp. Neurol.* 43:1-12.

Komiya, Y. and Austin, L. (1975): Axoplasmic flow of protein in the sciatic nerve
of mice with experimentally induced myopathy. *Exp. Neurol.* 47:307-315.

Konishi, S. and Otsuka, M. (1974): The effects of substance P and other peptides   319
on spinal neurons of the frog. *Brain Res.* 65:397-410.

Korr, I.M. and Appeltauer, G.S.L. (1974): The time-course of axonal transport of   276
neuronal proteins to muscle. *Exp. Neurol.* 43:452-463.

Korr, I.M., Wilkinson, P.N., and Chornock, F.W. (1967): Axonal delivery of
neuroplasmic components to muscle cells. *Science* 155:342-345.

Kreuger, B.K., Forn, J., and Greengard, P. (1975): Dopamine-sensitive adenylate
cyclase and protein phosphorylation in the rat caudate nucleus. *In: Modern
Pharmacology-Toxicology, Vol. 3. Pre- and Postsynaptic Receptors.* Usdin, E.
and Bunney, W., Jr., eds. New York: Marcel Dekker, pp. 123-147.

Kreutzberg, G.W., ed. (1975): *Advances in Neurology, Vol. 12. Physiology and
Pathology of Dendrites.* New York: Raven Press.

Kreutzberg, G.W. and Kaiya, H. (1974): Exogenous acetylcholinesterase as tracer   286
for extracellular pathways in the brain. *Histochemie* 42:233-237.

Kreutzberg, G.W. and Schubert, P. (1971): Changes in axonal flow during
regeneration of mammalian motor nerves. *Acta Neuropathol.* 5(Suppl. 5):70-75.

Kreutzberg, G.W. and Schubert, P. (1975): The cellular dynamics of intraneuronal   282,283,
transport. *In: The Use of Axonal Transport for Studies of Neuronal Connec-*   285,308,
tivity. Cowan, W.M. and Cuénod, M., eds. New York: Elsevier, pp. 83-112.   359,387

Kreutzberg, G.W., Schubert, P., and Lux, H.D. (1975a): Neuroplasmic transport in   283,284,
axons and dendrites. *In: Golgi Centennial Symposium: Perspectives in Neuro-*   359
biology. Santini, M., ed. New York: Raven Press, pp. 161-166.

Kreutzberg, G.W., Schubert, P, Tóth, L., and Rieske, E. (1973): Intradendritic   283
transport to postsynaptic sites. *Brain Res.* 62:399-404.

Kreutzberg, G.W. and Tóth, L. (1974): Dendritic secretion: a way for the neuron to 286
communicate with the vasculature. *Naturwissenschaften* 61:37.

Kreutzberg, G.W., Tóth, L., and Kaiya, H. (1975b): Acetylcholinesterase as marker 283,287
for dendritic transport and dendritic secretion. *In: Advances in Neurology,
Vol. 12. Physiology and Pathology of Dendrites.* Kreutzberg, G.W., ed. New
York: Raven Press, pp. 269-287.

Kristensson, K., Ghetti, B., and Wiśniewski, H.M. (1974): Study on the propagation
of *Herpes simplex* virus (type 2) into the brain after intraocular injection. *Brain
Res.* 69:189-201.

Kristensson, K. and Olsson, Y. (1974): Retrograde transport of horseradish peroxidase in transected axons. I. Time relationships between transport and induction of chromatolysis. *Brain Res.* 79:101-110.

Kristensson, K. and Olsson, Y. (1975): Retrograde transport of horseradish peroxidase in transected axons. II. Relations between rate of transfer from the site of injury to the perikaryon and onset of chromatolysis. *J. Neurocytol.* 4:653-661.   302

Kristensson, K., Olsson, Y., and Sourander, P. (1974): Virus encephalitis: pathogenesis in the immature brain. *Dev. Med. Child Neurol.* 16:382-394.

Kristensson, K. and Sjöstrand, J. (1972): Retrograde transport of protein tracer in the rabbit hypoglossal nerve during regeneration. *Brain Res.* 45:175-181.

Krnjević, K. and Morris, M.E. (1974): An excitatory action of substance P on cuneate neurones. *Can. J. Physiol. Pharmacol.* 52:736-744.

Krygier-Brévart, V., Weiss, D.G., Mehl, E., Schubert, P., and Kreutzberg, G.W.   260,282
(1974): Maintenance of synaptic membranes by the fast axonal flow. *Brain Res.* 77:97-110.

Kuffler, S.W., Dennis, M.J., and Harris, A.J. (1971): The development of chemosensitivity in extrasynaptic areas of the neuronal surface after denervation of parasympathetic ganglion cells in the heart of the frog. *Proc. R. Soc. B* 177:555-563.

Künzle, H. (1975): Notes on the application of radioactive amino acids for the tracing of neuronal connections. *Brain Res.* 85:267-271.

Kupfer, C. and Downer, J.C. (1967): Ribonucleic acid content and metabolic   360
activity of lateral geniculate nucleus in monkey following afferent denervation. *J. Neurochem.* 14:257-263.

Kupfer, C. and Palmer, P. (1964): Lateral geniculate nucleus: Histological and   360
cytochemical changes following afferent denervation and visual deprivation. *Exp. Neurol.* 9:400-409.

Lake, N. and Jordan, L.M. (1974): Failure to confirm cyclic AMP as second   377
messenger for norepinephrine in rat cerebellum. *Science* 183:663-664.

Lake, N., Jordan, L.M., and Phillis, J.W. (1972): Mechanism of noradrenaline action 377
in cat cerebral cortex. *Nature New Biol.* 240:249-250.

Lake, N., Jordan, L.M., and Phillis, J.W. (1973): Evidence against cyclic adenosine 377
3',5'-monophosphate (AMP) mediation of noradrenaline depression of cerebral cortical neurones. *Brain Res.* 60:411-421.

Landis, D. (1971): Cerebellar cortical development in the staggerer mutant mouse.   370
In: Program and Abstracts, American Society for Cell Biology, 11th Annual Meeting. New Orleans, La, p. 159.

Landis, D.M. and Sidman, R.L. (1974): Cerebellar cortical development in the   370
staggerer mouse. *J. Neuropathol. Exp. Neurol.* 33:180. (Abstr.)

Landmesser, L. (1972): Pharmacological properties, cholinesterase activity and   235
anatomy of nerve-muscle junctions in vagus-innervated frog sartorius. *J. Physiol.* 220:243-256.

Neurosciences Res. Prog. Bull., Vol. 14, No. 3 433

Page

Landmesser, L. and Pilar, G. (1972): The onset and development of transmission in   295
the chick ciliary ganglion. *J. Physiol.* 222:691-713.

Landmesser, L. and Pilar, G. (1974a): Synapse formation during embryogenesis on   294,295,
ganglion cells lacking a periphery. *J. Physiol.* 241:715-736.   296,297

Landmesser, L. and Pilar, G. (1974b): Synaptic transmission and cell death during   294,295
normal ganglionic development. *J. Physiol.* 241:737-749.

Landmesser, L. and Pilar, G. (1976): Fate of ganglionic synapses and ganglion cell   297,299,
axons during normal and induced cell death. *J. Cell Biol.* 68:357-374.   300

Lapa, A.J., Albuquerque, E.X., and Daly, J. (1974): An electrophysiological study
of the effects of d-tubocurarine, atropine, and α-bungarotoxin on the
cholinergic receptor in innervated and chronically denervated mammalian
skeletal muscles. *Exp. Neurol.* 43:375-398.

Lapresle, J. and Hamida, M.B. (1970): The dentato-olivary pathway. Somatotopic
relationship between the dentate nucleus and the contralateral inferior olive.
Arch. Neurol. 22:135-143.

Larramendi, L.M.H. (1969): Analysis of synaptogenesis in cerebellum of the mouse.   369
In: Neurobiology of Cerebellar Evolution and Development. Llinás, R.R., ed.
Chicago: American Medical Association/Education and Research Foundation,
pp. 803-843.

Lasek, R.J. (1968): Axoplasmic transport in cat dorsal root ganglion cells as studied 274
with [^{3}H]-ℓ-leucine. *Brain Res.* 7:360-377.

Lasek, R.J., Gainer, H., and Przybylski, R.J. (1974): Transfer of newly synthesized   323
proteins from Schwann cells to the squid giant axon. *Proc. Nat. Acad. Sci.*
71:1188-1192.

Lashkov, V.F. (1945): On the trophic action of the glossopharyngeal nerve. *Bull.*   219
Acad. Sci. USSR 3:273-285.

LaVail, J.H. and LaVail, M.M. (1974): The retrograde intraaxonal transport of   302
horseradish peroxidase in the chick visual system: a light and electron
microscopic study. *J. Comp. Neurol.* 157:303-358.

LaVail, M.M. and LaVail, J.H. (1975): Retrograde intraaxonal transport of
horseradish peroxidase in retinal ganglion cells of the chick. *Brain Res.*
85:273-280.

LaVail, M.M. and Mullen, R.J. (1975): Studies on the etiology of inherited retinal   248
degeneration in mice and rats using experimental chimeras. *Jap. J. Ophthalmol.*
19:223-224. (Abstr.)

LaVail, M.M. and Mullen, R.J. (1976): Role of the pigment epithelium in inherited   248,404
retinal degeneration analyzed with experimental mouse chimeras. *Exp. Eye Res.*
(In press)

Law, P.K. and Atwood, H.L. (1972): Cross-reinnervation of dystrophic mouse
muscle. *Nature* 238:287-288.

Lebeda, F.J., Warnick, J.E., and Albuquerque, E.X. (1974): Electrical and   227,354
chemosensitive properties of normal and dystrophic chicken muscles. *Exp.*
Neurol. 43:21-37.

Le Douarin, N. (1973): A biological cell labelling technique and its use in experimental embryology. *Dev. Biol.* 30:217-222.

Le Douarin, N.M., Renaud, D., Teillet, M.A., and Le Douarin, G.H. (1975): Cholinergic differentiation of presumptive adrenergic neuroblasts in interspecific chimeras after heterotopic transplantations. *Proc. Nat. Acad. Sci.* 72:728-732.   326

Lentz, T.L. (1968): *Primitive Nervous Systems.* New Haven: Yale University Press.   220,221

Lentz, T.L. (1971): Nerve trophic function. *In vitro* assay of effects of nerve tissue on muscle cholinesterase activity. *Science* 171:187-189.   237

Lentz, T.L. (1972a): Development of the neuromuscular junction. III. Degeneration of motor end plates after denervation and maintenance in vitro by nerve explants. *J. Cell Biol.* 55:93-103.   241,376

Lentz, T.L. (1972b): A role of cyclic AMP in a neurotrophic process. *Nature New Biol.* 238:154-155.   376

Lentz, T.L. (1974a): Effect of brain extracts on cholinesterase activity of cultured skeletal muscle. *Exp. Neurol.* 45:520-526.   220,237, 240,390

Lentz, T.L. (1974b): Neurotrophic regulation at the neuromuscular junction. *Ann. N.Y. Acad. Sci.* 228:323-337.   237,238, 376,390

Lentz, T.L. (1975): Effect of denervation on muscle cyclic AMP in the newt. *Exp. Neurol.* 49:716-724.   376

Lentz, T.L., Rosenthal, J., and Mazurkiewicz, J.E. (1975): Cytochemical localization of acetylcholine receptors by means of peroxidase-labeled α-bungarotoxin. *In: Neuroscience Abstracts, Vol. I.* (Fifth Annual Meeting of the Society for Neuroscience, New York City, Nov. 2-6, 1975.) P. 627.   375

LeVay, S. (1975): Polyribosomes in visual cortex: effects of deprivation and anesthesia. *In: Neuroscience Abstracts, Vol. I.* (Fifth Annual Meeting of the Society for Neuroscience, New York City, Nov. 2-6, 1975.) P. 497.   396

Levi-Montalcini, R. (1950): The origin and development of the visceral system in the spinal cord of the chick embryo. *J. Morphol.* 86:253-283.   297

Levi-Montalcini, R. and Levi, G. (1943): Recherches quantitatives sur la marche due processus de différentiation des neurones dans les ganglions spinaux de l'embryon de poulet. *Arch. Biol. (Liege)* 54:189-206.   294

Levi-Montalcini, R., Aloe, L., Magnaini, E., Oesch, F., and Thoenen, H. (1975): Nerve growth factor induces volume increase and enhances tyrosine hydroxylase synthesis in chemically axotomized sympathetic ganglia of newborn rats. *Proc. Nat. Acad. Sci.* 72:595-599.   269

Levitan, I.B. and Barondes, S.H. (1974): Octopamine- and serotonin-stimulated phosphorylation of specific protein in the abdominal ganglion of *Aplysia californica. Proc. Nat. Acad. Sci.* 71:1145-1148.   381

Levitan, I.B., Madsen, C.J., and Barondes, S.H. (1974): Cyclic AMP and amine effects on phosphorylation of specific protein in abdominal ganglion of *Aplysia californica*; localization and kinetic analysis. *J. Neurobiol.* 5:511-525.   381

Lewis, D.M., Kean, C.J.C., and McGarrick, J.D. (1974): Dynamic properties of slow and fast muscle and their trophic regulation. *Ann. N.Y. Acad. Sci.* 228:105-120.

Lewis, P.R. and Shute, C.C. (1969): An electron-microscopic study of cholinesterase distribution in the rat adrenal medulla. *J. Microsc.* 89:181-193.

Linkhart, T.A., Yee, G.W., and Wilson, B.W. (1975): Myogenic defect in acetylcholinesterase regulation in muscular dystrophy of the chicken. *Science* 187:549-551.

Lisk, R.D. (1967): Sexual behavior: hormonal control. *In: Neuroendocrinology,* 309
Vol. 2. Martini, L. and Ganong, W.F., eds. New York: Academic Press, pp. 197-239.

Litchy, W.J. (1973): Uptake and retrograde transport of horseradish peroxidase in frog sartorius nerve *In vitro. Brain Res.* 56:377-381.

Llinás, R., Hillman, D.E., and Precht, W. (1973): Neuronal circuit reorganization in 367
mammalian agranular cerebellar cortex. *J. Neurobiol.* 4:69-94.

Loeser, J.D., Ward, A.A., Jr., and White, L.E., Jr. (1968): Chronic deafferentation 364
of human spinal cord neurons. *J. Neurosurg.* 29:48-50.

Loewi, O. (1921): Über humorale Übertragbarkeit der Herznervenwirkung. I. Mit- 218
teilung. *Pfluegers Arch.* 189:239-242. An English translation of this article can
be found in *Cellular Neurophysiology: A Source Book.* Cooke, I. and Lipkin,
M., eds. New York: Holt, Rinehart, and Winston, Inc., 1972, pp. 464-466.

Lømo, T. (1974): Neurotrophic control of colchicine effects on muscle? *Nature* 220,228,
249:473-474. 261

Lømo, T. and Rosenthal, J. (1972): Control of ACh sensitivity by muscle activity 228
in the rat. *J. Physiol.* 221:493-513.

Lømo, T. and Westgaard, R.H. (1975): Further studies on the control of ACh 237
sensitivity by muscle activity in the rat. *J. Physiol.* 252:603-626.

Lømo, T. and Westgaard, R.H. (1976): Control of ACh sensitivity in rat muscle 237
fibers. *Cold Spring Harbor Symp. Quant. Biol.* 40:263-274.

Lubińska, L. (1956): Outflow from cut ends of nerve fibres. *Exp. Cell Res.*
10:40-47.

Lux, H.D. and Schubert, P. (1975): Some aspects of the electroanatomy of 388
dendrites. *In: Advances in Neurology, Vol. 12. Physiology and Pathology of
Dendrites.* Kreutzberg, G.W., ed. New York: Raven Press, pp. 29-44.

Lux, H.D., Schubert, P., Kreutzberg, G.W., and Globus, A. (1970): Excitation and 307
axonal flow: autoradiographic study on motoneurons intracellularly injected
with a ^{3}H-amino acid. *Exp. Brain Res.* 10:197-204.

Lynch, G., Brecha, N., Cotman, C.W., and Globus, A. (1974): Spine loss and
regrowth in hippocampus following deafferentation. *Nature* 248:71-73.

Lynch, G. and Cotman, C.W. (1975): The hippocampus as a model for studying 327
anatomical plasticity in the adult brain. *In: The Hippocampus. Vol. 1, Structure
and Development. A Comprehensive Treatise.* Isaacson, R.L. and Pribram, K.H.,
eds. New York: Plenum Press, pp. 123-154.

Lynch, G., Deadwyler, S., and Cotman, C. (1973a): Postlesion axonal growth 330
produces permanent functional connections. *Science* 180:1364-1366.

Page

Lynch, G., Gall, C., Rose, G., and Cotman, C. (1976): Change in the distribution of   330,388
the dentate gyrus associational system following unilateral or bilateral lesions of
the entorhinal cortex. *Brain Res.* (In press)

Lynch, G., Matthews, D.A., Mosko, S., Parks, T., and Cotman, C. (1972): Induced   330
acetylcholinesterase-rich layer in rat dentate gyrus following entorhinal lesions.
Brain Res. 42:311-318.

Lynch, G., Rose, G., Gall, C., and Cotman, C.W. (1975a): The response of the   322,327,
dentate gyrus to partial deafferentation. *In: Golgi Centennial Symposium:*   328,329,
Perspectives in Neurobiology. Santini, M., ed. New York: Raven Press,   330,331
pp. 305-317.

Lynch, G., Smith, R.L., Browning, M.D., and Deadwyler, S. (1975b): Evidence for   261,283,
bidirectional dendritic transport of horseradish peroxidase. *In: Advances in*   332,333,
Neurology, Vol. 12. Physiology and Pathology of Dendrites. Kreutzberg, G.W.,   334
ed. New York: Raven Press, pp. 297-313.

Lynch, G., Stanfield, B., and Cotman, C.W. (1973b): Developmental differences in   330
post-lesion axonal growth in the hippocampus. *Brain Res.* 59:155-168.

Lynch, G., Stanfield, B., Parks, T., and Cotman, C.W. (1974): Evidence for selective
post-lesion axonal growth in the dentate gyrus of the rat. *Brain Res.* 69:1-11.

McArdle, J.J. and Albuquerque, E.X. (1973): A study of the reinnervation of fast   227
and slow mammalian muscles. *J. Gen. Physiol.* 61:1-23.

McArdle, J.J. and Albuquerque, E.X. (1975): Effects of ouabain on denervated and
dystrophic muscles of the mouse. *Exp. Neurol.* 47:353-356.

McComas, A.J. and Mrozek, K. (1967): Denervated muscle fibres in hereditary   354
mouse dystrophy. *J. Neurol. Neurosurg. Psychiatr.* 30:526-530.

McComas, A.J., Sica, R.E.P., Upton, A.R.M., and Petito, F. (1974a): Sick   354
motoneurons and muscle disease. *Ann. N.Y. Acad. Sci.* 228:261-279.

McComas, A.J., Upton, A.R., and Sica, R.E. (1974b): Myopathies: the neurogenic   354
hypothesis. *Lancet* 2:42.

McGeer, E.G., Searl, K., and Fibiger, H.C. (1975): Chemical specificity of
dopamine transport in the nigro-neostriatal projection. *J. Neurochem.*
24:283-288.

McIlwain, H. (1973): Adenosine in neurohumoral and regulatory roles in the brain.   388
In: Central Nervous System–Studies on Metabolic Regulation and Function.
Genazzani, E. and Herken, H., eds. Berlin: Springer-Verlag, pp. 1-11.

McIlwain, H. (1974): Adenosine 3':5'-cyclic monophosphate and its precursors in
the brain: a cyclase-containing adenine-uptake region. *Biochem. Soc. Trans.*
2:379-382. (Abstr.)

McIlwain, J. (1974): Regulatory significance of the release and action of adenine
derivatives in cerebral systems. *Biochem. Soc. Symp.* 36:69-85.

McMahon, D. (1974): Chemical messengers in development: a hypothesis. *Science*   401
185:1012-1021.

McQuarrie, I.G. and Grafstein, B. (1973): Axon outgrowth enhanced by a previous
nerve injury. *Arch. Neurol.* 29:53-55.

Page

Maeda, T., Tohyama, M., and Shimizu, N. (1974): Modification of postnatal   379
development of neocortex in rat brain with experimental deprivation of locus
coeruleus. *Brain Res.* 70:515-520.

Maeno, H., Reyes, P.L., Ueda, T., Rudolph, S.A., and Greengard, P. (1974):   381
Autophosphorylation of adenosine 3',5'-monophosphate-dependent protein
kinase from bovine brain. *Arch. Biochem. Biophys.* 164:551-559.

Maeno, H., Ueda, T., and Greengard, P. (1975): Adenosine 3':5'-monophosphate-   381
dependent protein phosphatase activity in synaptic membrane fractions. *J.
Cyclic Nucleotide Res.* 1:37-48.

Magendie, M. (1824): De l'influence de la cinquième paire de nerfs sur la nutrition   217
et les fonctions de l'oeil. *J. Physiol. Exp. Path.* 4:176-182.

Mains, R.E. and Patterson, P.H. (1973a): Primary cultures of dissociated sympa-   323
thetic neurons. I. Establishment of long-term growth in culture and studies of
differentiated properties. *J. Cell Biol.* 59:329-345.

Mains, R.E. and Patterson, P.H. (1973b): Primary cultures of dissociated   323
sympathetic neurons. II. Initial studies on catecholamine metabolism. *J. Cell
Biol.* 59:346-360.

Mains, R.E. and Patterson, P.H. (1973c): Primary cultures of dissociated sympa-   323
thetic neurons. III. Changes in metabolism with age in culture. *J. Cell Biol.*
59:361-366.

Margolis, G. and Kilham, L. (1968): Virus-induced cerebellar hypoplasia. *Res. Publ.*   366
Assoc. Res. Nerv. Ment. Dis. 44:113-146.

Margolis, G., Kilham, L., and Johnson, R.H. (1971): The parvoviruses and   366
replicating cells: Insights into the pathogenesis of cerebellar hypoplasia. *In:
Progress in Neuropathology, Vol. 1.* Zimmerman, H.M., ed. New York: Grune
and Stratton, Inc., pp. 168-201.

Marin-Padilla, M. (1972): Structural abnormalities of the cerebral cortex in human
chromosomal aberrations: A Golgi study. *Brain Res.* 44:625-629.

Marin-Padilla, M. (1974): Structural organization of the cerebral cortex (motor
area) in human chromosomal aberrations. A Golgi study. I. D. (13-15) trisomy,
Patau syndrome. *Brain Res.* 66:375-391.

Massing, W. and Fleischhauer, K. (1973): Further observation on vertical bundles of
dendrites in the cerebral cortex of the rabbit. *Z. Anat. Entwicklungsgesch.*
141:115-123.

Mastaglia, F.L. and Walton, J.N. (1971): Histological and histochemical changes in
skeletal muscle from cases of chronic juvenile and early adult spinal muscular
atrophy (the Kugelberg-Welander syndrome). *J. Neurol. Sci.* 12:15-44.

Matthews, M.R. and Raisman, G. (1972): A light and electron microscopic study of   305
the cellular response to axonal injury in the superior cervical ganglion of the rat.
Proc. R. Soc. B 181:43-79.

Miani, N. (1971): Transport of S-100 protein in mammalian nerve fibers and   280
transneuronal signals. *Acta Neuropathol.* 5(Suppl. 5):104-108.

Miledi, R. (1960): The acetylcholine sensitivity of frog muscle fibers after complete   220
or partial denervation. *J. Physiol.* 151:1-23.

Miledi, R. (1975): Transmitter release from Schwann cells. *In: Molecular Neurobiology in Vitro.* (European Molecular Biology Organization Intensive Study Program, Cologne, Mar. 2-8.) Cologne: W.S. Druck, p. 72.   322

Miledi, R. and Slater, C.R. (1970): On the degeneration of rat neuromuscular junctions after nerve section. *J. Physiol.* 207:507-528.   235,260, 274

Molotkov, V. (1925): The trophic function of the nervous system as the basis of pathological processes in surgery. *J. Physiol. U.S.S.R.* 8:No. 5-6. (Russian)   221

Monard, D., Solomon, F., Rentsch, M., and Gysin, R. (1973): Glia-induced morphological differentiation in neuroblastoma cells. *Proc. Nat. Acad. Sci.* 70:1894-1897.   327

Monard, D., Stockel, K., Goodman, R., and Thoenen, H. (1975): Distinction between nerve growth factor and glial factor. *Nature* 258:444-445.   327

Morales, R. and Duncan, D. (1975): Specialized contacts of astrocytes with astrocytes and with other cell types in the spinal cord of the cat. *Anat. Rec.* 182:255-266.

Morest, D.K. and Jean-Baptiste, M. (1975): Degeneration and phagocytosis of synaptic endings and axons in the medial trapezoid nucleus of the cat. *J. Comp. Neurol.* 162:135-155.   358,359

Morgenroth, V.H., III, Hegstrand, L.R., Roth, R.H., and Greengard, P. (1975): Evidence for involvement of protein kinase in the activation by adenosine $3':5'$-monophosphate of brain tyrosine 3-monooxygenase. *J. Biol. Chem.* 250:1946-1948.

Morrell, F. (1961): Lasting changes in synaptic organization produced by continuous neuronal bombardment. *In: Brain Mechanisms and Learning.* Fessard, A., Gerard, R.W., Konorski, J., and Delafresnaye, J.F., eds. Oxford: Blackwell Scientific Publications, pp. 375-392.   364

Morrell, F. and Tsuru, N. (1974): Development of spontaneous hypersynchrony in the hippocampal cortex of the bullfrog, *Rana catesbeiana. Biol. Bull.* 147:492. (Abstr.)   365

Morrell, F. and Tsuru, N. (1976): Kindling in the frog: development of spontaneous epileptiform activity. *Electroencephalogr. Clin. Neurophysiol.* 40:1-11.   365

Morrell, F., Tsuru, N., Hoeppner, T.J., Morgan, D., and Harrison, W.H. (1975): Secondary epileptogenesis in frog forebrain: effect of inhibition of protein synthesis. *Can. J. Neurological Sci.* 2:407-416.   365

Moskowitz, M.A., Weiss, B.F., Lytle, L.D., Munro, H.N., and Wurtman, R.J. (1975): d-Amphetamine disaggregates brain polysomes via a dopaminergic mechanism. *Proc. Nat. Acad. Sci.* 72:834-836.   307,394

Mueller, R.A., Otten, U., and Thoenen, H. (1974): The role of adenosine cyclic $3',5'$-monophosphate in reserpine-initiated adrenal medullary tyrosine hydroxylase induction. *Mol. Pharmacol.* 10:855-860.   391

Mueller, R.A., Thoenen, H., and Axelrod, J. (1969): Inhibition of trans-synaptically increased tyrosine hydroxylase activity by cycloheximide and actinomycin D. *Mol. Pharmacol.* 5:463-469.   393

Mullen, R.J. (1975): Neurological mutants: use of chimeras to determine site of gene action. *Genetics* 80(Suppl.):56.   248,250

Neurosciences Res. Prog. Bull., Vol. 14, No. 3   **439**

Page

Mullen, R.J. and LaVail, M.M. (1976): Inherited retinal dystrophy: primary defect   404
in pigment epithelium determined with experimental rat chimeras. *Science*
192:799-801.

Munro, H.N., Roel, L., and Wurtman, R.J. (1973): Inhibition of brain protein   394
synthesis by doses of L-dopa that disaggregate brain polyribosomes. *J. Neural
Transm.* 34:321-323.

Murphy, R.A., Pantazis, N.J., Arnason, B.G.W., and Young, M. (1975): Secretion of
a nerve growth factor by mouse neuroblastoma cells in culture. *Proc. Nat. Acad.
Sci.* 72:1895-1898.

Musick, J. and Hubbard, J.I. (1972): Release of protein from mouse motor nerve   276
terminals. *Nature* 237:279-281.

Nadler, J.V., Cotman, C.W., and Lynch, G.S. (1973): Altered distribution of
choline acetyltransferase and acetylcholinesterase activities in the developing rat
dentate gyrus following entorhinal lesion. *Brain Res.* 63:215-230.

Nadler, J.V., Cotman, C.W., and Lynch, G.S. (1974): Biochemical plasticity of
short-axon interneurons: increased glutamate decarboxylase activity in the
denervated area of rat dentate gyrus following entorhinal lesion. *Exp. Neurol.*
45:403-413.

Naftolin, F., Ryan, K.J., and Petro, Z. (1972): Aromatization of androstenedione   313
by the anterior hypothalamus of adult male and female rats. *Endocrinology*
90:295-298.

Narahashi, T., Albuquerque, E.X., and Deguchi, T. (1971): Effects of batracho-   231
toxin on membrane potential and conductance of squid giant axons. *J. Gen.
Physiol.* 58:54-70.

Nelson, P.G. (1976): Central nervous system synapses in cell culture. *Cold Spring   325
Harbor Symp. Quant. Biol.* 40:359-371.

Nicholson, J.L. and Altman, J. (1972): Synaptogenesis in the rat cerebellum: 317
Effects of early hypo- and hyperthyroidism. *Science* 176:530-531.

Nicoll, R.A. and Barker, J.L. (1971a): Excitation of supraoptic neurosecretory cells   320
by angiotensin II. *Nature New Biol.* 233:172-174.

Nicoll, R.A. and Barker, J.L. (1971b): The pharmacology of recurrent inhibition in   320
the supraoptic neurosecretory system. *Brain Res.* 35:501-511.

Noon, J.P., McAfee, D.A., Roth, R.H., and Greengard, P. (1973): Norepinephrine
release from nerve terminals in the rabbit superior cervical ganglion. *The
Pharmacologist* 15:216. (Abstr.)

Norr, S.C. (1973): *In vitro* analysis of sympathetic nerve on neuron differentiation   326
from chick neural crest cells. *Dev. Biol.* 34:16-38.

Nurse, C.A. and O'Lague, P.H. (1975): Formation of cholinergic synapses between   325
dissociated sympathetic neurons and skeletal myotubes of the rat in cell culture.
Proc. Nat. Acad. Sci. 72:1955-1959.

Oakley, B. (1970): Reformation of taste buds by crossed sensory nerves in the rat's   219
tongue. *Acta Physiol. Scand.* 79:88-94.

  Page

O'Brien, R.A.D. (1975): Transport of cholinergic enzymes in regenerating   308
peripheral nerve. *J. Physiol.* 252:62P-63P.

Ochs, S. (1972): Rate of fast axoplasmic transport in mammalian nerve fibres. *J.*   270,274
Physiol. 227:627-645.

Ochs, S. (1974): Systems of material transport in nerve fibers (axoplasmic   260
transport) related to nerve function and trophic control. *Ann. N.Y. Acad. Sci.*
228:202-223.

Ochs, S. and Smith, C.B. (1971): Effect of temperature and rate of stimulation on   307
fast axoplasmic transport in mammalian nerve fibres. *Fed. Proc.* 30:665.
(Abstr.)

Ochs, S. and Worth, R. (1975): Batrachotoxin block of fast axoplasmic transport in   231
mammalian nerve fibers. *Science* 187:1087-1089.

Oger, J., Arnason, B.G.W., Pantazis, N., Lehrich, J., and Young, M. (1974):
Synthesis of nerve growth factor by L and 3T3 cells in culture. *Proc. Nat. Acad.*
Sci. 71:1554-1558.

Oh, T.H. (1975): Neurotrophic effects: characterization of the nerve extract that   242,376
stimulates muscle development in culture. *Exp. Neurol.* 46:432-438.

Okada, Y. and Kuroda, Y. (1975): Inhibitory action of adenosine and adenine
nucleotides on the postsynaptic potential of olfactory cortex slices of the guinea
pig. *Proc. Jap. Acad.* 51:491-494.

O'Lague, P.H., MacLeish, P.R., Nurse, C.A., Claude, P., Furshpan, E.J., and Potter,   322,326
D.D. (1976): Physiological and morphological studies on developing sympathetic neurons in dissociated cell culture. *Cold Spring Harbor Symp. Quant. Biol.*
40:399-407.

O'Lague, P.H., Obata, K., Claude, P., Furshpan, E.J., and Potter, D.D. (1974):   322,325
Evidence for cholinergic synapses between dissociated rat sympathetic neurons
in cell culture. *Proc. Nat. Acad. Sci.* 71:3602-3606.

Olmstead, J.M.D. (1920): The nerve as a formative influence in the development of   219
taste-buds. *J. Comp. Neurol.* 31:465-468.

Olson, L. and Malmfors, T. (1970): Growth characteristics of adrenergic nerves in   336,345,
the adult rat. Fluorescence histochemical and ^{3}H-noradrenaline uptake studies   349
using tissue transplantations to the anterior chamber of the eye. *Acta Physiol.*
Scand. 348(Suppl.):1-112.

Oppenheim, R.W., Chu-Wang, I.-W., and Foelix, R.F. (1975): Some aspects of
synaptogenesis in the spinal cord of the chick embryo: A quantitative electron
microscopic study. *J. Comp. Neurol.* 161:383-418.

Orkand, R.K. (1975): Physiology of neuroglia and neuron-glia interactions. *In:*   322
Molecular Neurobiology In Vitro. (European Molecular Biology Organization
Intensive Study Program, Cologne, Mar. 2-8.) Cologne: W.S. Druck, pp. 46-50.

Orkand, R.K., Nicholls, J.G., and Kuffler, S.W. (1966): Effect of nerve impulses on   322
the membrane potential of glial cells in the central nervous system of amphibia.
J. Neurophysiol. 29:788-806.

Neurosciences Res. Prog. Bull., Vol. 14, No. 3   **441**

Page

Otsuka, M., Konishi, S., and Takahashi, T. (1975): Hypothalamic substance P as a   319
candidate for transmitter of primary afferent neurons. *Fed. Proc.*
34:1922-1928.

Otten, U., Mueller, R.A., Oesch, F., and Thoenen, H. (1974a): Location of an   391
isoproterenol-responsive cyclic AMP pool in adrenergic nerve cell bodies and its
relationship to tyrosine 3-monooxygenase induction. *Proc. Nat. Acad. Sci.*
71:2217-2221.

Otten, U., Mueller, R.A., and Thoenen, H. (1974b): Evidence against a causal   390,391
relationship between increase in c-AMP and induction of tyrosine hydroxylase
in the rat adrenal medulla. *Naunyn-Schmiedebergs Arch. Pharmakol.*
285:233-242.

Otten, U., Mueller, R.A., and Thoenen, H. (1975): Effect of hypophysectomy on   391
c-AMP changes in rat adrenal medulla evoked by catecholamines and carbamylcholine. *Naunyn-Schmiedebergs Arch. Pharmakol.* 289:157-170.

Otten, U., Oesch, F., and Thoenen, H. (1973a): Dissociation between changes in   316,391
cyclic AMP and subsequent induction of TH in the rat superior cervical ganglion
and adrenal medulla. *Naunyn-Schmiedebergs Arch. Pharmakol.* 280:129-140.

Otten, U., Paravicini, U., Oesch, F., and Thoenen, H. (1973b): Time requirement   393
for the single steps of trans-synaptic induction of tyrosine hydroxylase in the
peripheral sympathetic nervous system. *Naunyn-Schmiedebergs Arch. Pharmakol.* 280:117-127.

Otten, U. and Thoenen, H. (1975): Circadian rhythm of tyrosine hydroxylase   315
induction by short-term cold stress: Modulatory action of glucocorticoids in
newborn and adult rats. *Proc. Nat. Acad. Sci.* 72:1415-1419.

Otten, U. and Thoenen, H. (1976): Selective induction of tyrosine hydroxylase in   317
sympathetic ganglia in organ culture: role of glucocorticoids as modulators. *Mol.
Pharmacol.* (In press)

Palacios Prü, E.L. and Mendoza Briceño, R.V. (1972): An unusual relationship   370
between glial cells and neuronal dendrites in olfactory bulbs of *Desmodus
rotundus. Brain Res.* 36:404-408.

Palay, S.L., Billings-Gagliardi, S., and Chan-Palay, V. (1974): Neuronal perikarya   396
with dispersed, single ribosomes in the visual cortex of *Macaca mulatta. J. Cell
Biol.* 63:1074-1089.

Paravicini, U., Stoeckel, K., and Thoenen, H. (1975): Biological importance of   262
retrograde axonal transport of nerve growth factor in adrenergic neurons. *Brain
Res.* 84:279-291.

Patterson, P.H. and Chun, L.Y. (1974): The influence of non-neuronal cells on   322,325
catecholamine and acetylcholine synthesis and accumulation in cultures of
dissociated sympathetic neurons. *Proc. Nat. Acad. Sci.* 71:3607-3610.

Patterson, P.H., Reichardt, L.F., and Chun, L.L.Y. (1976): Biochemical studies on   324,325,
the development of primary sympathetic neurons in cell culture. *Cold Spring*   326
Harbor Symp. Quant. Biol. 40:389-397.

Pavans de Ceccaty, M. (1974): The origin of the integrative systems: a change in   220
view derived from research on coelenterates and sponges. *Perspect. Biol. Med.*
17:379-390.

Pavlov, I.P. (1885): Zur Frage über die Innervation der Herzens. *Zweite vorläufige*   221
Mitteilung. Centrbl. Med. Wiss. 23:65-67.

Pavlov, I.P. (1952): *Works on Physiology of Digestion.* Moscow: U.S.S.R. Academy   218
of Medicine.

Payton, B.W., Bennett, M.V.L., and Pappas, G.D. (1969): Permeability and   290
structure of junctional membranes at an electrotonic synapse. *Science*
166:1641-1643.

Pearson, J., Axelrod, F., and Dancis, J. (1974): Current concepts of dysautonomia: 374
neuropathological defects. *Ann. N.Y. Acad. Sci.* 228:288-300.

Pelletier, G., Labrie, F., Arimura, A., and Schally, A.V. (1974): Electron   318
microscopic immunohistochemical localization of growth-hormone-release inhibiting hormone (somatostatin) in the rat median eminence. *Am. J. Anat.*
140:445-450.

Peter, J.B. (1971): Histochemical, biochemical and physiological studies of skeletal   236
muscle and its adaptation to exercise. *In: Contractility of Muscles and Related*
Processes. Podolsky, R.J., ed. Englewood Cliffs, N.J.: Prentice Hall,
pp. 161-173.

Peterson, A.C. (1974): Chimaera mouse study shows absence of disease in   246,249,
genetically dystrophic muscle. *Nature* 248:561-564.   404

Peterson, A.C. (1975): Neuromuscular analysis of dystrophic ↔ normal mouse
chimaeras. *In: Recent Advances in Myology.* (Proceedings of the Third
International Congress on Muscle Diseases.) Bradley, W.G., Gardner-Medwin, D.,
Walton, J.N., and Harris, J.B., eds. Amsterdam: Excerpta Medica, pp. 125-131.

Pfaff, D. and Keiner, M. (1973): Atlas of estradiol-concentrating cells in the central   309
nervous system of the female rat. *J. Comp. Neurol.* 151:121-158.

Phillis, J.W. and Limacher, J.J. (1974): Substance P excitation of cerebral cortical   319
Betz cells. *Brain Res.* 69:158-163.

Piatt, J. (1946): The influence of the peripheral field on the development of the   297
mesencephalic V nucleus in amblystoma. *J. Exp. Zool.* 102:109-141.

Pilar, G., Chiappinelli, V., Uchimura, H., and Giacobini, E. (1974): Changes of
acetylcholinesterase (AChE) and cholineacetyltransferase (ChAc) correlated
with the formation of cholinergic synapses in the chick embryo. *The*
Physiologist 17:307. (Abstr.)

Pilar, G. and Landmesser, L. (1975): Normal and induced neuron death in ganglia   295,297
during embryogenesis. *In: Neuroscience Abstracts, Vol. I.* (Fifth Annual
Meeting of the Society for Neuroscience, New York City, Nov. 2-6, 1975.)
P. 750.

Pilar, G. and Landmesser, L. (1976): Ultrastructural differences during embryonic   295,297,
cell death in normal and peripherally deprived ciliary ganglia. *J. Cell Biol.*   298
68:339-356.

Pinching, A.J. and Powell, T.P.S. (1971): Ultrastructural features of transneuronal   356
cell degeneration in the olfactory system. *J. Cell Sci.* 8:253-287.

Page

Plum, F., Gjedde, A., and Samson, F. (1976): Neuroanatomical functional mapping   405
as determined by the radioactive 2-deoxyglucose method. *Neurosciences Res.
Prog. Bull.* (In press)

Polz-Tejera, G., Schmidt, J., and Karten, H.J. (1975): Autoradiographic localisation   404
of α-bungarotoxin-binding sites in the central nervous system. *Nature* 258:
349-351.

Prasad, K.N. and Hsie, A.W. (1971): Morphologic differentiation of mouse   396
neuroblastoma cells induced in vitro by dibutyryl adenosine 3':5'-cyclic
monophosphate. *Nature New Biol.* 233:141-142.

Prestige, M.C. (1965): Cell turnover in the spinal ganglia of *Xenopus laevis* tadpoles.   294
J. Embryol. Exp. Morph. 13:63-72.

Prestige, M.C. (1967a): The control of cell number in the lumbar spinal ganglia   294,297
during the development of *Xenopus laevis* tadpoles. *J. Embryol. Exp. Morph.*
17:453-471.

Prestige, M.C. (1967b): The control of cell number in the lumbar ventral horns   294,297
during the development of *Xenopus laevis* tadpoles. *J. Embryol. Exp. Morph.*
18:359-387.

Prestige, M.C. (1970): Differentiation, degeneration, and the role of the periphery: 222,294
quantitative considerations. *In: The Neurosciences: Second Study Program.*
Schmitt, F.O., editor-in-chief. New York: Rockefeller University Press,
pp. 73-82.

Price, D.L. (1974): Trophic functions of the neuron. VI. Other trophic systems.   222
The influence of the periphery on spinal motor neurons. *Ann. N.Y. Acad. Sci.*
228:355-363.

Purpura, D.P. (1974): Dendritic spine "dysgenesis" and mental retardation. *Science*
186:1126-1128.

Raisman, G. (1969): Neuronal plasticity in the septal nuclei of the adult rat. *Brain*   327
Res. 14:25-48.

Raisman, G. (1973): Electron microscopic studies of the development of new
neurohaemal contacts in the median eminence of the rat after hypophysectomy.
Brain Res. 55:245-261.

Raisman, G. (1974): Evidence for a sex difference in the neuropil of the rat   312,314
preoptic area and its importance for the study of sexually dimorphic function.
Res. Publ. Assoc. Res. Nerve Ment. Dis. 52:42-51.

Raisman, G. and Field, P.M. (1973a): A quantitative investigation of the   349
development of collateral reinnervation after partial deafferentation of the
septal nuclei. *Brain Res.* 50:241-264.

Raisman, G. and Field, P.M. (1973b): Sexual dimorphism in the neuropil of the   309,310,
preoptic area of the rat and its dependence on neonatal androgen. *Brain Res.*   311,312
54:1-29.

Raisman, G., Field, P.M., Ostberg, A.J., Iversen, L.L., and Zigmond, R.E. (1974): A
quantitative ultrastructural and biochemical analysis of the process of
reinnervation of the superior cervical ganglion in the adult rat. *Brain Res.*
71:1-16.

Page

Rakic, P. (1975): Local circuit neurons. *Neurosciences Res. Prog. Bull.* 13:291-446.   222

Rakic, P. and Sidman, R.L. (1973a): Organization of cerebellar cortex secondary to   367
deficit of granule cells in weaver mutant mice. *J. Comp. Neurol.* 152:133-162.

Rakic, P. and Sidman, R.L. (1973b): Sequence of development abnormalities   367
leading to granule cell deficit in cerebellar cortex of weaver mutant mice. *J.
Comp. Neurol.* 152:103-132.

Rakic, P. and Sidman, R.L. (1973c): Weaver mutant mouse cerebellum: Defective   367
neuronal migration secondary to abnormality of Bergmann glia. *Proc. Nat.
Acad. Sci.* 70:240-244.

Rall, W. (1959): Branching dendritic trees and motoneuron membrane resistivity.
Exp. Neurol. 1:491-527.

Ramirez, B. and Luco, J.V. (1973): Some physiological and biochemical features of
striated muscles reinnervated by preganglionic sympathetic fibers. *J. Neurobiol.*
4:525-533.

Ramón y Cajal, S. (1928): *Degeneration and Regeneration of the Nervous System,*   218
Vol. I. (Translated and edited by R.M. May.) Cambridge: Oxford University
Press.

Rathbone, M.P., Beresford, B., Plach, N.R., and Yacoob, C. (1976): The role of
cyclic AMP in neurotrophic regulation of muscle cholinesterase. *Fed. Proc.*
35:697. (Abstr.)

Rathbone, M.P., Beresford, B., and Yacoob, C. (1974): Characterization of a factor   390
from nerve tissue that prevents post-denervation loss of cholinesterase in
cultured muscle. *Excerpta Med. Int. Congr. Series* 334:1. (Abstr.)

Rathbone, M., Beresford, B., and Yacoob, C. (1975a): Characterization of a factor   241,242,
from nerve tissue that prevents post-denervation loss of the cholinesterase in   243,376
cultured muscle. *In: Recent Advances in Myology.* (Proceedings of the Third
International Congress on Muscle Diseases.) Bradley, W.G., Gardner-Medwin, D.,
Walton, J.N., and Harris, J.B., eds. Amsterdam: Excerpta Medica, pp. 6-15.

Rathbone, M.P., Haslam, R.J., and Beresford, B. (1973): The role of cyclic   241,390
nucleotides in neurotrophic effects. *Canada Physiol.* 4:46. (Abstr.)

Rathbone, M.P., Stewart, P.A., and Vetrano, F. (1975b): Dystrophic spinal cord   241,245,
transplants induce abnormal thymidine kinase activity in normal muscles.   246
Science 189:1106-1107.

Razumovsky, V.I. (1884): Atrophic bone processes after neurotomy. Ph.D.   221
Dissertation, Levshin Surgical Clinic, Medical Faculty of Kazan. (Russian)

Razumovsky, V.I. (1887): *On Causes of Death After Surgical Operations and
Wounds.* Kazan: Kazan Birj. and Listka.

Renaud, L.P. and Martin, J.B. (1975): Thyrotropin releasing hormone (TRH):   319
depressant action on central neuronal activity. *Brain Res.* 86:150-154.

Renaud, L.P., Martin, J.B., and Brazeau, P. (1975): Depressant action of TRH,   318
LH-RH and somatostatin on activity of central neurones. *Nature* 255:233-235.

Richman, D.P., Stewart, R.M., Hutchinson, J.W., and Caviness, V.S., Jr. (1975):   362
Mechanical model of brain convolutional development. *Science* 189:18-21.

Neurosciences Res. Prog. Bull., Vol. 14, No. 3 445

Page

Rieske, E., Schubert, P., and Kreutzberg, G.W. (1975): Transfer of radioactive 287,288, material between electrically coupled neurons of the leech central nervous 289 system. *Brain Res.* 84:365-382.

Riley, C.M. (1974): Familial dysautonomia: clinical and pathophysiological aspects. 374 *Ann. N.Y. Acad. Sci.* 228:283-287.

Riviera-Domingues, M., Mettler, F.A., and Noback, C.R. (1974): Origin of 370 cerebellar climbing fibers in the Rhesus monkey. *J. Comp. Neurol.* 155:331-336.

Rodbell, M., Birnbaumer, L., and Pohl, S.L. (1971): Hormones, receptors, and 378 adenyl cyclase activity in mammalian cells. *In: The Role of Adenyl Cyclase and Cyclic 3',5'-AMP in Biological Systems.* Washington, D.C.: Fogarty International Center Proceedings. U.S. Government Printing Office, p. 59.

Rodbell, M., Lin, M.C., Salomon, Y., Londos, C., Harwood, J.P., Martin, B.R., 378 Rendell, M., and Berman, M. (1975): Role of adenine and guanine nucleotides in the activity and response of adenylate cyclase systems to hormones. Evidence for multisite transition states. *In: Advances in Cyclic Nucleotide Research, Vol. 5.* Drummond, G.I., Greengard, P., and Robison, G.A., eds. New York: Raven Press, pp. 3-29.

Roel, L.E., Schwartz, S.A., Weiss, B.F., Munro, H.N., and Wurtman, R.J. (1974): In 307,394 vivo inhibition of rat brain protein synthesis by L-dopa. *J. Neurochem.* 23:233-239.

Rogers, J.G., Siggers, D.C., Boyer, S.H., Margolis, L., Dorkin, H., Baterjec, S.P., and 374 Shooter, E.M. (1975): Serum nerve growth factor levels in familial dysauto- nomia. *Soc. Pediatr. Res.* 384. (Abstr.)

Rogers, L.A. and Cowan, W.M. (1973): The development of the mesencephalic 294 nucleus of the trigeminal nerve in the chick. *J. Comp. Neurol.* 147:291-320.

Roisen, F.J., Murphy, R.A., Pichichero, M.E., and Braden, W.G. (1972): Cyclic 396,397 adenosine monophosphate stimulation of axonal elongation. *Science* 175:73-74.

Rose, G., Lynch, G., and Cotman, C.W. (1976): Hypertrophy and redistribution of 329 astrocytes in the deafferented dentate gyrus. *Brain Res. Bull.* 1:87-92.

Rose, S.P.R. and Sinha, A.K. (1974): Incorporation of ^{3}H-lysine into a rapidly labelling neuronal protein fraction in visual cortex is suppressed in dark reared rats. *Life Sci.* 15:223-230.

Rudolph, S.A. and Greengard, P. (1974): Regulation of protein phosphorylation 381,383, and membrane permeability by β-adrenergic agents and cyclic adenosine 384 3':5'-monophosphate in the avian erythrocyte. *J. Biol. Chem.* 249:5684-5687.

Salafsky, B. and Stirling, C.A. (1973): Altered neural protein in murine muscular dystrophy. *Nature New Biol.* 246:126-128.

Salvaterra, P.M. and Moore, W.G. (1973): Binding of (^{125}I)-αbungarotoxin to 404 particulate fractions of rat and guinea pig brain. *Biochem. Biophys. Res. Commun.* 55:1311-1318.

Samaha, F.J., Guth, L., and Albers, R.W. (1970): The neural regulation of gene 236 expression in the muscle cell. *Exp. Neurol.* 27:276-282.

Page

Samuel, S. (1860): *Die trophischen Nerven. Ein Beitrag zur Physiologie und*   217
Pathologie. Leipzig.

Sandbank, U. and Bubis, J.J. (1974): *The Pathology of Synapses. A Review of the*   364
Lesions of Synapses. Los Angeles: Brain Information Service/Brain Research
Institute, University of California.

Sattin, A. and Rall, T.W. (1970): The effect of adenosine and adenine nucleotides   387
on the adenosine 3′,5′-phosphate content of guinea pig cerebral cortex slices.
Mol. Pharmacol. 6:13-23.

Scheibel, M.E., Lindsay, R.D., Tomiyasu, U., and Scheibel, A.B. (1975): Progressive   363
dendritic changes in aging human cortex. *Exp. Neurol.* 47:392-403.

Scheibel, M.E. and Scheibel, A.B. (1973): Dendrite bundles as sites for central
programs: An hypothesis. *Int. J. Neuroscience* 6:195-202.

Schmitt, F.O. (1970): Promising trends in neuroscience. *Nature* 227:1006-1009.   261

Schrier, B.K. and Thompson, E.J. (1974): On the role of glial cells in the   322
mammalian nervous system. *J. Biol. Chem.* 249:1769-1780.

Schubert, P. and Kreutzberg, G.W. (1974): Axonal transport of adenosine and   387
uridine derivatives and transfer to postsynaptic neurons. *Brain Res.* 76:526-530.

Schubert, P. and Kreutzberg, G.W. (1975a): [^{3}H] Adenosine, a tracer for neuronal   282,387
connectivity. *Brain Res.* 85:317-319.

Schubert, P. and Kreutzberg, G.W. (1975b): Dendritic and axonal transport of   282,285,
nucleoside derivatives in single motoneurons and release from dendrites. *Brain*   387,389
Res. 90:319-323.

Schubert, P. and Kreutzberg, G.W. (1975c): Parameters of dendritic transport. *In:*   282,285,
Advances in Neurology, Vol. 12. Physiology and Pathology of Dendrites.   389
Kreutzberg, G.W., ed. New York: Raven Press, pp. 255-268.

Schubert, P. and Kreutzberg, G.W. (1976): Communication between the neuron
and the vessels. *In: The Cerebral Vessel Wall.* Cervos Navarro, J., ed. New York:
Raven Press. (In press)

Schubert, P., Kreutzberg, G.W., and Lux, H.D. (1972): Neuroplasmic transport in   282
dendrites: effect of colchicine on morphology and physiology of motoneurones
in the cat. *Brain Res.* 47:331-343.

Schubert, P., Lee, K., West, M., Deadwyler, S., and Lynch, G. (1976): Stimulation-
dependent release of ^{3}H-adenosine derivatives from central axon terminals to
target neurones. *Nature* 260:541-542.

Schubert, P., Lux, H.D., and Kreutzberg, G.W. (1971): Single cell isotope injection   282
technique, a tool for studying axonal and dendritic transport. *Acta Neuropath-*
ol. 5:179-186.

Schwab, M.E. and Thoenen, H. (1976): Electron microscopic evidence for a   285
transsynaptic migration of tetanus toxin in spinal cord motoneurons: an
autoradiographic and morphometric study. *Brain Res.* 105:213-227.

Segal, M and Bloom, F.E. (1974a): The action of norepinephrine in the rat   377
hippocampus. I. Iontophoretic studies. *Brain Res.* 72:79-97.

Page

Segal, M. and Bloom, F.E. (1974b): The action of norepinephrine in the rat   377
hippocampus. II. Activation of the input pathway. *Brain Res.* 72:99-114.

Seil, F.J. and Herndon, R.M. (1970): Cerebellar granule cells *in vitro*. A light and   370
electron microscope study. *J. Cell Biol.* 45:212-220.

Seitelberger, F. (1971): Neuropathological conditions related to neuroaxonal   364
dystrophy. *Acta Neuropathol.* 5(Suppl. 5):17-29.

Sherlock, D.A., Field, P.M., and Raisman, G. (1975): Retrograde transport of
horseradish peroxidase in the magnocellular neurosecretory system of the rat.
Brain Res. 88:403-414.

Shieh, P. (1951): The neoformation of cells of preganglionic type in the cervical   297
spinal cord of the chick embryo following its transplantation to the thoracic
level. *J. Exp. Zool.* 117:359-395.

Shorey, M.L. (1909): The effect of the destruction of peripheral areas on the   222,294,
differentiation of the neuroblasts. *J. Exp. Zool.* 7:25-63.   355

Sidman, R.L. (1968): Development of interneuronal connections in brains of   367
mutant mice. *In: Physiological and Biochemical Aspects of Nervous Integration.*
Carlson, F.D., ed. Englewood Cliffs, N.J.: Prentice-Hall, Inc., pp. 163-193.

Sidman, R.L. (1972): Cell interactions in developing mammalian central nervous   370
system. *In: Cell Interactions. Proceedings of the Third Lepetit Colloquium.*
Silvestri, L.G., ed. Amsterdam: North-Holland Publishing Co., pp. 1-13.

Sidman, R.L., Green, M.C., and Appel, S.H. (1965): *Catalog of the Neurological*   367,369
Mutants of the Mouse. Cambridge, Mass.: Harvard University Press.

Sidman, R.L. and Rakic, P. (1973): Neuronal migration, with special reference to   322
developing human brain: a review. *Brain Res.* 62:1-35.

Siggins, G.R., Battenberg, E.F., Hoffer, B.J., Bloom, F.E., and Steiner, A.L. (1973):   378
Noradrenergic stimulation of cyclic adenosine monophosphate in rat Purkinje
neurons: an immunocytochemical study. *Science* 179:585-588.

Siggins, G.R., Hoffer, B.J., and Bloom, F.E. (1969): Cyclic 3',5'-adenosine   377
monophosphate: possible mediator for the response of cerebellar Purkinje cells
to microelectrophoresis of norepinephrine. *Science* 165:1018-1020.

Siggins, G.R., Hoffer, B.J., and Bloom, F.E. (1971a): Prostaglandin-norepinephrine   377
interactions in brain: microelectrophoretic and histochemical correlates. *Ann.*
N.Y. Acad. Sci. 180:302-323.

Siggins, G.R., Hoffer, B.J., and Bloom, F.E. (1971b): Studies on norepinephrine-   377
containing afferents to Purkinje cells of rat cerebellum. III. Evidence for
mediation of norepinephrine effects by cyclic 3',5'-adenosine monophosphate.
Brain Res. 25:535-553.

Siggins, G.R., Hoffer, B.J., Oliver, A.P., and Bloom, F.E. (1971c): Activation of a   377
central noradrenergic projection to cerebellum. *Nature* 233:481-483.

Siggins, G.R., Hoffer, B.J., and Ungerstedt, U. (1974): Electrophysiological   377
evidence for involvement of cyclic adenosine monophosphate in dopamine
responses of caudate neurons. *Life Sci.* 15:779-792.

Page

Siggins, G.R., Oliver, A.P., Hoffer, B.J., and Bloom, F.E. (1971d): Cyclic adenosine   377
monophosphate and norepinephrine: effects on transmembrane properties of
cerebellar Purkinje cells. *Science* 171:192-194.

Silinsky, E.M. and Hubbard, J.I. (1973): Release of ATP from rat motor nerve   276
terminals. *Nature* 243:404-405.

Singer, M. (1952): The influence of the nerve in the regeneration of the amphibian   219,220,
extremity. *Q. Rev. Biol.* 27:169-200.   226

Singer, M. (1974): Neurotrophic control of limb regeneration in the newt. *Ann.*   220
N.Y. Acad. Sci. 228:308-322.

Sjöqvist, F. (1963): The correlation between the occurrence and localization of   326
acetylcholinesterase-rich cell bodies in the stellate ganglion and the outflow of
cholinergic sweat secretory fibers to the forepaw of the cat. *Acta Physiol.*
Scand. 57:339-351.

Sjöstrand, J. and Frizell, M. (1975): Retrograde axonal transport of rapidly   308
migrating proteins in peripheral nerves. *Brain Res.* 85:325-333.

Sloboda, R.D., Rudolph, S.A., Rosenbaum, J.L., and Greengard, P. (1975): Cyclic   381,384,
AMP-dependent endogenous phosphorylation of a microtubule-associated pro-   385,386
tein. *Proc. Nat. Acad. Sci.* 72:177-181.

Smith, A.A. and Hui, F.W. (1973): Unmyelinated nerves in familial dysautonomia.   373
Neurology 23:8-11.

Smith, A.D., De Potter, W.P., Moerman, E.J., and De Schaepdryver, A.F. (1970):   276
Release of dopamine β-hydroxylase and chromogranin A upon stimulation of
the splenic nerve. *Tissue and Cell* 2:547-568.

Smith, A.R. and Wolpert, L. (1975): Nerves and angiotensin in amphibian   219,225
regeneration. *Nature* 257:224-225.

Smith, B.H. (1968): Neuroplasmic transport of bioelectrical activity in the nervous
system of the cockroach, *Periplaneta americana*. Ph.D. Thesis, Massachusetts
Institute of Technology, Cambridge, Mass.

Smith, B.H. (1971): Axoplasmic transport in the nervous system of the cockroach,
Periplaneta americana. *J. Neurobiol.* 2:107-118.

Smith, R.S. (1973): Microtubule and neurofilament densities in amphibian spinal   274
root nerve fibres: relationship to axoplasmic transport. *Can. J. Physiol.*
Pharmacol. 51:798-806.

Somjen, G.G. (1975): Electrophysiology of neuroglia. *Annu. Rev. Physiol.*   322,323
37:163-190.

Sotelo, C. (1973): Permanence and fate of paramembranous synaptic speciali-   367
zations in "mutants" and experimental animals. *Brain Res.* 62:345-351.

Sotelo, C. and Changeux, J.P. (1974): Transsynaptic degeneration "en cascade" in   370
the cerebellar cortex of staggerer mutant mice. *Brain Res.* 67:519-526.

Specht, S. and Grafstein, B. (1973): Accumulation of radioactive protein in mouse   276,280
cerebral cortex after injection of ^{3}H-fucose into the eye. *Exp. Neurol.*
41:705-722.

Neurosciences Res. Prog. Bull., Vol. 14, No. 3   449

                                                            Page

Speransky, A.D. (1943): *A Basis for the Theory of Medicine*. (Translated from   218,221
Russian by C.P. Dott and A.A. Subkov.) New York: International Publishers.

Stein, B.E. and Magalhães-Castro, B. (1975): Effects of neonatal cortical lesions
upon the cat superior colliculus. *Brain Res.* 83:480-485.

Sternberg, S.S. and Philips, F.S. (1958): 6-Aminonicotinamide and acute degenera-   234
tive changes in the central nervous system. *Science* 127:644-646.

Stewart, O., Cotman, C.W., and Lynch, G.S. (1974): Growth of a new fiber   330
projection in the brain of adult rats: re-innervation of the dentate gyrus by the
contralateral entorhinal cortex following ipsilateral entorhinal lesions. *Exp.
Brain Res.* 20:45-66.

Stöckel, K., Guroff, G., Schwab, M., and Thoenen, H. (1976): The significance of   264
retrograde axonal transport for the accumulation of systemically administered
nerve growth factor (NGF) in the rat superior cervical ganglion. *Brain Res.* (In
press)

Stöckel, K., Paravicini, U., and Thoenen, H. (1974): Specificity of the retrograde   262,265
axonal transport of nerve growth factor. *Brain Res.* 76:413-421.

Stöckel, K., Schwab, M., and Thoenen, H. (1975a): Comparison between the   262,263,
retrograde axonal transport of nerve growth factor and tetanus toxin in motor,   267,294
sensory and adrenergic neurons. *Brain Res.* 99:1-16.

Stöckel, K., Schwab, M., and Thoenen, H. (1975b): Specificity of retrograde   260,262,
transport of nerve growth factor (NGF) in sensory neurons: a biochemical and   266,294
morphological study. *Brain Res.* 89:1-14.

Stöckel, K. and Thoenen, H. (1975a): Retrograde axonal transport of nerve growth   262,274
factor: specificity and biological importance. *Brain Res.* 85:337-341.

Stöckel, K. and Thoenen, H. (1975b): Specificity of the retrograde axonal   262,265,
transport of nerve growth factor (NGF). *In: Symposium on Nerve Growth   268,274
Factor*. (Sixth International Congress on Pharmacology, Helsinki, Finland, July
20-25, 1975.) New York: Pergamon Press, p. 344. (Abstr.)

Stumpf, W.E. and Sar, M. (1971): Estradiol concentrating neurons in the amygdala.   309
Proc. Soc. Exp. Biol. Med. 136:102-106.

Taleisnik, S., Caligaris, L., and Astrada, J.J. (1971): Feedback effects of gonadal   309
steroids on the release of gonadotropins. *In: Hormonal Steroids*. James, V.H.T.
and Martini, L., eds. Amsterdam: Excerpta Medica, pp. 699-707.

Taleisnik, S., Velasco, M.E., and Astrada, J.J. (1970): Effect of hypothalamic
deafferentation on the control of luteinizing hormone secretion. *J. Endocrinol.*
46:1-7.

Tang, B.Y., Komiya, Y., and Austin, L. (1974): Axoplasmic flow of phospholipids
and cholesterol in the sciatic nerve of normal and dystrophic mice. *Exp. Neurol.*
43:13-20.

Terry, L.C., Bray, G.M., and Aguayo, A.J. (1974): Schwann cell multiplication in
developing rat unmyelinated nerves—a radioautographic study. *Brain Res.*
69:144-148.

Page

Thoenen, H. and Otten, U. (1976): Cyclic nucleotides and transsynaptic enzyme   391
induction: Lack of correlation between initial cAMP increase, changes in
cAMP/cGMP ratio and subsequent induction of tyrosine hydroxylase in the
adrenal medulla. *In: Chemical Tools in Catecholamine Research.* Göteborg,
Sweden. (In press)

Thornton, C.S. (1968): Amphibian limb regeneration. *Adv. Morphog.* 7:205-249.   219,226

Thornton, C.S. (1970): Amphibian limb regeneration and its relation to nerves.   226
Am. Zool. 10:113-118.

Torrey, T.W. (1934): The relation of taste buds to their nerve fibers. *J. Comp.*   219
Neurol. 59:203-220.

Trabucchi, M., Cheney, D.L., Susheela, A.K., and Costa, E. (1975): Possible defect
in cholinergic neurons of muscular dystrophic mice. *J. Neurochem.* 24:417-423.

Turner, C., Cooper, E., MacIntyre, L., and Diamond, J. (1975): Specificity of nerve
sprouting in salamander skin. *Canada Physiol.* 6:64. (Abstr.)

Turner, C., Fried, J.A., Cooper, E., and Diamond, J. (1976): Neuronal transport in
salamander nerves and its blockage by colchicine. *Brain Res.* (In press)

Ueda, T., Maeno, H., and Greengard, P. (1973): Regulation of endogenous   381,382,
phosphorylation of specific proteins in synaptic membrane fractions from rat   383
brain by adenosine 3':5'-monophosphate. *J. Biol. Chem.* 248:8295-8305.

Ueda, T., Rudolph, S.A., and Greengard, P. (1975): Solubilization of a phospho-   381
protein and its associated cyclic AMP-dependent protein kinase and phosphoprotein phosphatase from synaptic membrane fractions, and some kinetic
evidence for their existence as a complex. *Arch. Biochem. Biophys.*
170:492-503.

Vale, W., Rivier, C., Palkovits, M., Saavedra, J.M., and Brownstein, M. (1974):   318
Ubiquitous brain distribution of inhibitors of adenohypophysial secretion.
Endocrinology 94:128. (Abstr.)

Valverde, F. (1971): Rate and extent of recovery from dark rearing in the visual   356
cortex of the mouse. *Brain Res.* 33:1-11.

Van Wijngaarden, G.K. and Bethlem, J. (1973): Benign infantile spinal muscular
atrophy. A prospective study. *Brain* 96:163-170.

Varon, S. (1975a): Nerve growth factor and its mode of action. *Exp. Neurol.*   323
48(No. 3, Part 2):75-92.

Varon, S. (1975b): Neurons and glia in neural cultures. *Exp. Neurol.* 48(No. 3, Part 323
2):93-134.

Varon, S. and Raiborn, C. (1972): Dissociation fractionation, and culture of chick 323
embryo sympathetic ganglionic cells. *J. Neurocytol.* 1:211-221.

Varon, S. and Saier, M. (1975): Culture techniques and glial-neuronal interrelationships in vitro. *Exp. Neurol.* 48(No. 3, Part 2):135-162.

Velasco, M.E. and Taleisnik, S. (1969): Release of gonadotropins induced by   309
amygdaloid stimulation in the rat. *Endocrinology* 84:132-139.

Page

Walton, G.M. and Gill, G.N. (1973): Adenosine 3',5'-monophosphate and protein   396
kinase dependent phosphorylation of ribosomal protein. *Biochemistry*
12:2604-2611.

Warnick, J.E., Albuquerque, E.X., and Sansone, F.M. (1971): The pharmacology of   231
batrachotoxin. I. Effects on the contractile mechanism and on neuromuscular
transmission of mammalian skeletal muscle. *J. Pharmacol. Exp. Ther.*
176:497-510.

Watson, W.E. (1970): Some metabolic responses of axotomized neurones to
contact between their axons and denervated muscle. *J. Physiol.* 210:321-343.

Watson, W.E. (1974): Physiology of neuroglia. *Physiol. Rev.* 54:245-271.   323

Weiss, B.F., Leibschutz, J.L., Wurtman, R.J., and Munro, H.N. (1975): Participa-   394
tion of dopamine- and serotonin-receptors in the disaggregation of brain
polysomes by L-dopa and L-5-HTP. *J. Neurochem.* 24:1191-1195.

Weiss, B.F., Munro, H.N., Ordonez, L.A., and Wurtman, R.J. (1972): Dopamine: 394
mediator of brain polysome disaggregation after L-dopa. *Science* 177:613-616.

Weiss, B.F., Munro, H.N., and Wurtman, R.J. (1971): L-Dopa: disaggregation of   394,395
brain polysomes and elevation of brain tryptophan. *Science* 173:833-835.

Weiss, B.F., Roel, L.E., Munro, H.N., and Wurtman, R.J. (1974): L-Dopa,   394
polysomal aggregation and cerebral synthesis of protein. *In: Aromatic Amino
Acids in the Brain.* (Ciba Foundation Symposium 22.) Amsterdam: Excerpta
Medica, pp. 325-334.

Weiss, B.F., Wurtman, R.J., and Munro, H.N. (1973): Disaggregation of brain   395
polysomes by L-5-hydroxytryptophan: mediation by serotonin. *Life Sci.*
13:411-416.

Weller, W.L. and Johnson, J.I. (1975): Barrels in cerebral cortex altered by receptor
disruption in newborn, but not in five-day-old mice (Cricetidae and muridae).
Brain Res. 83:504-508.

Westrum, L.E. (1974): Electron microscopy of deafferentation in the spinal   364
trigeminal nucleus. *Adv. Neurol.* 4:53-71.

Whittaker, V.P., Dowdall, M.J., Dowe, G.H.C., Facino, R.M., and Scotto, J. (1974):   276
Proteins of cholinergic synaptic vesicles from the electric organ of *torpedo:*
characterization of a low molecular weight acidic protein. *Brain Res.*
75:115-131.

Wiesel, T.N. and Hubel, D.H. (1963a): Effects of visual deprivation on morphology   356
and physiology of cells in the cat's lateral geniculate body. *J. Neurophysiol.*
26:970-993.

Wiesel, T.N. and Hubel, D.H. (1963b): Single-cell responses in striate cortex of   356
kittens deprived of vision in one eye. *J. Neurophysiol.* 26:1003-1017.

Wiesel, T.N. and Hubel, D.H. (1974): Reorganization of ocular dominance columns   345
in monkey striate cortex. *In: Program and Abstracts, Society for Neuroscience.
Fourth Annual Meeting.* St. Louis, Mo., p. 478.

Page

Zieglgänsberger, W. and Reiter, Ch. (1974): Interneuronal movement of procion
yellow in cat spinal neurones. *Exp. Brain Res.* 20:527-530.

Zimmer, J. (1973): Extended commissural and ipsilateral projections in postnatally   330
deentorhinated hippocampus and fascia dentata demonstrated in rats by silver
impregnation. *Brain Res.* 64:293-311.

Zimmer, J. (1974): Proximity as a factor in the regulation of aberrant axonal   330
growth in the postnatally deafferented fascia dentata. *Brain Res.* 72:137-142.

Zukin, S.R., Young, A.B., and Snyder, S.H. (1975): Development of the synaptic
glycine receptor in chick embryo spinal cord. *Brain Res.* 83:525-530.

NEUROANATOMICAL FUNCTIONAL MAPPING BY THE RADIOACTIVE 2-DEOXY-D-GLUCOSE METHOD

*Based on an NRP Conference
held October 20, 1975, and updated by participants*

by

Fred Plum
New York Hospital
Cornell Medical Center
New York, New York

Albert Gjedde
Institute of Medical Physiology
Copenhagen, Denmark

Fred E. Samson
R. Smith Center for Mental Retardation
University of Kansas Medical Center
Kansas City, Kansas

Yvonne M. Homsy
NRP Writer-Editor

CONTENTS

PARTICIPANTS

Robert C. Collins
Department of Neurology
Washington University
   School of Medicine
660 S. Euclid Avenue
St. Louis, Missouri 63110

Thomas E. Duffy
Departments of Neurology and
   Biochemistry
Cornell University Medical College
1300 York Avenue
New York, New York 10021

Mac V. Edds, Jr.*
Neurosciences Research Program
165 Allandale Street
Jamaica Plain, Massachusetts 02130

Edward V. Evarts
Laboratory of Neurophysiology
National Institute of Mental Health
9000 Rockville Pike
Bethesda, Maryland 20014

Albert Gjedde
Department A
Institute of Medical Physiology
Juliane Mariesvej 28
DK-2100 Copenhagen, Denmark

Ann M. Graybiel
Department of Psychology, E10-104A
Massachusetts Institute of Technology
Cambridge, Massachusetts 02139

David H. Hubel
Department of Neurobiology
Harvard Medical School
25 Shattuck Street
Boston, Massachusetts 02115

Manfred L. Karnovsky
Department of Biological Chemistry
Harvard Medical School
25 Shattuck Street
Boston, Massachusetts 02115

John S. Kauer
Department of Physiology
Yale University School of Medicine
333 Cedar Street
New Haven, Connecticut 06510

Seymour S. Kety
Psychiatric Research Laboratories
Massachusetts General Hospital
Boston, Massachusetts 02114

Vernon B. Mountcastle
Department of Physiology
The Johns Hopkins University
   School of Medicine
725 North Wolfe Street
Baltimore, Maryland 21205

Walle J.H. Nauta
Department of Psychology, E10-104
Massachusetts Institute of Technology
Cambridge, Massachusetts 02139

Fred Plum
Department of Neurology
New York Hospital
Cornell Medical Center
525 East 68th Street
New York, New York 10021

Charles E. Polletti
Department of Neurosurgery
Massachusetts General Hospital
Boston, Massachusetts 02114

*Deceased November 29, 1975

Martin Reivich
Department of Neurology
University of Pennsylvania
    School of Medicine
Philadelphia, Pennsylvania 19174

Fred E. Samson
R. Smith Center for Mental Retardation
University of Kansas Medical Center
Kansas City, Kansas 66103

Francis O. Schmitt
Neurosciences Research Program
165 Allandale Street
Jamaica Plain, Massachusetts 02130

Frank R. Sharp
Department of Neurology
University of California at
    San Francisco
San Francisco, California 94143

Gordon M. Shepherd
Department of Physiology
Yale University School of Medicine
333 Cedar Street
New Haven, Connecticut 06510

Louis Sokoloff
Laboratory of Cerebral Metabolism
Building 36, Room 1A-27
National Institute of Mental Health
9000 Rockville Pike
Bethesda, Maryland 20014

Torsten Wiesel
Department of Neurobiology
Harvard Medical School
25 Shattuck Street
Boston, Massachusetts 02115

Frederic G. Worden
Neurosciences Research Program
165 Allandale Street
Jamaica Plain, Massachusetts 02130

Richard J. Wurtman
Department of Nutrition and
    Food Science, 56-245
Massachusetts Institute of
    Technology
Cambridge, Massachusetts 02139

*Note: NRP Work Session and Conference reports are reviewed and revised by participants prior to publication.

I. INTRODUCTION

The purpose of this conference was two-fold: to discuss some recent advances in the neuroanatomical mapping of functional activity in the brain, in particular the use of the radioactive 2-deoxy-D-glucose (DG) method for identifying those brain regions where activity changes during different functional states, and to explore the potential of the method for the studies of brain and behavior. The $[1\text{-}^{14}C]\text{-}2\text{-deoxy-D-}$ glucose ($[^{14}C]DG$) method, developed by Sokoloff, Reivich, Kennedy, and their colleagues (see Kennedy et al., 1975, for the first major publication of this procedure), stems from earlier work by Kety and colleagues (Landau et al., 1955; Reivich et al., 1969) on the localization of cerebral blood flow changes.*

A structural analogue of glucose, DG differs from glucose only by lacking an oxygen atom on the second carbon atom. Earlier studies with this compound established that DG readily enters tissues and cells and that at sufficiently high concentrations it inhibits the transport and utilization of glucose (Wick et al., 1957; Laszlo et al., 1958). It was also found that DG is phosphorylated by hexokinase from brain and tumor cells (Sols and Crane, 1954; Woodward and Hudson, 1954). It is generally thought that DG is phosphorylated to 2-deoxyglucose-6-phosphate (DG-6-P) and is not metabolized further; at least, it is not a substrate for glucose-6-phosphate dehydrogenase (G-6-Pase) or phosphohexose isomerase (Sols and Crane, 1954).

In a study of the effects of DG on the metabolism of brain slices, Tower (1958) concluded that its inhibitory action (at 10 mM concentration) on glycolysis was primarily due to a depletion of available adenosine triphosphate (ATP) for the hexose-catalyzed phosphorylation of glucose. It should be noted that the $[^{14}C]DG$ method discussed at the conference involves only "trace" amounts of DG, and that any of its inhibitory effects on metabolism is considered inconsequential. Furthermore, the method is applicable to conscious as well as to anesthetized experimental animals.

The current interest in this method arises from the fact that, under controlled conditions, it provides a powerful tool for mapping

*Also, a manuscript entitled "The $[^{14}C]$deoxyglucose method for the measurement of local cerebral glucose utilization" by L. Sokoloff, M. Reivich, C. Kennedy, M.H. Des Rosiers, C. Patlak, K. Pettigrew, O. Sakurada, and M. Shinohara, which will be a detailed report on the theory, procedures, and quantitative values obtained by the method, is in preparation.

levels of activity or function in neuroanatomical areas in intact animals. Experimentally induced local changes in functional activity produce focal *evoked metabolic responses* that the method can reveal. Since the information is obtained from density patterns by autoradiography of serial sections, all regions of the brain can be mapped simultaneously. In other words, the technique provides a radioisotopic "stain" for functional activity.

In the kinetic model developed by Sokoloff and colleagues, the rate of glucose consumption per gm of tissue can be estimated. Since a number of assumptions are necessary, the accuracy of the calculated values rests primarily on the validity of the assumptions. Local glucose utilization in both normal conscious and thiopental-anesthetized rats has been calculated by the [14C]DG method, and the values were found to be compatible with average metabolic rates determined by other methods.

The principles of the [14C]DG method, modified to employ tomographic scanning, may prove to be of great importance in neurological diagnosis, such as in the localization of brain lesions. Moreover, this technique has the potential for mapping the amount of functional activity in small brain regions, hitherto inaccessible, during different states of activity. It is hoped that this report will help catalyze research in this area and lead to an understanding of brain functions in both their normal and disordered states.

II. HISTORICAL OVERVIEW: F. Plum

The relationship between form and function in the nervous system has always had a central place in neuroscience. Progress has been considerable since 1906 when the awarding of the Nobel Prize to both Ramón y Cajal and Golgi made explicit the two conflicting interpretations—Ramón y Cajal believed that neuronal connectivity is modifiable by functional activity (e.g., physical exercise, piano playing, etc.) during adulthood whereas Golgi felt that connectivities are permanently set after development. Recent work, best represented by Wiesel's and Hubel's (1974) demonstration in the monkey that regional, cerebral physiological processes are able to produce focal structural changes, has shown Ramón y Cajal's interpretation to be the more correct one. Thus, neurobiology has moved from an overemphasis on the rigidity and separateness of neurons to an understanding of their involvement as mutable elements in systems and networks that act as pathways, and not as barriers, to interaction.

The initial description of the nervous system as a system of connections rather than as divisions was provided by Sherrington's (1891) reflex arc. This era of reflex analysis of the nervous system witnessed developments of the brain tissue-slice technique by Stilling (1842) and useful methods of tissue staining by Weigert (1882, 1884) for myelin and neuroglia, by Nissl (1885) for intracellular matter, by Golgi (1873) and Ramón y Cajal (1909) for individual neurons, and by Ehrlich (1886) for whole tissue slices.

Demonstration and comprehension of the neuron as a "cable" were made possible by (1) degeneration methods introduced by Waller (1850, 1852) and later refined by Gudden (1870), Nissl (1895), Marchi and Algeri (1885, 1886), (2) by retrograde or inverse Wallerian degeneration developed by Klippel and Durante (1895; Klippel, 1896) among others, (3) as well as by the identification of developing myelin sheaths in the study of tracts by Flechsig (1876). While these and other studies from the period before the turn of the century prepared the way for much of our understanding of neurochemistry and neuroanatomy, the ultimate standards for degenerative mapping of neuronal tracts were set by the Nauta-Gygax method (1951).

Progress in understanding neuronal functional relationships was impeded by the tedious and slow improvements of methods of qualitative and quantitative study of the brain. Histochemistry was the logical extension of the broad studies of the chemical properties of stains by German chemists and pharmacologists. Although histochemistry in the hands of investigators interested in brain function rather than form did not yield the desired answers to questions about enzymatic and structural changes during neuronal function and pathology, it has produced the dramatic fluorescent visualization of putative transmitters and transmitter-linked tracts (Falck et al., 1962; Hökfelt, 1967).

Comprehension of the function-morphology relationship was further advanced by the discovery that axonal transport processes can be studied with labeled amino acids by autoradiography and with horseradish peroxidase by light or electron microscopy (Grafstein, 1969; Cowan et al., 1972; LaVail and LaVail, 1972). When these techniques were combined with the recording of electrical activity of evoked potentials and with mapping by the spread of intracellularly injected Procion yellow (Stretton and Kravitz, 1968), the histologist was able to observe the entire neuron from which electrical recordings are obtained.

Measurements of energy supply and of the rate of its utilization by determining whole-brain and regional cerebral blood flow and metabolic rates, initiated by Kety and Schmidt (1945), were based to a large extent on the calculations carried out by Kety (1951, 1960). The use of autoradiography in measuring cerebral blood flow (Landau et al., 1955; Kety, 1960; Reivich et al., 1969) and the advances made by the adaptation of positron-emitting isotopes to the noninvasive study of cerebral blood flow and uptake rates in humans by computerized tomography (Raichle et al., 1975) have introduced some degree of correlation, but the exact relation of flow to function has yet to be solved.

The determination of the rate of $[^{14}C]DG$ phosphorylation in brain tissue slices promises to provide the missing link between the form and function of neuronal networks and thus give a partial answer to the question: How does the brain work? As Greenfield and Meyer (1963) so admirably put it in a somewhat different context: " . . . in the past [neuroanatomy and neurophysiology] have suffered through being tied to too few special techniques. The rapid growth of neurochemistry and the development of ultramicroscopes impose a heavy task on the [neurologist] who will be responsible for integrating these developments with established techniques. Since a single worker cannot hope to acquire expert knowledge in all these new fields, arrangements must be made to include specialists in the [neurological] laboratory. Many [neurologists] now appoint biochemists in their departments. Such teams will succeed, however, only to the extent that the specialists have a basic understanding of each other's province."

III. [1-^{14}C]-2-DEOXY-D-GLUCOSE METHOD FOR MEASURING LOCAL CEREBRAL GLUCOSE UTILIZATION

Mathematical Analysis and Determination of the "Lumped" Constants: L. Sokoloff

The quantitative or qualitative estimation of the rates of glucose utilization in various structural components of the brain by the [1-^{14}C]-2-deoxy-D-glucose method is based on the rate of phosphorylation of [^{14}C]DG in local regions of cerebral tissues following an intravenous pulse of the radioactive tracer. This method grew out of earlier studies in which regional cerebral blood flow was visualized by autoradiography of brain slices after injection of [^{14}C]antipyrine (Reivich et al., 1969). It was possible to quantify regional blood flow by making the appropriate analysis of the density patterns, as shown by Kety and colleagues (Landau et al., 1955; Kety, 1960). A similar technique was sought to measure cerebral energy metabolism, for which a suitable radioactive substrate is necessary. The primary substrates, oxygen and glucose, are unsuitable because of their short biological half-lives. Certain special properties of DG make it particularly appropriate for this purpose: It is transported from the blood into the brain by the same carrier that transports glucose, and in the brain it is phosphorylated by hexokinase. Unlike glucose, however, it is not converted to fructose-6-phosphate but is essentially "trapped" in the location where it is phosphorylated by the hexokinase. The half-life of [^{14}C]DG-6-P is 9 hours in gray matter and 15 hours in white matter.

In order to achieve as fine a resolution and as broad a representation of the various cerebral structures as possible, the quantitative autoradiographic technique used to measure the [^{14}C]antipyrine content in tissue in the measurement of local cerebral blood flow (Reivich et al., 1969) was selected to measure the [^{14}C]DG-6-P concentration in the cerebral tissues. The autoradiographs provide a pictorial representation of the relative rates of glucose phosphorylation in the various cerebral regions throughout the entire brain. The quantitation is arrived at by means of an equation derived from a kinetic model that considers the relationship between the rates of phosphorylation of DG and glucose by hexokinase. Briefly stated, the technique involves the administration of a pulse of [^{14}C]DG via a femoral venous catheter and killing the animal 45 min later. In the interval, timed samples of arterial blood are taken for the determination of the plasma concentration curves for [^{14}C]DG and glucose. The brain is frozen in Freon 12, chilled to $-75°C$ with liquid nitrogen, and cut into 20-μm sections. Autoradiographs are then prepared and the optical densities corresponding to specific cerebral structures are measured with a densitometer.

The details of the theoretical analysis have been published elsewhere (Sokoloff, 1975a,b), but the key assumptions involved are as follows: (1) A steady state for glucose (i.e., a constant plasma glucose concentration and a constant rate of tissue glucose consumption) is maintained throughout the procedure; (2) there are homogeneous tissue compartments within which the precursor concentrations of [^{14}C]DG and glucose are uniform and exchange directly with the plasma; and (3) tracer concentrations of [^{14}C]DG (i.e., molecular concentrations of free [^{14}C]DG) are essentially equal to zero. Mathematical analysis of the model leads to the following equation:

$$R_i = \frac{C_i^*(T) - k_1^* e^{-(k_2^* + k_3^*)T} \int_0^T C_p^* e^{(k_2^* + k_3^*)t} \, dt}{\left(\dfrac{\lambda \cdot V_{max}^* \cdot K_m}{\phi \cdot V_{max} \cdot K_m^*} \right) \left[\int_0^T (C_p^*/C_p) \, dt - e^{-(k_2^* + k_3^*)T} \int_0^T (C_p^*/C_p) e^{(k_2^* + k_3^*)t} \, dt \right]}$$

where

R_i = glucose consumption per gm of tissue

$C_i^*(T)$ = total concentration of [^{14}C]DG and [^{14}C]DG-6-P (determined by quantitative autoradiography) in the tissues at time, T

C_p^* = arterial plasma [^{14}C]DG concentration

C_p = arterial plasma glucose concentration

k_1^* = rate constant for transport of [^{14}C]DG from plasma to tissue precursor pool

k_2^* = rate constant for transport of [^{14}C]DG from tissue back to plasma

k_3^* = rate constant for phosphorylation of [^{14}C]DG

λ = ratio of distribution volume of [^{14}C]DG to that of glucose in the tissue

ϕ = fraction of glucose that, once phosphorylated, is glycolytically and oxidatively metabolized

K_m^* = Michaelis-Menten kinetic constant of hexokinase for [^{14}C]DG

$V_{max}^* =$ maximum velocity of hexokinase for $[^{14}C]DG$

$K_m =$ Michaelis-Menten constant of hexokinase for glucose

$V_{max} =$ maximum velocity of hexokinase for glucose

The rate constants are determined experimentally, and the λ, ϕ, and enzyme kinetic constants are conveniently grouped to constitute a single "lumped" constant (shown in the denominator of the equation). This lumped constant can be shown mathematically to equal the asymptotic value of the product of the ratio of the cerebral extraction ratio of $[^{14}C]DG$ to that of glucose and the ratio of the relative concentrations of $[^{14}C]DG$ and glucose in arterial blood and plasma-specific activities when the arterial $[^{14}C]DG$ concentration is maintained constant. In the rat the lumped constant has been determined from arterial and cerebral venous blood samples drawn during an intravenous infusion schedule that maintains a constant arterial plasma $[^{14}C]DG$ concentration (see Table 1).

TABLE 1

Values for Lumped Constant in Conscious and
Thiopental-Anesthetized Albino Rats
[Sokoloff et al.*]

	Conscious	Thiopental anesthesia	Overall lumped constant
Mean	0.464	0.512	0.483
Standard deviation	±0.099	0.118	±0.107
Standard error	±0.026	0.039	±0.022
No. of animals	15	9	24
Significance of difference: $0.4 > p > 0.3$			

*Sokoloff, Reivich, Kennedy, Des Rosiers, Patlak, Pettigrew, Sakurada, and Shinohara: "The $[^{14}C]$deoxyglucose method for the measurement of local cerebral glucose utilization," manuscript in preparation.

Improved Resolution of the $[1\text{-}^{14}C]$-2-Deoxy-D-Glucose Technique and Tissue Localization: F.R. Sharp

Improved Resolution

One continuing problem that besets techniques for the measurement of brain glucose consumption is what proportion of the total brain glucose uptake is accounted for by the uptake of individual glial, synaptic, and neuronal elements. One possible approach to the solution of this problem would be to improve the resolution of the $[^{14}C]DG$ technique. In addition, improved resolution might eventually make possible the mapping of specific synapses, glia, and/or neuronal perikarya that have altered their $[^{14}C]DG$ uptake in relation to functional activity.

The resolution of the $[^{14}C]DG$ technique has been improved somewhat by utilizing $[^3H]$-2-deoxy-D-glucose ($[^3H]DG$) and a modified Appleton technique for diffusible substances (Rogers, 1973; Sharp, 1976b) in the following ways: Frozen sections of rat brain, 10 μm thick, are cut at $-12°C$ in a cryostat, picked up onto frozen, emulsion-coated slides under a safelight, and kept frozen in sealed black boxes at $-20°C$ for 2 weeks. The slides are then developed, fixed, and counterstained with thionin, and grain counts of the various tissue elements are carried out. Technical factors that limit the use of this method include possible diffusion of DG-6-P and limited penetration of ^3H through the tissue.

The resulting autoradiographs revealed that silver grains (representing mainly $[^3H]DG$-6-P) were located over gray (Figure 1, B to F) as well as over white matter (Figure 1A). Cervical cord gray matter in the resting rat had, on the average, 2.4 times the grain density as white matter (Table 2). In gray matter the grain density over neuronal perikarya was slightly greater or about equal to the grain density over immediately surrounding neuropil (Figure 1D and Figure 2); there were from 2% to 20% more grains per unit area over neuronal perikarya than over the adjacent neuropil (Table 2). Although grain counts over glia were not done, it appeared that glia tended to have grain densities similar to those of the surrounding neuropil in gray matter, and white matter oligodendroglia tended to have grain densities similar to those of the surrounding white matter.

The observation that neuronal perikarya have only slightly greater grain densities than those of the surrounding neuropil throughout CNS gray matter implies that the glucose uptake of neuronal perikarya is similar to that of its immediately surrounding neuropil. Using this generalization, an estimate of what proportion of gray matter glucose uptake is accounted for by the uptake of neuronal perikarya and neuropil can be made. For example, on a volume basis, cervical cord gray matter is 85% neuropil and 10% neuronal perikarya (Mayhew and Momoh, 1974). Using the grain counts for cervical cord in Table 2, it can be estimated that 82% of cervical cord glucose uptake is accounted for by the *neuropil* and 13% by the *neuronal perikarya*. Since in most CNS areas the gray matter is composed predominantly of

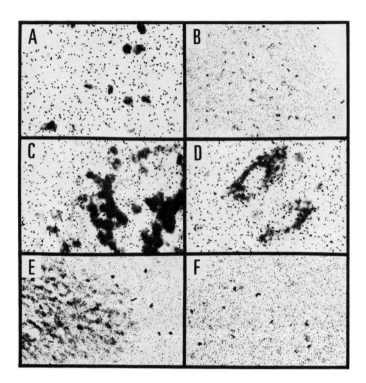

Figure 1. [³H]-2-Deoxy-D-glucose nuclear emulsion autoradiographs of thionin-stained brain sections of a resting, restrained rat. The silver grains represent mainly [³H]DG-6-P. Note that silver grains are located over cell bodies, neuropil, and white matter. A. White matter of cervical cord. ×1000. B. Dorsal horn of cervical cord. ×400. C. Cerebellum. ×1000. D. Nucleus reticularis gigantocellularis. ×1000. E. Hippocampus. ×400. F. Auditory cortex. ×400. [Sharp, 1976b]

TABLE 2

Averaged Grain Counts of [³H]-2-Deoxy-D-Glucose Autoradiographs
in Four Resting, Awake Rats [Sharp]

Structure	Grain count
White matter of cervical cord	7.3 ± 0.8
Neuronal perikarya of ventral horn of cervical cord	17.2 ± 1.8
Neuropil of ventral horn of cervical cord	16.9 ± 1.7
Neuronal perikarya of nucleus reticularis gigantocellularis	13.9 ± 1.4
Neuropil of nucleus reticularis gigantocellularis	12.6 ± 1.3
Neuronal perikarya of inferior olive	20.5 ± 2.1
Neuropil of inferior olive	17.8 ± 1.8
Neuronal perikarya of hippocampus	13.1 ± 1.4
Neuropil of hippocampus	10.8 ± 1.1

All counts were done under oil within a 400-μ^2 area. The 95% confidence limits are given.

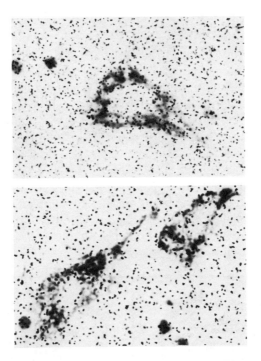

Figure 2. [³H]-2-Deoxy-D-glucose nuclear emulsion autoradiographs of thionin-stained sections of the ventral horn of the lumbar spinal cord of a resting, restrained rat. Note the similar density of silver grains over the cell bodies of the motor neurons and the surrounding neuropil. ×1000. [Sharp]

neuropil, the bulk of gray matter glucose uptake must be accounted for by the neuropil (Sharp, 1976b).

The finding that glucose uptake is highly active in the neuropil is compatible with the observation of high-affinity transport of deoxyglucose in synaptosomes (Diamond and Fishman, 1973). It is also compatible with the suggestion by Lowry and co-workers (1954) that the bulk of brain oxidative metabolism is accounted for by cell processes and nerve terminals. This was based on the finding of similar oxidative enzyme activities in the granular and molecular layers of Ammon's horn.

That neuropil accounts for much of the DG uptake of gray matter has important implications. The DG technique may well serve as an indicator of activity-related changes in neuropil glucose uptake—in short, as a "neuropil stain" of functional activity. If resolution can be improved even further, it might eventually be possible to study functionally related changes at individual synapses.

Tissue Localization

Additional evidence concerning the distribution of DG in the neuropil and neuronal perikarya has been obtained by comparison of histological sections with routine $[^{14}C]DG$ autoradiographs. Figure 3A shows a Nissl-stained (thionin) rat brain section in which mainly neuronal perikarya are seen. The $[^{14}C]DG$ X-ray film autoradiograph in Figure 3D, however, demonstrates that $[^{14}C]DG$ uptake occurs in regions of the neuropil, neuronal perikarya, and white matter. In neuronal perikarya regions (for example, in the granular layer of the cerebellum), the optical density is either slightly greater or very similar to the optical density in neuropil areas (for example, in the molecular layer of the cerebellum). This observation is consistent with the finding of similar grain counts over neuronal perikarya and neuropil noted in the previous section.

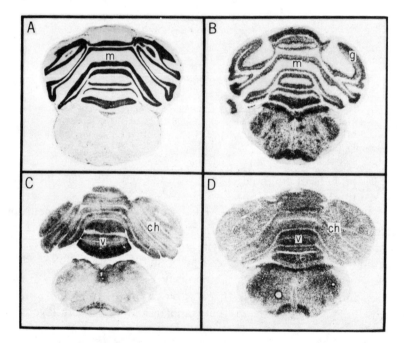

Figure 3. A. Nissl-stained section (thionin) of the pons and cerebellum of rat brain. B. X-ray film autoradiograph of the pons and cerebellum of rat brain obtained by perfusion with formaldehyde 45 min after administration of $[^{14}C]$glucose. C. X-ray film autoradiograph obtained by perfusion with glutaraldehyde 45 min after intravenous administration of $[^{14}C]$glucose to the rat. D. $[^{14}C]DG$ autoradiograph of pons and cerebellum of rat brain obtained by sacrificing the rat 45 min after administration of $[^{14}C]DG$. ch = cerebellar hemisphere; g = granular layer of cerebellum; m = molecular layer of cerebellum; v = vermis of cerebellum. [Sharp]

Although most of the glucose normally metabolized by the brain is converted into ATP, CO_2, and water, a small proportion of the glucose does go into the formation of amino acids, peptides, glycoprotein and other proteins, glycogen, as well as other derivatives. Therefore, independent methods were used to show that the derivatives of metabolized glucose are found in neuropil regions as well as in the neuronal perikarya. To do this, the following two sets of experiments were performed: In the first instance, rats were given [^{14}C]glucose intravenously and 45 min later perfused with 10% formalin. The brains were soaked in formalin for 3 weeks, cut, and then autoradiographed (see Figure 3B). It is apparent that the formalin-fixed derivatives of [^{14}C]glucose occur primarily in neuronal perikarya and glia. Since it is believed that formalin fixes protein and since protein is formed primarily in the cell bodies of neurons and glia, this result might be expected. The second series of experiments were done by using 1.25% glutaraldehyde-1% formalin as the perfusate instead of 10% formalin as in the above experiments (see Figure 3C for a typical autoradiograph). It is apparent that glutaraldehyde-formaldehyde-fixed derivatives of [^{14}C]glucose occur over regions of the neuronal perikarya and neuropil in a distribution somewhat similar to that seen in [^{14}C]DG autoradiographs (see Figure 3D). Since it is thought that glutaraldehyde may fix amino acids, peptides, and glycogen as well as proteins, glutaraldehyde appears to be fixing these derivatives of [^{14}C]glucose in about the same proportions over neuropil as over neuronal perikarya.

IV. APPLICATION OF THE 2-DEOXY-D-GLUCOSE METHOD TO THE COUPLING OF CEREBRAL METABOLISM AND BLOOD FLOW: M. Reivich and L. Sokoloff

Coupling between the metabolism and blood flow of a tissue in a given functional state has concerned physiologists for many years. Although the results of most past studies in this area have supported the existence of such a flow-metabolism couple in brain, they have been largely inferential in nature. Recent efforts to find a functional role for the rich innervation that surrounds cerebral vessels have emphasized the paucity of definitive experiments that link blood flow to a purely metabolic signal in brain tissue (Reivich, 1974; Ingvar and Lassen, 1975). The advent of the $[^{14}C]DG$ method has made it possible to attack this problem more directly.

For the relation of oxygen metabolism to cerebral blood flow, the noninvasive indicator exchange method described by Kety and Schmidt (1945) has been applied to various species, including man. Studies of various functional and disease states indicate that the rate of oxygen metabolism varies widely among different species, being highest in rat (Norberg and Siesjö, 1974a,b; Gjedde et al., 1975b) and lower among the higher mammals but roughly similar in dog, nonhuman primate, and man. The findings indicate that blood flow and metabolism change in parallel with each other in many functional states, but the couple can vary widely in conditions where drugs or disease directly affects the responses of either the brain, the vascular bed, or both. The DG method has made the measurement of regional metabolism in experimental animals feasible; moreover, in conjunction with the tools for measuring regional blood flow (Landau et al., 1955), this method will make possible a deeper understanding of the circumstances, as well as the extent of coupling, of blood flow and cerebral metabolism.

Local cerebral blood flow has been measured by the $[^{14}C]$anti-pyrine technique, and local cerebral glucose utilization has been measured by the $[^{14}C]DG$ method in the same cerebral structures of the conscious and anesthetized rat (Des Rosiers et al., 1974; Reivich, 1974). The results demonstrated a remarkably close correlation between local blood flow and glucose consumption ($r = 0.974$) in the conscious rat (Figure 4). Depression in energy metabolism produced by thiopental anesthesia resulted in proportionate decreases in local blood flow, and the close correlation between local blood flow and metabolism was maintained (Des Rosiers et al., 1974). These results indicate an adjustment of the blood flow to local metabolic demands.

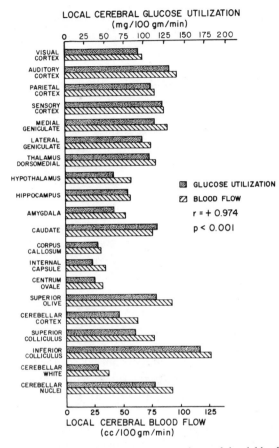

Figure 4. Correlation between local glucose consumption and local blood flow in various regions of the brain in awake rats. The values for local cerebral glucose utilization were calculated on the assumption of a lumped constant of 0.483. [Adapted from Reivich, 1974]

V. RELATION OF CENTRAL NERVOUS SYSTEM GLUCOSE
METABOLISM TO NEURONAL STRUCTURE

Sciatic Nerve Stimulation: F.R. Sharp and L. Sokoloff

Autoradiographs obtained by the $[^{14}C]$ DG method (Sokoloff et al., 1974;Sokoloff, 1975a,b) provide a pictorial representation of the relative rates of glucose uptake in brain regions. In other words, the darker the area on an autoradiograph (the greater the optical density), the greater is the glucose uptake of that area. Thus, it seemed appropriate to use the $[^{14}C]$ DG method to test the hypothesis that local alterations of brain glucose consumption accompany alterations of local CNS activity. The technique revealed not only regional increases due to sciatic nerve stimulation but also the anatomical distribution in which these glucose uptake changes occurred (Sharp, 1974; Kennedy et al., 1975).

$[^{14}C]$ DG was administered intravenously as a pulse (16.7 μCi/ 100 gm body weight) to anesthetized rats, and the sciatic nerve was stimulated at 50 cps for 45 min. The animal was then sacrificed with sodium pentobarbital, and the lumbar spinal cord was rapidly removed and frozen. Frozen sections, 20-μm thick, were immediately cut on a cryostat, quickly dried on a hot plate, and autoradiographed (Reivich et al., 1969).

Sciatic nerve stimulation caused large increases of glucose uptake in the ipsilateral dorsal horn of the lumbar spinal cord, as shown by autoradiography in Figures 5 and 6D. Increases in optical density in

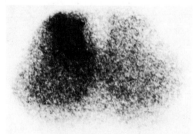

Figure 5. Autoradiograph of the lumbar cord of an anesthetized rat subjected to unilateral electrical stimulation of sciatic nerve. Note the increased optical density in the ipsilateral dorsal horn gray, ventral horn gray, and white matter as compared with the unstimulated side. [Kennedy et al., 1975]

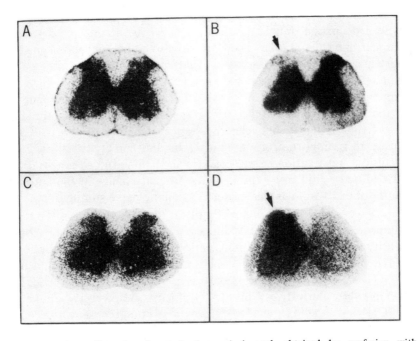

Figure 6. A. Autoradiograph of rat lumbar spinal cord obtained by perfusion with glutaraldehyde-formaldehyde 45 min after injection of [^{14}C]glucose into the anesthetized, unstimulated rat. B. Autoradiograph prepared as that in A, except that the sciatic nerve was stimulated for 45 min. The arrow points to the decreased optical density in the dorsal horn ipsilateral to the side of stimulation. C. Autoradiograph of rat lumbar spinal cord obtained by sacrifice of the animal 45 min after injection of [^{14}C]DG into the anesthetized, unstimulated rat. D. Autoradiograph prepared as that in C, except that the sciatic nerve was stimulated for 45 min. The arrow points to the increased optical density in the dorsal horn ipsilateral to the side of stimulation. [Sharp, 1976a]

the white matter and ventral horn gray matter ipsilateral to the side of stimulation were also seen. The [^{14}C]DG autoradiographs of control rats, which were anesthetized but not stimulated, reveal that the optical densities of the two dorsal horns were similar, as shown in Figure 6C.

The demonstration that stimulation of the sciatic nerve increases the total glucose uptake of the ipsilateral dorsal horn suggested that stimulation of the sciatic nerve might also alter the small fraction of glucose incorporated into amino acids, peptides, and glycoproteins, as well as other proteins. To demonstrate such an alteration, another technique was used in which [^{14}C]glucose, rather than [^{14}C]DG, was given intravenously, and the sciatic nerve was stimulated for 45 min. The animal was perfused with 1.25% glutaraldehyde-1% formalin, the lumbar cord was removed and soaked in the perfusate, and sections were cut and autoradiographed (Sharp, 1976a). Of twelve rats, six showed decreased optical density ipsilateral to the side of sciatic nerve stimulation (Figure 6B). There were also small decreases in white matter and ventral horn gray matter ipsilateral to the side of stimulation. In the other six rats in which the sciatic nerve was stimulated, there was no effect. A typical autoradiograph (Figure 6A) of the lumbar cord from a control rat, anesthetized but not stimulated, shows the similarity between the optical densities of the two dorsal horns. It is important to note that in another study 10% formalin perfusion and fixation *alone,* performed 45 min after administration of [^{14}C]glucose, did not exhibit any signficant change in the autoradiographs of eight animals that underwent sciatic nerve stimulation.

The area of *decreased* optical density after [^{14}C]glucose administration (Figure 6B) is similar to the region of *increased* optical density after [^{14}C]DG administration. Sciatic nerve stimulation resulted in similar anatomical distributions of both the increase in [^{14}C]DG uptake and the decrease in glutaraldehyde-formaldehyde-precipitated derivatives of [^{14}C]glucose. However, unlike the [^{14}C]DG technique, the [^{14}C]glucose method at present is unreliable, since only six out of twelve rats showed an effect. In spite of such problems, the use of both techniques has revealed that functionally related changes of two *different* aspects of glucose metabolism appear to occur in approximately the same anatomical regions (Sharp, 1976a).

The decrease of glutaraldehyde-formaldehyde-fixed derivatives of [^{14}C]glucose in the dorsal horn ipsilateral to the side of sciatic nerve stimulation suggests decreased anabolic activity associated with massive neuronal excitation. Other workers have found that electrical stimulation of brain slices decreased the incorporation of [^{14}C]glucose into protein (Orrego and Lipmann, 1967). There are also indications that the brain damage that results from excessive neuronal activity in neonate and infantile epilepsy may be related to decreased protein synthesis (Wasterlain and Plum, 1973b; Wasterlain, 1974).

Olfactory Stimulation: G.M. Shepherd

The olfactory bulb was one of the first regions of the mammalian brain to be described in detail in terms of local circuit neurons and their synaptic interactions and central connections (Rall et al., 1966; Shepherd, 1972; Rakic, 1975). In brief (see Figure 7), the arrangement consists of olfactory fibers coming from the nose and

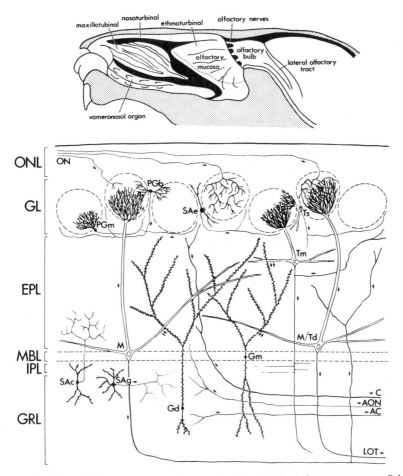

Figure 7. *Above:* Schematic diagram of head of a rabbit showing olfactory structures. *Below:* Schematic diagram of neuronal organization of olfactory bulb. AC = fibers from anterior commissure; AON = fibers from anterior olfactory nucleus; C = centrifugal fibers; EPL = external plexiform layer; Gd = granule cell with cell body in deep layers; GL = glomerular layer; Gm = granule cell with cell body in mitral body layer; GRL = granule layer; IPL = internal plexiform layer; LOT = lateral olfactory tract. Main layers of bulb are indicated at left; M = mitral cell; MBL = mitral body layer; M/Td = displaced mitral or deep tufted cell; ON = olfactory nerves; ONL = olfactory nerve layer; PGb = periglomerular cell with biglomerular dendrites; PGm = periglomerular cell with monoglomerular dendrites; SAc = short-axon cell of Ramón y Cajal; SAe = short-axon cell with extraglomerular dendrites; SAg = short-axon cell of Golgi; Tm = middle tufted cell; Ts = superficial tufted cell. [Shepherd, 1972]

terminating in the glomeruli of the olfactory bulb where they synapse with the principal relay cells, the mitral (and tufted) cells, which send their axons to the olfactory cortex of the rhinencephalon. The mitral

cells have both primary and secondary dendrites that form dendrodendritic synapses along much of their length with the dendrites of
interneurons.

     The olfactory bulb contains two main types of interneurons: In
the outer glomerular layer, periglomerular (PG) short-axon cells have
dendrites that terminate in tufts inside the glomeruli and make single or
reciprocal synapses with the dendritic tufts of the mitral cells. In the
deeper, external plexiform layer, granule cells (which lack axons) have
dendritic trees that ramify and have reciprocal synapses between their
dendritic spines and the secondary dendrites of the mitral cells. The
mitral cells are believed to be excitatory to the granule cells, and the
granule cells inhibitory to the mitral cells, through these synapses (Rall
et al., 1966). There is evidence that PG cells, possibly acting through
dopamine, are also inhibitory to mitral cells; granule cell inhibition may
be mediated by γ-aminobutyric acid.

     The layers of cell bodies and synaptic neuropil in the olfactory
bulb are organized in several distinct layers, as can be seen in Figure 7.
From the surface, these are the olfactory nerve layer, glomerular layer,
external plexiform layer, mitral body layer, internal plexiform layer,
and granule layer. This distinct lamination and the fact that specific
excitatory and inhibitory actions have been identified at the main types
of synaptic connections led to the olfactory bulb's being selected for a
detailed analysis of the relation of localized metabolic activity to
neuronal structure. The procedure is as follows: Rats in sealed jars were
studied at rest, with or without one nostril closed by suture, and during
exposure to specific odors, e.g., amyl acetate (a banana-like odor) and
camphor. During the test period they were injected with a pulse of
$[^{14}C]$ DG in the manner described above by Sokoloff. The brains were
then removed and frozen, and the olfactory bulbs and telencephalon
were sectioned and autoradiographed. Selected sections were then
stained with thionin for detailed comparison with the autoradiographic
patterns.

     The olfactory bulbs of rats with nostrils open only to ambient
room air showed three main layers of different glucose uptake
(Figure 8B, right bulb): an outer light layer that corresponds to the
olfactory nerve layer, a middle dense band that extends from the
glomerular layer superficially to the granule layer centrally, and a
center that, by comparison, is also light. The histological section from
which this autoradiograph was produced is shown in Figure 8A (right
bulb). In some of the controls exposed to room air, small densities,

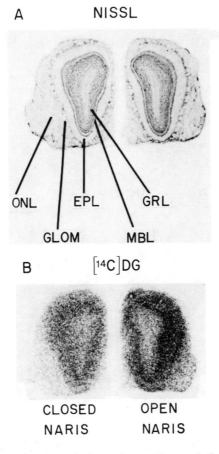

Figure 8. A. Thionin-stained Nissl sections of rat olfactory bulb. B. Autoradiograph of sections in A. Left nostril was sutured shut 24 hours prior to the administration of [^{14}C] DG. EPL = external plexiform layer; GLOM = glomerular layer; GRL = granule layer; MBL = mitral body layer; ONL = olfactory nerve layer. [Sharp et al., 1975]

roughly the size of a small group of glomeruli, were occasionally visible over the glomerular layer.

     Closure of one nostril 1 day prior to the experiment caused a general decrease of density in the bulb on that side (Figure 8B, left bulb). There was also a slightly decreased density in the olfactory nerve layer, indicating a reduced glucose consumption in these layers.

     Exposure of the rat to the fruitlike odor of amyl acetate resulted in the appearance of two main areas of increased glucose consumption: one area appeared over the lateral and dorsolateral aspects of the bulb, extending from the anterior to the middle of the

A   NISSL

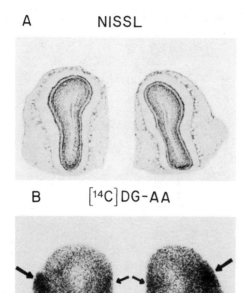

B   [¹⁴C]DG-AA

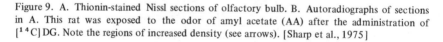

Figure 9. A. Thionin-stained Nissl sections of olfactory bulb. B. Autoradiographs of sections in A. This rat was exposed to the odor of amyl acetate (AA) after the administration of [¹⁴C]DG. Note the regions of increased density (see arrows). [Sharp et al., 1975]

bulb, and the other over the medial aspect of the bulb, extending from the middle to the posterior of the bulb (Figure 9). These results were generally reproducible in different animal experiments. Exposure to the odor of camphor resulted in a different density pattern; it was more localized over the dorsal region of the bulb.

The thionin-stained sections of the bulb (Figure 9A) showed that the increased densities occurred primarily in the glomerular layer and extended into the olfactory nerve and external plexiform layers. The olfactory nerve layer consists of many millions of unmyelinated fibers, 0.2 μm in diameter, and glia. The absence of nerve cell bodies and synapses in this layer indicates that neuronal activity near, as well as at the site of, the synaptic terminals may be associated with an increased glucose consumption, and it confirms that considerable energy is required by unmyelinated fibers compared to myelinated fibers. In addition, the density of the glomerular layer may provide a

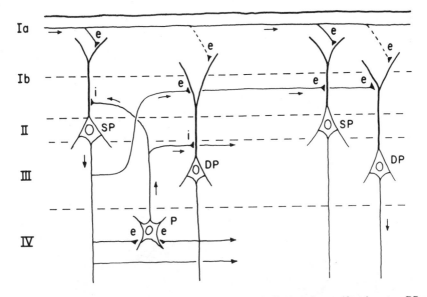

Figure 10. Schematic diagram of synaptic organization of olfactory (prepyriform) cortex. DP = deep pyramidal cell; e = excitatory action; i = inhibitory action; P = polymorphic cell; SP = superficial pyramidal cell. Abbreviations for layers are explained in the text. [Haberly and Shepherd, 1973]

specific model for the energy demands of a dense synaptic system somewhat similar to the motor end plate.

Stimulation of the olfactory nerves in rabbits under pentothal anesthesia (1 volley every 4 sec for the 45-min period following [^{14}C] DG injection) demonstrated the presence of localized regions of glucose consumption; these regions were consistent with the topography of localized olfactory nerve projections shown by Land and co-workers (1970).

The olfactory bulb projects by way of the lateral olfactory tract to the olfactory cortex (prepyriform cortex). A schematic diagram of synaptic connections postulated within the prepyriform cortex is shown in Figure 10. There are several distinct histological layers, which include the tract itself most superficially, the terminals of the tract (Ib), the superficial pyramidal cells (II), the deep pyramidal cells (III), and the polymorphic cells (IV) centrally. It is believed that within these layers, short- and long-axon collaterals of pyramidal cells form excitatory connections, and polymorphic cells form inhibitory connections. The [^{14}C] DG autoradiographs revealed a superficial transparent

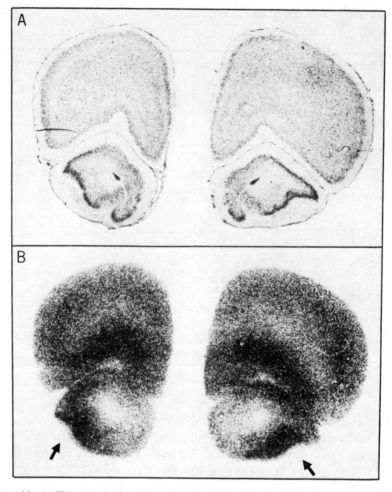

Figure 11. A. Thionin-stained sections through anterior telencephalon. B. Autoradiographs of sections in A. Note low density over lateral olfactory tracts (see arrows) and high density in underlying prepyriform cortex. [Sharp, Kauer, and Shepherd]

layer coinciding with the tract, and a deeper dense band that contains the plexiform layer and extends into the deeper pyramidal and polymorphic cell layers (Figure 11).

Visual Stimulation: L. Sokoloff

The visual system in the rat is 80% to 85% crossed at the optic chiasma, and unilateral enucleation removes most of the sensory input, which derives from either retinal stimulation by light or spontaneous retinal ganglion cell discharge to the central visual structures of the contralateral side. In the conscious rat studied 4 to 24 hours after

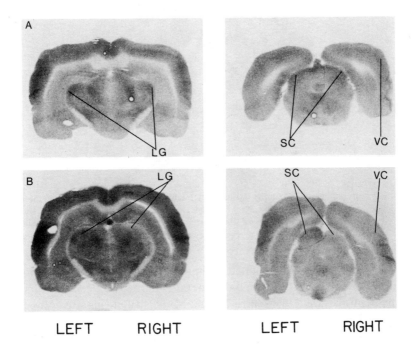

Figure 12. Effects of unilateral enucleation on local cerebral glucose utilization in the lateral geniculates (LG), superior colliculi (SC), and visual cortex (VC) of the conscious rat. A. Control. B. Left eye removed. [Kennedy et al., 1975]

unilateral enucleation, there were marked decrements in $[^{14}C]$ DG-6-P accumulation in the contralateral superior colliculus, lateral geniculate body, and visual cortex as compared to the ipsilateral side. These effects were observed whether the remaining eye was stimulated repetitively with a photoflash or the animal was maintained in normal room light (Figure 12B). In the rat with both eyes intact, no asymmetry was observed (Figure 12A).

In the monkey, in which the visual pathways are approximately 50% crossed at the optic chiasm (Brouwer and Zeeman, 1926; Polyak, 1932), unilateral enucleation produced no asymmetry in the optical densities corresponding to the superior colliculi, lateral geniculate, and most areas of the visual cortex. There were, however, two small areas of the striate cortex which exhibited asymmetry. One, which is situated in the most rostral portion of the mushroom-like area of the deep calcarine cortex (Figure 13), receives only monocular input from the extreme nasal portion of the contralateral retina (Brouwer and Zeeman, 1926; Polyak, 1932).

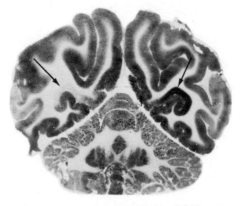

Figure 13. Autoradiographic demonstration of monocular input to the dorsal lip of the most rostral portion of the mushroom-like area of the calcarine cortex in the rhesus monkey. The left occipital cortex is on the left side of the figure. The left eye was enucleated. Note the asymmetry in the mushrooms of the two sides (see arrows) with the diminished optical density contralateral to the enucleated eye. [Kennedy et al., 1975]

Thus, it can be concluded that unilateral enucleation removes all input to this area on the contralateral side, and, indeed, autoradiographs demonstrate a marked reduction of density at this site compared to the ipsilateral side.

The other area of asymmetry is located in a portion of striate cortex that may correspond to the "blind" spots of the visual fields. This area receives no input from the portion of the contralateral retina occupied by the optic disc, but it is fully innervated from the area of the ipsilateral retina that corresponds to the same spot in the visual field. Hence, unilateral enucleation does not alter the input to the contralateral cortical locus of the "blind" spot but removes all input to the ipsilateral locus. On the other hand, the surrounding striate cortex loses 50% of its input when either eye is removed. The neuroanatomical relationships are such that unilateral enucleation would be expected to reduce the input to the striate cortex of both sides by one-half, except in the loci for the "blind" spot where input is unaffected on the contralateral side and completely interrupted on the ipsilateral side.

In autoradiographs prepared from primates studied in the conscious state 24 hours after unilateral enucleation, a contralateral cortical locus in the deep-folded portion of the calcarine cortex appeared very dark compared to its surrounding striate cortex, whereas the same locus on the ipsilateral side was almost "blank," indicating markedly lower glucose consumption compared to the surrounding cortex (Figure 14). Other evidence suggests that the cortical locus of the "blind" spot is approximately in this area (Daniel and Whitteridge, 1961). Qualitatively similar though quantitatively less pronounced

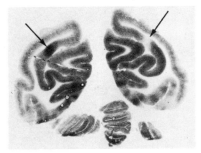

Figure 14. Localization of visual cortical representation of the "blind spots" of the visual fields in the rhesus monkey. The dark spot (see arrow) is in the visual cortex contralateral to the enucleated eye; the "blank" spot (see arrow) is in the ipsilateral occipital cortex. [Kennedy et al., 1975]

differences between the two sides were obtained when visual input to one eye was blocked with an opaque plastic disc instead of enucleation; the lesser contrast between the two sides probably reflects the persistence of spontaneous discharges from the retinal ganglion cells of the occluded eye (Hughes and Maffei, 1965).

The autoradiographs from monkeys with unilateral enucleation or obstructed vision also exhibited another interesting aspect of the structural and functional organization of the visual cortex. The areas corresponding to the visual cortex were permeated by alternating dark and light bands traversing perpendicularly through the visual cortex (Figure 15). These bands were not seen in blindfolded monkeys or in

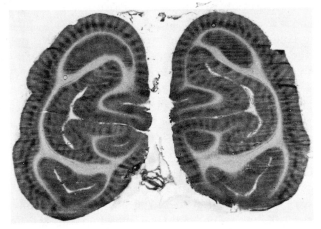

Figure 15. Autoradiographic visualization by means of the [^{14}C]DG method of the ocular dominance columns of Hubel and Wiesel (1972; Wiesel et al., 1974) in the rhesus monkey. One eye was enucleated; the other eye was stimulated by an illuminated, black-white, rotating geometric pattern. [Sokoloff, 1975b]

TABLE 3

A Comparison of Properties of Ocular Dominance Columns Observed
with Various Methods [Kennedy, Des Rosiers, and Sokoloff]

	Methods		
	Nauta degeneration*	Autoradiography† L [6-³H] fucose + L-[³H] proline	Autoradiography [¹⁴C]-2-Deoxy-D-glucose
Mode of induction	Lesion produced in a locus of a single layer of the lateral geniculate body	Labeled material injected into one eye. Autoradiographs made 3 weeks later	Labeled material given intravenously. Autoradiographs made from brain frozen 40 min later
Layers involved	Mainly IVc but also IVa and IVb. Also I, depending on locus or lesion in lateral geniculate	Mainly IVc; traces in IVa	Greatest density in IVc, but all cortical layers affected
Width of columns	0.25–0.5 mm	0.3–0.5 mm	0.4–0.5 mm; rarely as small as 0.2 mm
Columns deleted by	Lesion involving adjacent layers of lateral geniculate		
Columns absent in		Sections made in deep rostral (monocular) region of striate cortex	Sections made in deep rostral (monocular) region and cortical locus of retinal blind spot

*Hubel and Wiesel (1972).
†Wiesel and co-workers (1974).

monkeys with both eyes intact, and they resembled very closely the pattern of visual cortical organization for ocular dominance described by Hubel and Wiesel (1969, 1972) (Table 3).

The columns represent the pronounced vertical cellular organization of the sensory areas of the cerebral cortex that were described anatomically by Lorente de No (1934) and electrophysiologically by Mountcastle (1957), Mountcastle and Powell (1959), Hubel and Wiesel (1962), and Abeles and Goldstein (1970). This led Werner (1970) and Spinelli (1970) to suggest a process for somesthetic feature analysis in which "each cortical column comes to constitute an engram by virtue of its specific sensitivity to one pattern of neural activity, a 'list' of interresponse times of a firing neuron or the wave form that describes the envelope of the firing pattern" (Pribram, 1971, p. 127). Jones and co-workers (1975), likewise, demonstrated that commissural and corticocortical fibers arising and terminating in the somatic sensory cortex of primates originate and terminate in vertical bands or functional units based on afferent input.

Auditory Stimulation: L. Sokoloff

[^{14}C]DG has also been used to map the central auditory pathways of rat brain. Autoradiographs of brains of rats exposed to ambient laboratory noise showed high optical densities in regions that mediate hearing, i.e., the auditory cortex, medial geniculate body, inferior colliculus, lateral lemniscus, superior olive, and layer IV of the auditory cortex. When the external auditory canals were occluded and the rats were kept in sound-proof conditions, the optical densities of these regions decreased markedly (Figure 16). Unilateral occlusion resulted in marked asymmetry of optical density in the inferior colliculus, which shows decreased density on the contralateral side, in agreement with neuroanatomical observations (Osen, 1972).

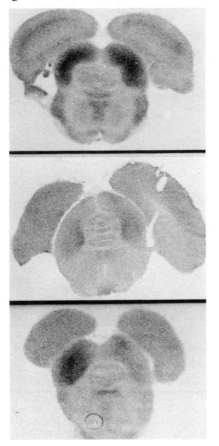

Figure 16. [^{14}C]DG autoradiographic visualization of the effects of altered auditory input on the local glucose utilization of some central auditory structures in the conscious albino rat. *Upper figure:* normal conscious rat. *Middle figure:* both external auditory canals were obstructed with wax and the animal was placed in a sound-proof room. *Lower figure:* only one auditory canal (contralateral to the side of the brain with reduced optical density in auditory structures) was obstructed. Note the inferior colliculi, lemnisci, and superior olives. [Des Rosiers, Kennedy, and Sokoloff]

Vestibular Stimulation: F.R. Sharp

These experiments were designed to determine whether vestibular stimulation would induce localized changes of $[^{14}C]DG$ uptake in the appropriate CNS structures. Continuous vestibular stimulation was achieved by placing rats, previously injected with $[^{14}C]DG$, in restrainers attached to a motorized rotating wheel and spinning them in the vertical plane for 45 min. Control rats were injected and placed in identical restrainers on the benchtop for 45 min.

Regional increases of $[^{14}C]DG$ uptake occurred in rotating (Figure 17, B and D) compared to resting (Figure 17, A and C) rats in the following structures: vestibular nuclei, flocculi, nodulus, ventral uvula, and accessory parafloculi (Sharp, 1976b). The regions of increased optical density correlated best with the major sites of

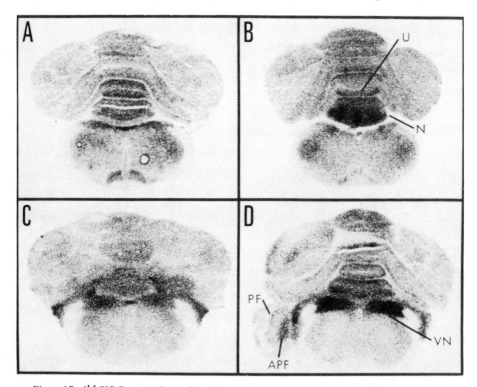

Figure 17. $[^{14}C]DG$ autoradiographs of the pons and cerebellum at two different levels of resting rats (A) and (C) and of rats that were rotated in the vertical plane (B) and (D). APF = accessory parafloculus; N = nodulus; PF = parafloculus; U = uvula; VN = vestibular nuclei. [Sharp, 1976b]

A   NISSL

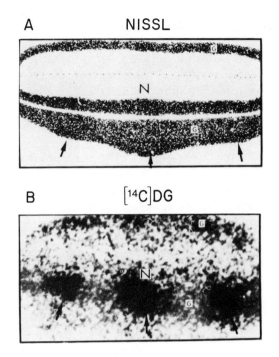

B   [¹⁴C]DG

Figure 18. A. Thionin-stained Nissl section of the dorsal and ventral folia of the nodulus similar to the one used to obtain the autoradiograph in B. The dotted line indicates the junction of the molecular layer of the dorsal folium of the nodulus and the molecular layer of the ventral folium of the nodulus. The three arrows indicate slight thickenings of the granular layer of the nodulus. B. [¹⁴C]DG autoradiograph in the region identical to that shown in A. The three arrows indicate three spots of increased optical density that occurred in the nodulus related to rotation. The three spots correspond to the three thickenings of the nodular granular layer shown in A (see arrows). G = granular layer; N = nodulus. [Sharp, 1976b]

termination of primary vestibular afferents. The changes in the cerebellum occurred both in the neuronal perikarya-rich granular layer and in the neuropil-rich molecular layer.

Autoradiographs of the vermis of the cerebellum from both control (Figure 17A) and rotating rats (Figure 17, B and D) showed dark horizontal bands of increased optical density alternating with lighter ones. Comparison of a thionin-stained Nissl section of the nodulus of the vermis in Figure 18A with a [¹⁴C]DG autoradiograph of the nodulus in Figure 18B revealed that the darker bands on the autoradiographs correspond to the granular layer while the lighter bands correspond to the molecular layers.

Three discrete spots of increased optical density in the nodulus were seen in all rotating animals (two rotating animals are represented in Figure 17, B and C). One spot was located in the center of the nodulus and the other two on either side. Comparison of autoradiographs with identical histological sections showed that the three spots correspond to three anatomical thickenings in the granular layer of the nodulus. Reconstructions showed that the three spots run longitudinally the entire length of the nodular granular layer, thereby dividing the granular layer of the nodulus into at least seven separate longitudinal zones of differing glucose uptake.

The seven metabolic zones in the granular layer of the nodulus of the rotating rat most likely represent a pattern of CNS activity related to rotation. The metabolic subdivision of the nodulus into longitudinal zones is in basic agreement with the anatomical subdivision of other areas of the vermis into longitudinal zones based on cerebellar morphology and corticogenesis (Korneliussen, 1968a,b,c), climbing fiber system projections (Oscarsson, 1965, 1969), and the spinocerebellar projection to the anterior lobe and simple lobule (Voogd et al., 1969).

Other experiments in which the $[^{14}C]DG$ technique can be used to study the vestibular system include: (1) unilateral destruction of the vestibular apparatus, (2) rotation in one plane of the semicircular canals, (3) stimulation of the vestibular nerves, and (4) determination of the effects of linear or angular acceleration.

General Motor Activity: F.R. Sharp

Swimming Rats

In these experiments the $[^{14}C]DG$ method was used to detect those areas of the brain in which glucose uptake was altered in swimming as compared with resting rats (Sharp, 1976b). Resting rats, injected with $[^{14}C]DG$ and restrained in clear Plexiglass holders, were placed in the bottom of an empty 10-gallon tank. Other rats without swimming experience were injected with $[^{14}C]DG$ and allowed to swim for 45 min in a similar tank filled with lukewarm water.

The optical densities obtained from autoradiography of the brains of swimming rats were 27% to 150% higher than those of resting rats. The largest increases due to swimming were in the vermis (150%) and paraflocculus (140%) of the cerebellum. Large increases were also found in the ventral tegmental nucleus (125%), cervical cord gray

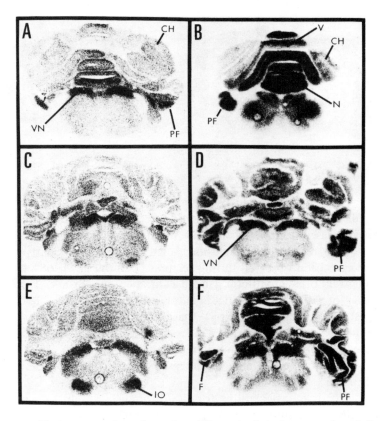

Figure 19. [^{14}C]DG autoradiographs at three different levels in the pons and cerebellum of resting rats (A), (C), and (E) and of swimming rats (B), (D), and (F). CH = cerebellar hemisphere; F = flocculus; IO = inferior olive; N = nodulus; PF = paraflocculus; VN = vestibular nuclei. [Sharp, 1976a]

(106%), ventral nuclei of the thalamus (95%) and vestibular nuclei (89%). Only small changes were found in the inferior colliculi (27%) and posterior cerebellar hemispheres (39%).

Typical autoradiographs of the pons and cerebellum at three different coronal levels in the resting rat are demonstrated in Figure 19, A, C, and E. For comparison, the typical patterns of altered [^{14}C]DG uptake of the pons and cerebellum at three different levels in the swimming rat are shown in Figure 19, B, D, and F. In the swimming rat the increases of optical density of the vermis and paraflocculus were much greater than the increases in the posterior cerebellar hemispheres or paramedian zones. Swimming and resting rats showed differences in most areas of the brain, including the frontal cortex and caudato-putamen (Figure 20).

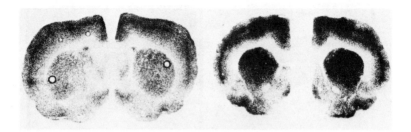

Figure 20. [^{14}C]DG autoradiographs at the level of the caudatoputamen and prefrontal cortex in a resting rat (at the left) and a swimming rat (at the right). [Sharp]

The changes in glucose uptake seen in the swimming rat may be related to stress and/or to the motor activity involved in swimming. That increased functional activity results in increased brain glucose uptake is a reasonable conclusion, since increases in oxidative metabolism have been observed during seizures (Plum et al., 1968), electrical stimulation of sympathetic ganglia (Larrabee and Bronk, 1952), and changes of firing rate of single neurons (Giacobini, 1969). It has been suggested by Sokoloff (1969) that stress per se need not increase cerebral oxygen consumption; but, if the degree of stress is of such a nature that pressor levels of circulating epinephrine are attained, then cerebral metabolic rate may be increased (King et al., 1952; Sensenbach et al., 1953).

Possible explanations for the differences in glucose uptake in the various structures of the swimming rat might include the following: those factors mediating stress affect various structures differently; different maximal rates of glucose uptake occur in different structures; or, different structures are not functionally driven to the same extent. The finding that glucose uptake in the cerebellar vermis is higher than that in the paramedian zones of the swimming rat is consonant with a cerebellar theory that postulates vermal control of whole-body movement and paramedian control of individual limb movement (Chambers and Sprague, 1955).

Behaving Monkey

The [^{14}C]DG technique has also been applied to the study of behaving monkeys. A water-deprived monkey, who was trained to squeeze a rubber bulb as rapidly as possible for 45 min, averaged 100 squeezes per min and received a juice reward every ninth squeeze. He was also required to keep the other hand constantly clenched. Autoradiographs revealed several discrete regions of increased optical density in the orbitofrontal and prefrontal areas contralateral to the rapidly squeezing hand. Bilateral increases of optical density in the face, pharyngeal, and "hand" regions of pre- and postcentral cortices were observed, the "hand" area of cortex contralateral to the rapidly squeezing hand having a greater optical density than the ipsilateral one. There were discrete regions of increased optical density in the cerebellar hemispheres, both ipsilateral to the rapidly squeezing hand and ipsilateral to the clenched hand.

The results indicate that regional increases of glucose uptake occur in the brain of the awake primate trained to do a specific task. By studying alterations of glucose uptake in specific brain structures or sets of structures with changes of behavior, the mapping of those structures that *are* involved in a given behavior may be possible. By careful analysis of the behaviors that "turn on a structure," it may be possible to ascribe certain functions to that structure.

Unanswered Questions

Although the previous sections of this *Bulletin* demonstrated that the $[^{14}C]DG$ technique holds considerable promise for mapping functional pathways, a host of unanswered questions arise regarding the use of this technique for "metabolic mapping." Will structures far removed from the primary sensory input increase their glucose uptake with appropriate changes of behavior? Can all brain structures be shown to increase or decrease their glucose uptake? What is the effect of diffusely projecting brain pathways on brain glucose utilization? What is the relationship between cell firing rate and release of excitatory or inhibitory transmitters with changes of brain glucose uptake? What are the brain compartments (neuronal, glial, synaptic, etc.) that change their uptake and to what degree do they do so? Will the technique be applicable to invertebrates? How sensitive is the method?

Some answers to these questions are already becoming available. For example, most of the gray structures in the brains of swimming and anesthetized rats do change their $[^{14}C]DG$ uptake whereas the brains of resting rats do not, and the behaving monkey experiment provides some preliminary evidence that structures far removed from the initial sensory input can increase their glucose utilization.

The question of what effect diffusely projecting systems have on brain glucose uptake has been probed by making lesions in ascending catecholaminergic pathways. It was found that unilateral destruction of ascending dopaminergic pathways results in an ipsilateral depression of forebrain glucose uptake in the caudatoputamen, frontal cortex, and other structures (Schwartz et al., 1976). The normal rate of forebrain glucose uptake in the awake, restrained rat appears to depend on intact dopaminergic fibers. The effects of lesions of other central pathways remain to be determined.

The mammalian brain is unique in that under normal circumstances most of its energy is derived from glucose. Therefore, the $[^{14}C]DG$ uptake of a brain region can be viewed as an index of that region's *total metabolic work,* and alterations of $[^{14}C]DG$ uptake associated with alterations of behavior could be viewed as changes of such a region's metabolic work. It is important to note that changes in cell firing rates seen with alterations of behavior are not necessarily measures of changes of metabolic work. For example, increased release of an inhibitory neurotransmitter will decrease the firing rates of cells in a particular region of the neuropil; but, if the total metabolic work of that region should increase, then the $[^{14}C]DG$ uptake would increase as well. On the other hand, increased release of excitatory neurotransmitter might also require increased metabolic work, in which case both $[^{14}C]DG$ uptake and cell firing rates would increase. It is possible that changes of metabolic work detectable with the $[^{14}C]DG$ technique might occur without any changes in cell firing rates at all. In this way, the technique, particularly when combined with other more classical methods, may prove very useful for helping us to understand the brain.

VI. REGIONAL CEREBRAL GLUCOSE CONSUMPTION RATES IN SOME EXPERIMENTAL STATES

Anesthetics: M. Reivich and L. Sokoloff

The depression of local cerebral glucose utilization in some selected structures of thiopental-anesthetized rats has been determined, as shown in Table 4 (Sokoloff, 1975a). In studies conducted with Shapiro and Greenberg, Reivich and Sokoloff determined the regional rates of cerebral glucose consumption in rhesus monkeys anesthetized with halothane, pentobarbital, or phencyclidine and compared their findings with those obtained from awake animals (see Shapiro et al., 1975). Significant differences in the action of these three anesthetics were noted: (1) Halothane (0.9%) caused a reduction in metabolism in almost all structures except the vestibular nuclei where regional glucose metabolism was increased. A progressive depression in cortical metabolism appeared to occur in a rostral-caudal direction. However, such a gradient did not exist in the awake state, nor was this gradient observed

TABLE 4

Normal Values for Local Cerebral Glucose Utilization
in Some Selected Structures of Conscious and
Thiopental-Anesthetized Albino Rats
[Sokoloff, 1975a]

Structure	Mean glucose utilization (μmoles/100 gm/min)		Percent difference
	Unanesthetized (8 rats)	Anesthetized* (3 rats)	
Visual cortex	95	65	−31
Auditory cortex	148	80	−45
Thalamus	106	54	−49
Medial geniculate	119	63	−47
Lateral geniculate	98	47	−51
Hypothalamus	67	37	−45
Inferior colliculus	185	129	−30
Superior colliculus	91	57	−37
Pontine gray matter	60	42	−30
Cerebral white matter	44	26	−43

*All reductions from normal in the anesthetized state are statistically significant ($p < 0.05$).

in animals under pentobarbital anesthesia. (2) Pentobarbital caused a greater and more uniform reduction in gray matter structures. In white matter areas, both halothane and pentobarbital produced a relatively uniform decrease in metabolism of approximately 40%. Differential regional effects were also apparent in the basal ganglia where halothane had no effect, whereas pentobarbital reduced glucose consumption in the putamen and caudate nucleus by approximately 35%. (3) Phencyclidine (1 mg per kg administered intramuscularly), a convulsant, caused increases of 10% to 50% in the consumption of glucose except in the inferior colliculus, pontine nuclei, and cerebellar gray matter, where significant decreases were observed. These studies confirm the observation that the phosphorylation rate of the inferior colliculus is usually very brisk under normal conditions. These observations may also point to a selective vulnerability of specific structures that have high regional metabolic rates for glucose.

Focal Seizures: R.C. Collins

Since the discovery of Walker and colleagues (1945) that the topical application of penicillin to the cortex causes intense focal seizures, many workers have explored the electrical spread of focal convulsions through the brain with depth electrodes. From the motor cortex there is rapid activation into the contralateral cortex, ipsilateral thalamus, extrapyramidal pathways, and cerebellum (Udvarhelyi and Walker, 1965). Following the injection of [^{14}C]DG during focal penicillin seizures, Kennedy and co-workers (1975) noted an increase in [^{14}C]DG phosphorylation in discrete areas in the ipsilateral basal ganglia and thalamus, as well as in the seizure focus (Figure 21). These regions also have increased blood flow under the same experimental conditions (Ueno et al., 1975), reflecting the tight couple between electrical activity, metabolism, and circulation in the brain (Plum et al., 1974).

The injection of 25 units of penicillin in 0.2 μl of artificial cerebrospinal fluid 500 μm into the motor cortex of the rat resulted in repetitive single-spike discharges that were maximal over the seizure focus (Figure 22). They lasted 60 to 90 min and were synchronous with contralateral motor jerks. A reasonable steady state was obtained with approximately 35 spikes per min during [^{14}C]DG circulation. Autoradiography (Figure 23) revealed a well-defined focus of increased

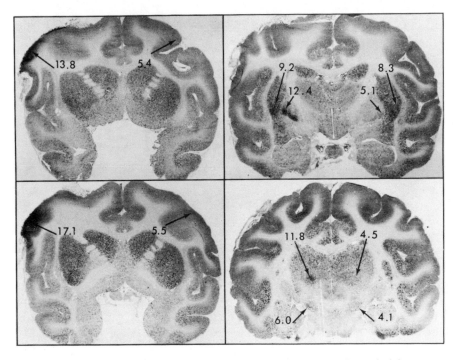

Figure 21. Effects of focal seizures produced by local injection of penicillin to the left motor cortex on local cerebral glucose utilization in the conscious rhesus monkey (left side of figure). The numbers (see arrows) represent the local rates of glucose utilization in mg of glucose/100 gm of tissue/min. [Adapted from Kennedy et al., 1975]

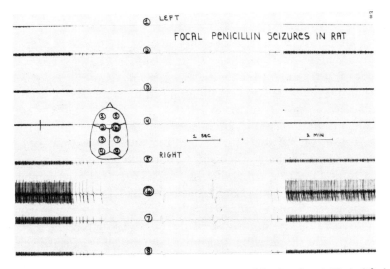

Figure 22. Electroencephalogram in focal penicillin seizures. 25 units of penicillin in 0.2 μl of CSF were injected into the right motor cortex ⑥ . With each spike discharge there were synchronous jerks of the left face, head, and forepaw. [Collins]

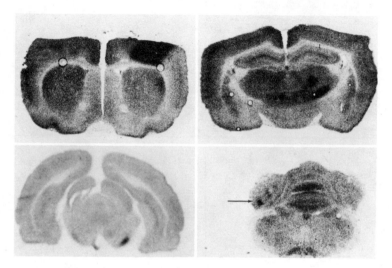

Figure 23. [^{14}C]DG autoradiography during unilateral focal penicillin seizures. *Upper left:* increased activity in seizure focus and outer rim of caudate/putamen. *Upper right:* activity in thalamic nuclei, parafascicularis, and ventralis. *Lower left:* increased activity in right substantia nigra. *Lower right:* focal activation (see arrow) in contralateral posterior inferior cerebellar folium. [Collins et al., 1976]

[^{14}C]DG phosphorylation at the site of maximum electrical discharge and in discrete areas of the ipsilateral thalamus (nucleus ventralis, nucleus parafascicularis), caudate/putamen, globus pallidus, substantia nigra, and contralateral cerebellar cortex.

Injections of larger amounts of penicillin resulted in more intense seizures that progressed sequentially to bilateral convulsions. The cortex surrounding the focus, as well as the contralateral "mirror" cortex, displayed increased activity arranged in columns. These columns resembled those noted in the occipital cortex by Hubel and Wiesel and the columns described by Lorente de Nó (see the discussion in the above section on "Visual stimulation"). Associated with the bilateral seizure spread was bilateral increased [^{14}C]DG phosphorylation in the medial frontal cortex, medial thalamic nuclei (particularly rhomboideus and reuniens), cingulate gyri, lateral amygdaloid nuclei, substantia nigra, and cerebellum (Figure 24).

According to Collins, use of the [^{14}C]DG method has allowed a demonstration of the functional anatomy involved as focal discharges spread to bilateral convulsions (Collins et al., 1976). In the cortex, cortical columns are progressively involved in epileptic activity, while in the diencephalon there is recruitment òf medial thalamic nuclei.

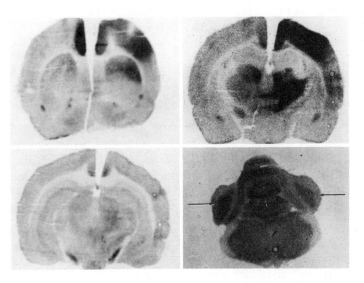

Figure 24. [^{14}C]DG autoradiography during focal penicillin seizures with bilateral spread. *Upper left:* large seizure focus (right) with capture of cortical columns, bilateral medial frontal cortex, cingulate gyri, and bilateral caudate/putamen and globus pallidus. *Upper right:* increased activity in lateral ventral basal thalamus and new activation of medial thalamus. *Lower left:* bilateral substantia nigra. *Lower right:* bilayeral cerebellum (see arrows), left > right. [Collins et al., 1976]

Activation of the medial thalamofrontal cortical system indicates that this may be the important pathway in the generalization of seizures, as was first postulated by Penfield (Penfield and Jasper, 1954) when he referred to it as the "centrencephalon." This concept has been more recently modified by Goldring (1972).

VII. APPLICATION OF THE DEOXYGLUCOSE METHOD TO HUMAN CEREBRAL DYSFUNCTION

The Use of [2-^{18}F] Fluoro-2-Deoxy-D-Glucose in Man: M. Reivich

Application of the deoxyglucose method to man requires the following: (1) a suitable tracer labeled with γ-emitting radionuclide must be used to enable detection of the activity through the skull; (2) the distribution of activity within the brain must be determined with three-dimensional resolution; (3) the tracer utilized must fulfill the criteria met by deoxyglucose; and (4) the radiation exposure must be safe.

It was decided to use ^{18}F-labeled 2-fluoro-2-deoxy-D-glucose ([^{18}F] FDG) as the tracer since ^{18}F emits positrons that can be detected through the skull. Preliminary studies* have been performed in collaboration with Sokoloff and Greenberg, utilizing ^{14}C-labeled 2-fluoro-2-deoxy-D-glucose ([^{14}C] FDG).† The tracer was incubated in a reaction mixture containing ATP and purified hexokinase, and the reaction products were separated and identified by thin-layer chromatography. The results showed that 2-fluoro-2-deoxy-D-glucose is a suitable substrate for brain hexokinase and is phosphorylated to 2-fluoro-2-deoxy-D-glucose phosphate.

The results of a study in which the regional cerebral metabolic rate for glucose in the rat was measured with [^{14}C] FDG and then compared with the results obtained with [^{14}C] DG indicate that the attachment of fluorine to 2-deoxy-D-glucose does not drastically alter the properties of the molecule (see Table 5). The values obtained with [^{14}C] FDG were close to, but about 20% to 30% lower than, those obtained with [^{14}C] DG. This is most likely due to the fact that the lumped constant for [^{14}C] FDG is different than that for [^{14}C] DG, owing to the different Michaelis-Menten kinetic constants for these two compounds. The exact value for the lumped constant for [^{14}C] FDG needs to be determined.

In order to determine the distribution of 2-fluoro-2-deoxy-D-glucose in the brain with three-dimensional resolution, a transverse section scan device, such as that described by Kuhl and co-workers (1975) was used (see Figure 25). By means of this technique, the

---

*M. Reivich, L. Sokoloff, and J. Greenberg, unpublished studies.
†This compound was prepared by A. Wolf and J. Fowler at the Brookhaven National Laboratory.

TABLE 5

Local Cerebral Glucose Metabolism [Reivich] *

Structure	$[^{14}C]$-2-deoxy-D-glucose (8 rats)		$[^{14}C]$-2-fluoro-2-deoxy-D-glucose (1 rat)	
	mg/100 gm/min	μmoles/100 gm/min	mg/100 gm/min	μmoles/100 gm/min
Visual cortex	17.46	98.98	16.93	94.07
Auditory cortex	25.68	142.68	19.73	109.60
Lateral geniculate	17.52	97.33	14.69	81.63
Superior olive	21.46	119.23	18.74	104.13
Lateral lemniscus	16.63	92.37	13.43	74.61
Inferior colliculus	32.41	180.07	21.91	121.74
Superior colliculus	16.37	90.98	13.12	72.87
Centrum ovale	8.40	46.64	7.07	39.27
Internal capsule	7.83	43.49	5.49	30.50
Cerebellar white matter	8.23	45.70	6.10	33.90

*The rates of glucose consumption were calculated on the basis of the lumped constant for $[^{14}C]DG$ determined in the rat. The lumped constant for $[^{14}C]FDG$ has not yet been determined.

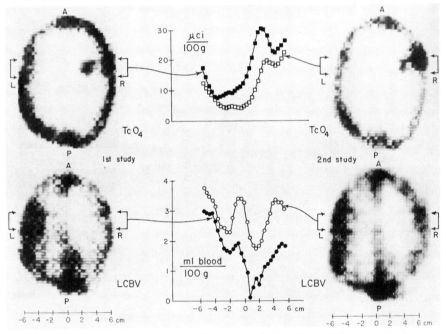

Figure 25. Section scans of a malignant glioma surrounded by edema. At the top of the figure, section scans of ^{99m}Tc pertechnetate (TcO_4) show the alteration of the blood-brain barrier. At the bottom, section scans of ^{99m}Tc-labeled red blood cells show LCBV. Initial studies are at the left (■, ●), and studies made 2 months later, after steroid therapy, are at the right (□, ○). The section scans of ^{99m}Tc-labeled red blood cells initially showed a large region of reduced LCBV due to compression of local microcirculation by edema. After steroid therapy, peritumor edema decreased and peritumor LCBV returned towards normal. The present resolution of this technique is a cube 1.6 cm on a side. A = anterior; L = left; LCBV = local cerebral blood volume; P = posterior; R = right; abscissas = the distance to the left and right of midline of brain section; midline is represented by zero. [Kuhl et al., 1975]

activity within a brain section can be determined quantitatively, and this information can be used in place of the autoradiograph obtained by the $[^{14}C]$ DG method. In the example of the resolution of the transverse section scanner shown in Figure 25, ^{99m} Tc-labeled erythrocytes were used to measure local cerebral blood volume in a patient with a brain tumor. From these preliminary studies it seems feasible to pursue further development of this technique for use in man.

VIII. POSSIBLE INVOLVEMENT OF CEREBRAL GLUCOSE-6-PHOSPHATASE IN 2-DEOXY-D-GLUCOSE PHOSPHORYLATION

Relationship of 2-Deoxy-D-Glucose Phosphorylation to Local Cerebral Energy Utilization: M.L. Karnovsky

Assumptions Concerning the DG Method

Interpreting the phosphorylation rate of regional cerebral glucose and correlating it with cerebral regional function hinge on the following major assumptions. (1) Glucose and DG share the same carrier-facilitated transfer mechanism across the blood-brain barrier and into neurons, as well as the same mechanism of phosphorylation. (2) The phosphorylation rates of glucose and DG are closely linked to the rate of energy use of the tissue. (3) The phosphorylation of glucose is in a steady state. (4) DG is converted only to DG-6-P, which is stable and not degradable, i.e., the label is not significantly removed from DG or DG-6-P. (5) The ^{14}C activity of the autoradiograph is distributed in the locus of phosphorylation of DG.

Since the conversion of DG-6-P to structural or storage components would not directly affect the quantification of [^{14}C]DG phosphorylation and would not be related to immediate energy use, it might tend to cause overestimations of cerebral metabolic rate or changes therein. On the other hand, the reversion of DG-6-P to DG would tend to cause underestimations of the actual phosphorylation rate. Until recently, glucose-6-phosphatase was believed not to be present in the brain to any extent, and, thus, the hexokinase reaction was considered virtually irreversible. However, recent evidence has been adduced that glucose-6-phosphatase is, indeed, present in rat brain (Anchors and Karnovsky, 1975). Because this enzyme can also catalyze the phosphorylation of glucose (as well as the dephosphorylation of DG-6-P), it can be considered as an alternative enzyme to hexokinase in forming DG-6-P (Nordlie, 1974). This is an even more tempting possibility when one considers that brain glucose-6-phosphatase is a membrane component of neurons; perhaps control of its activity is linked to the electrical activity of the cell membrane (Anchors and Karnovsky, 1975).

Glucose-6-Phosphatase in Brain and Its Possible
Role in the Phosphorylation of DG

Evidence indicating that glucose-6-phosphatase is present in brain and its possible role in initiating the steps for energy provision in different functional states is derived from studies of sleep. The method used is as follows: ^{32}P was injected into the lateral ventricle of sleeping or waking rats, which were decapitated after 30 to 40 min. The whole-brain homogenate was extracted to remove lipids and freed of small molecules with cold 5% trichloroacetic acid. The residue was then extracted with sodium dodecyl sulfate, and the extract was submitted to electrophoresis on polyacrylamide gels. The gels were sectioned and each disc was assayed for radioactivity (see Figure 26). A peak was noted at the band having a molecular weight of 28,000, and this peak's activity in sleeping rats exceeded 5-fold that in waking animals (Reich et al., 1973; Anchors and Karnovsky, 1975).

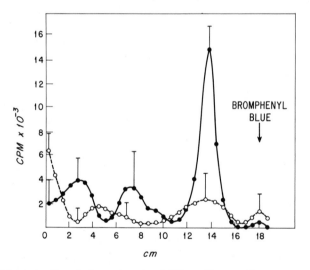

Figure 26. Polyacrylamide gel electrophoresis of ^{33}P- or ^{32}P-labeled proteins from brains of sleeping and waking animals. In four experiments, paired animals were infused intraventricularly with ^{33}P$_i$ or ^{32}P$_i$. Following the infusion, one animal of each pair was allowed to sleep (●) for 20 to 30 min while the control animal was kept awake (○). The animals were killed by immersion in liquid nitrogen. The frozen brains were extracted to remove lipids and acid-soluble compounds. Equal weights of the residues were combined and extracted with sodium dodecyl sulfate buffer. The extracts were submitted to electrophoresis on large 10% polyacrylamide gels. The distributions of radioactivities on the four gels were averaged by computer and plotted. The error bars at selected points represent standard deviations. [Anchors and Karnovsky, 1975]

Purification of the protein was also accomplished by removing myelin from rat brain, suspending the remaining material in deoxycholate, and passing the suspension through G-100- and diethylaminoethyl-Sephadex columns. A phosphoprotein was obtained from which phosphohistidine could be isolated, as confirmed by comparison of autoradiographs with phosphoamino acid standards after alkaline hydrolysis. The kinetics of hydrolysis of the phosphate from the intact phosphoprotein were consistent with this confirmation (Anchors and Karnovsky, 1975).

The enzymatic properties of the brain phosphoprotein were studied with different organic phosphates, and it was shown to be a phosphohydrolase, with a preference for glucose-6-phosphate (G-6-P) (Table 6), as well as a glucose-phosphotransferase (Table 7). The enzyme is present primarily in neurons and not in glia, as ascertained on preparations monitored by characteristic marker enzymes for those

TABLE 6

Phosphohydrolase Activities of the Purified Protein
[Anchors and Karnovsky, 1975]

$$(X - P + H_2O \approx X + P_i)$$

Substrate	Activity μmoles/min/mg
Glucose-6-phosphate	7.9 ± 0.5*
Inorganic pyrophosphate	1.8
β-Glycerophosphate	0.10
p-Nitrophenyl phosphate	0.11
5'-Adenosine monophosphate	0.21
Adenosine triphosphate	0.00

*Mean and standard deviation (3 experiments).

TABLE 7

Phosphotransferase Activities of the Purified Protein
[Karnovsky]

$$(Donor - P + glucose \approx donor + glucose - P)$$

Donor	Activity μmoles/min/mg
Inorganic pyrophosphate	4.2
Phosphoenol pyruvate	4.3
Adenosine triphosphate	2.3

cells. Determination of the subcellular distribution of the enzyme showed that it is mainly in the membrane (Anchors and Karnovsky, 1975).

In sleeping rats there was a 5-fold increase in the labeling of glucose-6-phosphatase with ^{32}P (Figure 26); however, during sleep the actual activity of the enzyme in whole brain increased only 20% to 25% of its activity in the brain of awake rats.* This finding could be due to the fact that the enzymatic measurements were made under standard conditions, and not under those that actually control the enzyme's activity in the brain. The latter conditions are reflected in the labeling experiments in vivo, since the phosphorylated enzyme is an intermediate in the transfer of phosphate to an organic acceptor or water. Nonetheless, the direct enzymatic measurements did show a change in activity with change in functional state (sleep vs waking).

Although the presence of glucose-6-phosphatase in rat brain and its potential participation in the *formation* of G-6-P (and DG-6-P) might modify the lumped constant of Sokoloff's quantification of the regional cerebral glucose use rate in that the familiar kinetic constants for hexokinase might not apply, the principle of the quantification itself would not be affected. Significant changes in glucose-6-phosphatase activity and kinetic properties, perhaps with changes of brain function, would require an independent assessment of the lumped constant with each change.

Karnovsky concluded that glucose-6-phosphatase, owing to its activity as a phosphotransferase and its presence in the neuronal membrane, may play an important role in what seems to be the crucial step (i.e., phosphorylation to G-6-P) in making glucose available for energy needs when the brain's functional state is changed.

*B. Lee, unpublished data.

ABBREVIATIONS

ATP	adenosine triphosphate
CSF	cerebrospinal fluid
DG	2-deoxy-D-glucose
[^{14}C]DG	[1-^{14}C]-2-deoxy-D-glucose
DG-6-P	2-deoxy-D-glucose-6-phosphate
[^{14}C]FDG	[^{14}C]-2-fluoro-2-deoxy-D-glucose
[^{18}F]FDG	[2-^{18}F]fluoro-2-deoxy-D-glucose
G-6-P	glucose-6-phosphate
G-6-Pase	glucose-6-phosphate dehydrogenase
[^{3}H]DG	[^{3}H]-2-deoxy-D-glucose
PG	periglomerular

BIBLIOGRAPHY

This bibliography contains two types of entries: (1) citations given or work alluded to in the report, and (2) additional references to pertinent literature by conference participants and others. Citations in group (1) may be found in the text on the pages listed in the right-hand column.

Page

Abeles, M. and Goldstein, M.H., Jr. (1970): Functional architecture in cat primary   488
auditory cortex: columnar organization and organization according to depth. *J.
Neurophysiol.* 33:172-187.

Anchors, J.M. and Karnovsky, M.L. (1975): Purification of cerebral glucose-6-   505,506,
phosphatase. An enzyme involved in sleep. *J. Biol. Chem.* 250:6408-6416.   507,508

Barker, J.N. (1966): Fetal and neonatal cerebral blood flow. *Am. J. Physiol.*
210:897-902.

Behrman, R.E. and Lees, M.H. (1971): Organ blood flows of the fetal, newborn and
adult rhesus monkey. *Biol. Neonate* 18:330-340.

Behrman, R.E., Lees, M.H., Peterson, E.N., de Lannoy, C.W., and Seeds, A.E.
(1970): Distribution of the circulation in the normal and asphyxiated fetal
primate. *Am. J. Obstet. Gynecol.* 108:956-969.

Brouwer, B. and Zeeman, W.P.C. (1926): The projection of the retina in the   485
primary optic neuron in monkeys. *Brain* 49:1-35.

Caveness, W.F. (1969): Ontogeny of focal seizures. *In: Basic Mechanisms of the
Epilepsies.* Jasper, H.H., Ward, A.A., Jr., and Pope, A., eds. Boston: Little,
Brown and Co., pp. 517-534.

Caveness, W.F., Ueno, H., and Kemper, T.L. (1976): Subcortical factors in
experimental Jacksonian seizures. *In: International Congress on Neuropathology, Vol. 2. Budapest, 1974.* Kornyey, S., Tariska, S., and Gosztonyi, G., eds.
Amsterdam: Excerpta Medica, pp. 29-34.

Chambers, W.W. and Sprague, J.M. (1955): Functional organization in the   494
cerebellum. Organization in longitudinal and cortico-nuclear zones and their
contribution to the control of posture, both extrapyramidal and pyramidal. *J.
Comp. Neurol.* 103:105-129.

Collins, R.C., Kennedy, C., Sokoloff, L., and Plum, F. (1976): Metabolic anatomy   500,501
of focal motor seizures. *Arch. Neurol.* 33:536-542.

Collins, R.C., Posner, J.B., and Plum, F. (1970): Cerebral energy metabolism during
electroshock seizures in mice. *Am. J. Physiol.* 218:943-950.

Cowan, W.M., Gottlieb, D.I., Hendrickson, A.E., Price, J.L., and Woolsey, T.A.   464
(1972): The autoradiographic demonstration of axonal connections in the
central nervous system. *Brain Res.* 37:21-51.

Daniel, P.M. and Whitteridge, D. (1961): The representation of the visual field on   486
the cerebral cortex in monkeys. *J. Physiol.* 159:203-221.

Des·Rosiers, M.H., Kennedy, C., Patlak, C.S., Pettigrew, K.D., Sokoloff, L., and   474
Reivich, M. (1974): Relationship between local cerebral blood flow and glucose
utilization in the rat. *Neurology* 24:389. (Abstr.)

Diamond, I. and Fishman, R.A. (1973): High-affinity transport and phosphoryla-   471
tion of 2-deoxy-D-glucose in synaptosomes. *J. Neurochem.* 20:1533-1542.

Dunnihoo, D.R. and Quilligan, E.J. (1973): Carotid blood flow distribution in the
in utero sheep fetus. *Am. J. Obstet. Gynecol.* 116:648-656.

Durante, G. (1898): Contribution à l'étude des dégénérescences propagées et en
particulier des altérations des cordons postérieurs consécutives aux lésions en
foyer de l'éncephale. *Rev. Neurol. (Paris)* 6:390-402.

Eckman, W.W., Phair, R.D., Fenstermacher, J.D., Patlak, C.S., Kennedy, C., and
Sokoloff, L. (1975): Permeability limitation in estimation of local brain blood
flow with [^{14}C] antipyrine. *Am. J. Physiol.* 229:215-221.

Ehrlich, P. (1886): Uber die Methylenblaureaction der lebenden Nervensubstanz.
Dtsch. Med. Wochenschr. 12:49-52.

Eklöf, B., Lassen, N.A., Nilsson, L., Norberg, K., Siesjö, B.K., and Torlöf, P.
(1974): Regional cerebral blood flow in the rat measured by the tissue sampling
technique; a critical evaluation using four indicators C^{14}-antipyrine, C^{14}-
ethanol, H^3-water and Xenon^{133}. *Acta Physiol. Scand.* 91:1-10.

Eklöf, B. and Siesjö, B.K. (1973): Cerebral blood flow in ischemia caused by
carotid artery ligation in the rat. *Acta Physiol. Scand.* 87:69-77.

Falck, B., Hillarp, N.-A., Thieme, G., and Torp, A. (1962): Fluorescence of   464
catechol amines and related compounds condensed with formaldehyde. *J.
Histochem. Cytochem.* 10:348-354.

Flechsig, P. (1896): *Die Leitungsbahnen im Gehirn und Rückenmark des Menschen*   463
auf Grund entwicklungsgeschichtlicher Untersuchungen. Leipzig: Engelmann.

Giacobini, E. (1969): Chemistry of isolated invertebrate neurons. *In: Handbook of*   494
Neurochemistry, Vol. 2. Structural Neurochemistry. Lajtha, A., ed. New York:
Plenum Press, pp. 195-239.

Gjedde, A., Andersson, J., and Eklöf, B. (1975a): Brain uptake of lactate,
antipyrine, water and ethanol. *Acta Physiol. Scand.* 93:145-149.

Gjedde, A., Caronna, J.J., Hindfelt, B., and Plum, F. (1975b): Whole-brain blood   474
flow and oxygen metabolism in the rat during nitrous oxide anesthesia. *Am. J.
Physiol.* 229:113-118.

Goldring, S. (1972): The role of prefrontal cortex in grand mal convulsion. *Arch.*   501
Neurol. 26:109-119.

Golgi, C. (1873): Sulla struttura della sostanza griglia dell cervello. *Gazz. Med. Ital.*   463
Lombarda 33:244-246.

Golgi, C. (1875): Sulla fina struttura dei bulba olfattoria. *Riv. Sper. Freniatria Med.
Legal.* 1:66-78.

Grafstein, B. (1969): Axonal transport: communication between soma and synapse.   464
In: Advances in Biochemical Psychopharmacology, Vol. 1. Costa, E. and
Greengard, P., eds. New York: Raven Press, pp. 11-25.

Greenfield, J.G. and Meyer, A. (1963): General pathology of the nerve cell and   464
neuroglia. *In: Greenfield's Neuropathology, 2nd Ed.* Blackwood, W., McMen-
emey, W.H., Meyer, A., Norman, R.M., and Russell, D.S., eds. Baltimore:
Williams and Wilkins, pp. 1-70.

Page

Gudden, B. von (1870): Experimentaluntersuchungen über das peripherische und   463
centrale Nervensystem. *Arch. Psychiatr. Nervenkr.* 2:693-723.

Haberly, L.B. and Shepherd, G.M. (1973): Current-density analysis of summed   483
evoked potentials in opossum prepyriform cortex. *J. Neurophysiol.* 36:789-802.

Hawkins, R.A., Miller, A.L., Cremer, J.E., and Veech, R.L. (1974): Measurement of
the rate of glucose utilization by rat brain in vivo. *J. Neurochem.* 23:917-923.

Hawkins, R.A., Miller, A.L., Nielsen, R.C., and Veech, R.L. (1973): The acute
action of ammonia on rat brain metabolism in vivo. *Biochem. J.* 134:1001-1008.

Hökfelt, T. (1967): The possible ultrastructural identification of tubero-   464
infundibular dopamine-containing nerve endings in the median eminence of the
rat. *Brain Res.* 5:121-123.

Hubel, D.H. and Wiesel, T.N. (1962): Receptive fields, binocular interaction and   488
functional architecture in the cat's visual cortex. *J. Physiol.* 160:106-154.

Hubel, D.H. and Wiesel, T.N. (1969): Anatomical demonstration of columns in the   488
monkey striate cortex. *Nature* 221:747-750.

Hubel, D.H. and Wiesel, T.N. (1972): Laminar and columnar distribution of   487,488
geniculo-cortical fibers in the macaque monkey. *J. Comp. Neurol.* 146:421-450.

Hughes, G.W. and Maffei, L. (1965): On the origin of the dark discharge of retinal   487
ganglion cells. *Arch. Ital. Biol.* 103:45-59.

Ingvar, D.H. and Lassen, N.A., eds. (1975): *Brain Work. The Coupling of Function,*   474
Metabolism and Blood Flow in the Brain. Copenhagen: Munksgaard.

Jones, E.G., Burton, H., and Porter, R. (1975): Commissural and cortico-cortical   488
"columns" in the somatic sensory cortex of primates. *Science* 190:572-574.

Kennedy, C., Des Rosiers, M.H., Jehle, J.W., Reivich, M., Sharpe, F., and Sokoloff,   461,476,
L. (1975): Mapping of functional neural pathways by autoradiographic survey of   485,486,
local metabolic rate with [^{14}C]deoxyglucose. *Science* 187:850-853.   487,498,
                                                                                    499

Kety, S. (1949): The physiology of the human cerebral circulation. *Anesthesiology*
10:610-614.

Kety, S.S. (1951): The theory and applications of the exchange of inert gas at the   464
lungs and tissues. *Pharmacol. Rev.* 3:1-41.

Kety, S.S. (1960): Measurement of local blood flow by the exchange of an inert,   464,466
diffusible substance. *Methods Med. Res.* 8:228-236.

Kety, S.S. and Schmidt, C.F. (1945): The determination of cerebral blood flow in   464,474
man by the use of nitrous oxide in low concentrations. *Am. J. Physiol.*
143:53-66.

Kety, S.S. and Schmidt, C.F. (1948): The nitrous oxide method for the
quantitative determination of cerebral blood flow in man: theory, procedure and
normal values. *J. Clin. Invest.* 27:476-483.

King, B.D., Sokoloff, L., and Wechsler, R.L. (1952): The effects of *l*-epinephrine   494
and *l*-nor-epinephrine upon cerebral circulation and metabolism in man. *J. Clin.*
Invest. 31:273-279.

Page

Klippel, M. (1896): Les neurones. Les lois fondamentales de leurs dégénérescences.   463
Arch. Neurol. 1(Series 2):417-440.

Klippel, M. and Durante, G. (1895): Des dégénérescences rétrogrades dans les nerfs   463
périphériques et les centres nerveux. *Rev. Med.* 15:1-31, 142-171, 343-354,
574-600, 655-684.

Korneliussen, H.K. (1968a): Comments on the cerebellum and its division. *Brain*   492
Res. 8:229-236.

Korneliussen, H.K. (1968b): On the morphology and subdivision of the cerebellar   492
nuclei of the rat. *J. Hirnforsch.* 10:109-122.

Korneliussen, H.K. (1968c): On the ontogenic development of the cerebellum   492
(nuclei, fissures, and cortex) of the rat, with special reference to regional
variations in corticogenesis. *J. Hirnforsch.* 10:379-412.

Kuhl, D.E., Reivich, M., Alavi, A., Nyary, I., and Staum, M.M. (1975): Local   502,503
cerebral blood volume determined by three-dimensional reconstruction of
radionuclide scan data. *Circ. Res.* 36:610-619.

Land, L.J., Eager, R.P., and Shepherd, G.M. (1970): Olfactory nerve projections to   483
the olfactory bulb in rabbit: demonstration by means of a simplified
ammoniacal silver degeneration method. *Brain Res.* 23:250-254.

Landau, W.M., Freygang, W.H., Jr., Rowland, L.P., Sokoloff, L., and Kety, S.S.   461,464,
(1955): The local circulation of the living brain; values in the unanesthetized and   466,474
anesthetized cat. *Trans. Am. Neurol. Assoc.* 80:125-129.

Larrabee, M.G. and Bronk, D.W. (1952): Metabolic requirements of sympathetic   494
neurons. *Cold Spring Harbor Symp. Quant. Biol.* 17:245-266.

Laszlo, J., Landau, B., Wight, K., and Burk, D. (1958): The effect of glucose   461
analogues on the metabolism of human leukemic cells. *J. Nat. Cancer Inst.*
21:475-483.

LaVail, J.H. and LaVail, M.M. (1972): Retrograde axonal transport in the central   464
nervous system. *Science* 176:1416-1417.

Lorente de Nó, R. (1934): Studies on the structure of the cerebral cortex.   488
II. Continuation of the study of the ammonic system. *J. Psychol. Neurol.*
46:113-117.

Lowry, O.H., Passoneau, J.V., Hasselberger, F.X., and Schulz, D.W. (1964): Effect
of ischemia on known substrates and cofactors of the glycolytic pathway in
brain. *J. Biol. Chem.* 239:18-30.

Lowry, O.H., Roberts, N.R., Leiner, K.Y., Wu, M.-L., Farr, A.L., and Albers, R.W.   471
(1954): The quantitative histochemistry of brain Ammon's horn. *J. Biol. Chem.*
207:39-49.

Makowski, E.L., Schneider, J.M., Tsoulos, N.G., Colwill, J.R., Battaglia, F.C., and
Meschia, G. (1972): Cerebral blood flow, oxygen consumption, and glucose
utilization of fetal lambs in utero. *Am. J. Obstet. Gynecol.* 114:292-303.

Marchi, V. and Algeri, G. (1885): Sulle degenerazioni discendenti consecutive a   463
lesioni della corteccia cerebrale. *Riv. Sper. Freniatria Med. Legal.* 11:492-494.

Neurosciences Res. Prog. Bull., Vol. 14, No. 4   515

Page

Plum, F., Howse, D.C., and Duffy, T.E. (1974): Metabolic effects of seizures. *Res. Publ. Assoc. Res. Nerv. Ment. Dis.* 53:141-157.   498

Plum, F., Posner, J.B., and Troy, B. (1968): Cerebral metabolic and circulatory responses to induced convulsions in animals. *Arch. Neurol.* 18:1-13.   494

Polyak, S. (1932): *The Main Afferent Fiber Systems of the Cerebral Cortex in Primates.* (University of California Publication in Anatomy, Vol. 2.) Berkeley: University of California Press, p. 203.   485

Pribram, K.H. (1971): *Languages of the Brain. Experimental Paradoxes and Principles in Neuropsychology.* Englewood Cliffs, N.J.: Prentice-Hall, Inc.   488

Purves, M.J. (1972): *The Physiology of the Cerebral Circulation.* Cambridge: Cambridge University Press.

Raichle, M.E., Larson, K.B., Phelps, M.E., Grubb, R.L., Jr., Welch, M.J., and Ter-Pogossian, M.M. (1975): In vivo measurement of brain glucose transport and metabolism employing glucose-^{11}C. *Am. J. Physiol.* 228:1936-1948.   464

Rakic, P. (1975): Local circuit neurons. *Neurosciences Res. Prog. Bull.* 13:291-446.   478

Rall, W., Shepherd, G.M., Reese, T.S., and Brightman, M.W. (1966): Dendro-dendritic synaptic pathway for inhibition in the olfactory bulb. *Exp. Neurol.* 14:44-56.   478,480

Ramón y Cajal, S. (1909): *Histologie du Système Nerveux de l'Homme et des Vértébrés, Vol. 2.* Paris: A. Maloine. (Reprinted in 1952 by Consejo Superior de Investigaciones Cientificas, Instituto Ramón y Cajal, Madrid.)   463

Reich, P., Geyer, S.J., Steinbaum, L., Anchors, M., and Karnovsky, M.L. (1973): Incorporation of phosphate into rat brain during sleep and wakefulness. *J. Neurochem.* 20:1195-1205.   506

Reivich, M. (1974): Blood flow metabolism couple in brain. *Res. Publ. Assoc. Res. Nerv. Ment. Dis.* 53:125-140.   474,475

Reivich, M., Jehle, J.W., Sokoloff, L., and Kety, S.S. (1969): Measurement of regional cerebral blood flow with antipyrine-^{14}C in awake cats. *J. Appl. Physiol.* 27:296-300.   461,464, 466,476

Rogers, A.W. (1973): *Technique of Autoradiography.* Amsterdam: Elsevier.   469

Roy, C.S. and Sherrington, C.S. (1890): On the regulation of the blood-supply of the brain. *J. Physiol.* 11:85-108.

Rudolph, A.M. and Heymann, M.A. (1967): The circulation of the fetus in utero. Method for studying distribution of blood flow, cardiac output and organ blood flow. *Circ. Res.* 21:163-184.

Schwartz, W.J., Sharp, F.R., Gunn, R.H., and Evarts, E.V. (1976): Lesions of ascending dopaminergic pathways decrease forebrain glucose uptake. *Nature* 261:155-157.   496

Sensenbach, W., Madison, L., and Ochs, L. (1953): A comparison of the effects of *l*-nor-epinephrine, synthetic *l*-epinephrine, and the U.S.P. epinephrine upon cerebral blood flow and metabolism in man. *J. Clin. Invest.* 32:226-232.   494

Page

Shapiro, H., Greenberg, J., Reivich, M., Shipko, E., Van Horn, K., and Sokoloff, L.   497
  (1975): Local cerebral glucose utilization during anesthesia. *In: Blood Flow and
  Metabolism in the Brain.* Harper, A.M., Jennett, W.B., Miller, J.A., and Rowan,
  J.O., eds. Edinburgh: Churchill Livingstone, pp. 42-43.

Sharp, F.R. (1974): Activity related 2-deoxy-D-glucose uptake in the central   476
  nervous system of the rat. *In: Program and Abstracts, Society for Neuroscience,
  Fourth Annual Meeting.* St. Louis, Mo., p. 422.

Sharp, F.R. (1976a): Activity-related increases of glucose utilization associated   477,478,
  with reduced incorporation of glucose into its derivatives. *Brain Res.*   493
  107:663-666.

Sharp, F.R. (1976b): Relative cerebral glucose consumption of neuronal perikarya   469,470,
  and neuropil determined with 2-deoxyglucose in resting and swimming rat. *Brain*   471,490,
  Res. (In press)   491,492

Sharp, F.R. (1976c): Rotation induced increases of glucose metabolism in rat
  vestibular nuclei and vestibulocerebellum. *Brain Res.* (In press)

Sharp, F.R., Kauer, J.S., and Shepherd, G.M. (1975): Local sites of activity-related 481,482
  glucose metabolism in rat olfactory bulb during olfactory stimulation. *Brain Res.*
  98:596-600.

Shepherd, G.M. (1972): Synaptic organization of mammalian olfactory bulb.   478,479
  Physiol. Rev. 52:864-917.

Sherrington, C.S. (1891): Note on the knee-jerk. *St. Thomas Hosp. Rep.*   463
  21:145-147.

Sokoloff, L. (1969): Cerebral circulation and behaviour in man: strategy and   494
  findings. *In: Psychochemical Research in Man.* Mandell, A.J. and Mandell, M.P.,
  eds. New York: Academic Press, pp. 237-252.

Sokoloff, L. (1975a): Determination of local cerebral glucose consumption. *In:*   467,476,
  Blood Flow and Metabolism in the Brain. Harper, A.M., Jennett, W.B., Miller,   497
  J.A., and Rowan, J.O., eds. Edinburgh: Churchill Livingstone, pp. 1-8.

Sokoloff, L. (1975b): Influence of functional activity on local cerebral glucose   476,487
  utilization. *In: Brain Work. The Coupling of Function, Metabolism and Blood
  Flow in the Brain.* Ingvar, D.H. and Lassen, N.A., eds. Copenhagen: Munksgaard,
  pp. 385-388.

Sokoloff, L. (1976): Measurement of local glucose utilization and its use in
  mapping local functional activity in the central nervous system. *In: Neurosurgi-
  cal Treatment in Psychiatry, Pain and Epilepsy.* (Proceedings of the IV World
  Congress of Psychiatric Surgery, Madrid, 1975.) Sweet, W.H., ed. Baltimore:
  University Park Press. (In press)

Sokoloff, L., Reivich, M., Patlak, C.S., Pettigrew, K.D., Des Rosiers, M., and   476
  Kennedy, C. (1974): The (^{14}C)deoxyglucose method for the quantitative
  determination of local cerebral glucose consumption. *Trans. Am. Soc. Neurochem.* 5:85. (Abstr.)

Sols, A. and Crane, R.K. (1954): Substrate specificity of brain hexokinase. *J. Biol.* 461
  Chem. 210:581-595.

Neurosciences Res. Prog. Bull., Vol. 14, No. 4 — 517

Page

Spinelli, D.N. (1970): OCCAM: a computer model for a content addressable memory in the central nervous system. *In: Biology of Memory.* Pribram, K.H. and Broadbent, D.E., eds. New York: Academic Press, pp. 293-306.

488

Stilling, B. (1842): *Untersuchungen über die Functionen Rückenmarks und der Nerven.* Leipzig: Wigand.

463

Stretton, A.O. and Kravitz, E.A. (1968): Neuronal geometry: determination with a technique of intracellular dye injections. *Science* 162:132-134.

464

Tower, D.B. (1958): The effects of 2-deoxy-D-glucose on metabolism of slices of cerebral cortex incubated *in vivo. J Neurochem.* 3:185-205.

461

Udvarhelyi, G.B. and Walker, A.E. (1965): Dissemination of acute focal seizures in the monkey. I. From cortical foci. *Arch. Neurol.* 12:333-356.

498

Ueno, H., Yamashita, Y., and Caveness, W.F. (1975): Regional cerebral blood flow pattern in focal epileptiform seizures in the monkey. *Exp. Neurol.* 47:81-96.

498

Voogd, J., Broere, G., and van Rossum, J. (1969): The medio-lateral distribution of the spinocerebellar projection in the anterior lobe and the simple lobule in the cat and a comparison with some other afferent fiber systems. *Psychiatr. Neurol. Neurochir.* 72:137-151.

Walker, A.E., Johnson, H.C., and Kollros, J.J. (1945): Penicillin convulsions. The convulsive effects of penicillin applied to the cerebral cortex of monkey and man. *Surg. Gynecol. Obstet.* 81:692-701.

498

Waller, A.V. (1850): Experiments on the section of the glossopharyngeal and hypoglossal nerves of the frog, and observations of the alterations produced thereby in the structure of their primitive fibres. *Phil. Trans. R. Soc.* 140:423-429.

463

Waller, A. (1852): Sur la reproduction des nerfs et sur la structure et les fonctions des ganglions spinaux. *Arch. Anat. Physiol. Wissensch. Med.* 392-401.

463

Wasterlain, C.G. (1974): Inhibition of cerebral protein synthesis by epileptic seizures without motor manifestations. *Neurology* 24:175-180.

478

Wasterlain, C.G. and Plum, F. (1973a): Retardation of behavioral landmarks after neonatal seizures in rats. *Trans. Am. Neurol. Assoc.* 98:320-321.

Wasterlain, C.G. and Plum, F. (1973b): Vulnerability of developing rat brain to electroconvulsive seizures. *Arch. Neurol.* 29:38-45.

478

Weigert, C. (1882): Ueber eine neue Untersuchungsmethode des Centralnervensystems. *Zentralbl. Med. Wiss.* 20:753-757, 772-774.

463

Weigert, C. (1884): Ausführliche Beschreibung der in No. 2 dieser Zeitschrift erwähnten neuen Färbungsmethode für das Centralnervensystem. *Fortschr. Med.* 2:190-191.

463

Werner, G. (1970): The topology of the body representation in the somatic afferent pathway. *In: The Neurosciences: Second Study Program.* Schmitt, F.O., editor-in-chief. New York: Rockefeller University Press, pp. 605-617.

488

Page

Wick, A.N., Drury, D.R., Nakada, H.I., and Wolfe, J.B. (1957): Localization of the   461
primary metabolic block produced by 2-deoxyglucose. *J. Biol. Chem.*
224:963-969.

Wiesel, T.N. and Hubel, D.H. (1974): Reorganization of ocular dominance columns   463
in monkey striate cortex. *In: Program and Abstracts, Society for Neuroscience,*
Fourth Annual Meeting. St. Louis, Mo., p. 478.

Wiesel, T.N., Hubel, D.H., and Lam, D.M.K. (1974): Autoradiographic demonstra-   487,488
tion of ocular-dominance columns in the monkey striate cortex by means of
transneuronal transport. *Brain Res.* 79:273-279.

Woodward, G.E. and Hudson, M.T. (1954): The effect of 2-deoxy-D-glucose on   461
glycolysis and respiration of tumor and normal tissues. *Cancer Res.* 14:599-605.

NAME INDEX

SUBJECT INDEX